HEART *of* WELLNESS

A SHORT HISTORY OF A NEW AGE

S. J. Spiegel

ISBN-10 Number: 0997554207
ISBN-13: 9780997554205
Library of Congress Number: 2016939732
LCCN Imprint Name: VaLPoSa Books, Florida, NY

Author and Copyright Holder: Steven J. Spiegel (registered © 2015, as revised © 2016)
Loosely based on a white paper written circa 2008
Original Art Work: Melissa Spiegel (registered © 2016)
Business Opportunities and Engagements: Spiegel Legal, LLC
Website: *www.SJSpiegel.com*

Dedicated to my parents Lynda and Albert, better known as Nana and Papa, on the occasion of my father's 80th birthday.

When I was growing up, my parents hoped I might be a doctor, like the ones I saw when I was sick. They didn't get their wish—I have no medical degree—but I learned a lot of lessons about wellness and healing from those kid visits to physicians.

The childhood lessons I learned were not the ones my parents intended, and may have disheartened me from medical schooling besides, though the education was invaluable. It taught me to proactively find better health in my life, which ultimately helped my children find better health in theirs. I hope those lessons can now benefit other families, maybe even help our health-care system find wellness for itself too. My mom and dad would like all that very much, but I'm still not the doctor they wanted me to be.

I remember drawing in a coloring book my parents gave me when I was a boy to encourage an interest in medicine. The book had anatomical pictures of organs and body parts, like the heart, and it taught me their names, shapes, and biological functions. It was fun to learn these new scientific things, but looking back, my favorite part was choosing the colors of the crayons.

My drawings were not particularly good, then or now, so my parents must have known early on that I would not be a painter either. My parents appreciate works of art and beauty, as do most caring people, so I know they will enjoy the wonderful drawing of the heart on the cover of this book, even more so because it is by their beautiful granddaughter Melissa. When Melissa was a child, Al and Lynda encouraged her to be a medical doctor too, and though that was not the path her life and career would take, her cover art shows that she understands some things about the complexion of a beating heart that no anatomical drawing could ever show.

Surely, the heart knows truths of unconditional love and its boundless beauty, which is a lesson my parents taught me, and why this dedication is to them.

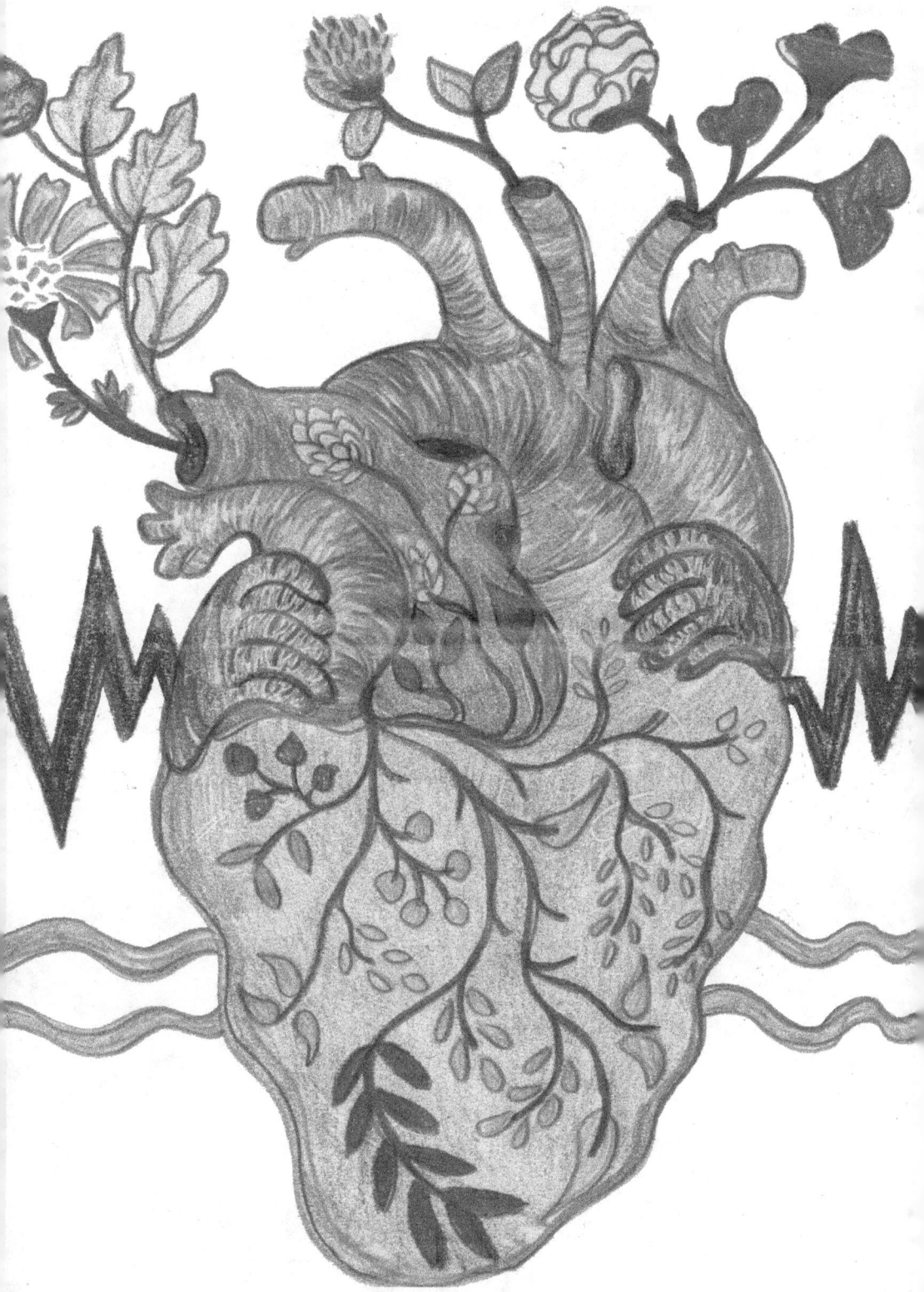

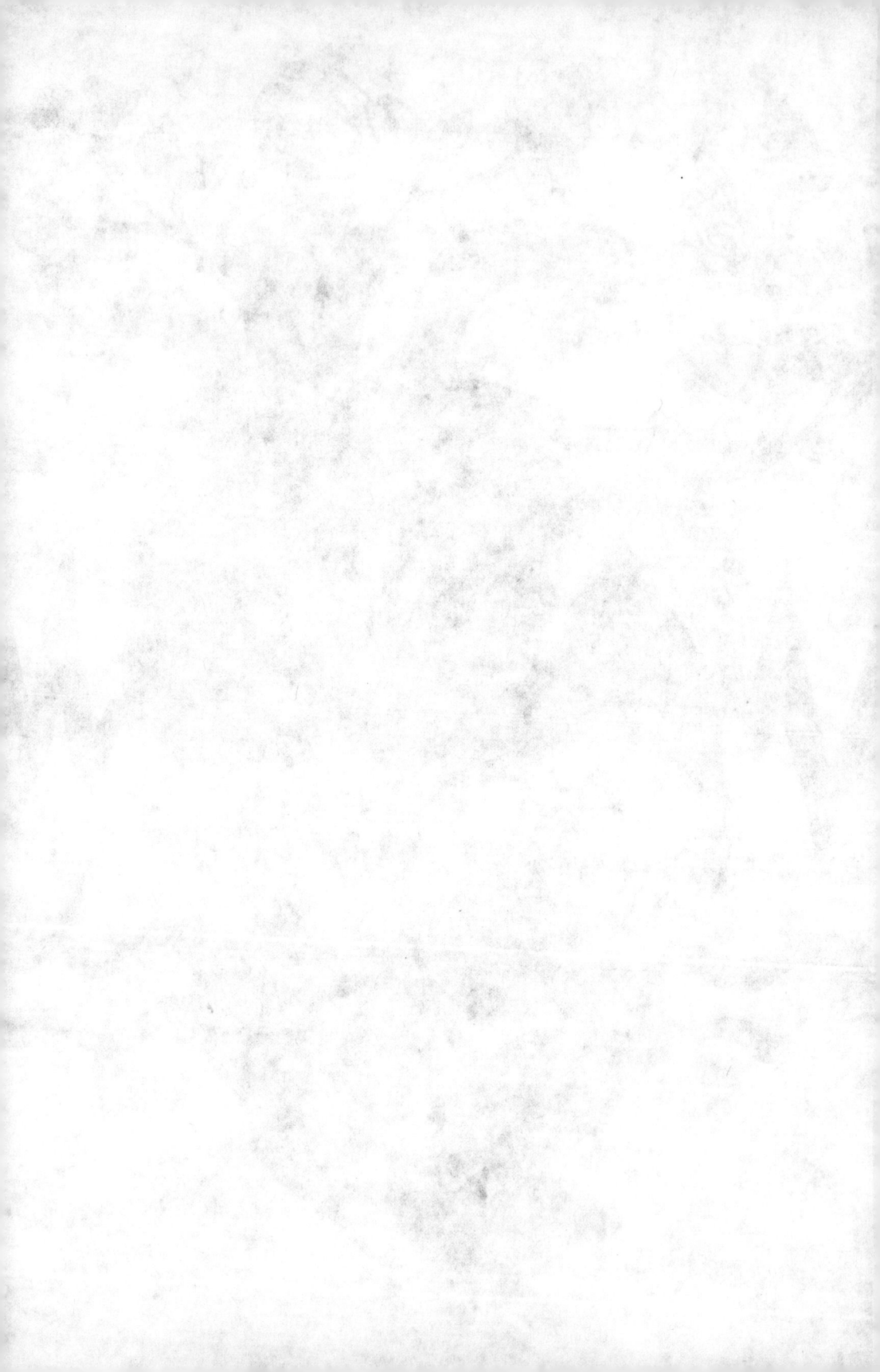

CONTENTS

Introduction

WHY WELLNESS?

This book is about *wellness*—what it means, why it matters, and how to find its heart.

The premise of this book is that:

(1) At some basic primal level, nearly everyone wants to feel well.
(2) Despite strong differences of opinion about how to achieve wellness or even what wellness means, there are simple truths at the heart of wellness.
(3) Applying these simple truths will promote wellness—no matter your circumstances or your path in life, no matter what else you (or your doctors) may be doing for good health and well-being, and no matter what your opinion is of *"wellness."*

Defining *wellness*—like many words that really matter in our lives—is not an easy task. The word has taken on many meanings. It has been used to describe a method of health care as well as a type of lifestyle; categories of foods as well as varieties of therapies. It has been explained as an emotional coping strategy, a workplace condition, a spiritual mindset, a physical regimen, and an eco-friendly balance. And that's just for starters...

With all these varied definitions of wellness, it's no surprise that the term is often misapplied. Sometimes the word has no real meaning, or it's just a catchy phrase used to sell things, that different people react differently to. Wellness can be complicated, and it can be controversial.

It can even agitate extreme opinions. At one extreme, critics call wellness an empty promise, which is impractical, filled with quack medicine, and devoid of scientific reason. These skeptics marginalize wellness, describing it as a fringe remnant of hippie counterculture or a New Age panacea without workable solutions for a real world. At the other extreme, supporters celebrate the good health and happiness wellness brings to people and the planet. Wellness zealots sharply contrast wellness to the failed approaches of big pharmaceuticals, highly processed foods, environmental destruction, corrupt politics, and religious hypocrisy. Our institutions and systems failed us, they argue, as they imagine wellness solutions for a world they want to manifest.

This book is not about those opinions.

Whatever your opinion, what is clear is that the impact of wellness has been practical, far-reaching, and worldwide. It has changed cultural attitudes, consumer tastes, our foods, and health care. It has altered how we look at the places we work and the environments we share. Commercially, it is big business, selling products and services in ever-growing numbers, spawning new industries, and remaking old ones.

More profoundly, wellness has moved our understanding of ourselves. It helps us see our health and happiness as involving not just our bodies, but our minds, emotions, and spirits as we slowly begin to understand the connections among them.

———

I have been asked why I write about wellness, given my career in business and law. The recurring and sometimes unspoken question seems to be: *What qualifies you to write such a book?*

One answer—though I don't think it's the only answer or even the best answer—is that for nearly a quarter century, I've explored diverse aspects of wellness in my career as an entrepreneur and attorney. Each of my business ventures—*adv*entures really—gave me new stories to tell and taught me new lessons about wellness. Although I'd say it is not my résumé or any job I had that qualifies me to write this book, my career may interest some readers who want to gauge my credibility or satisfy their curiosity.

I've been a part owner of a chain of local health and fitness centers, which offered exercise regimens, therapeutic treatments, and beauty services for their members, and I am still a part owner of an integrative homeopathic medicine company that makes a safe and effective natural pain relief cream (*Topricin*®—sold nationally in pharmacies, groceries, and online). I've been chairman of a manufacturer of a futuristic medical device that could spot diseased and dysfunctional areas of the body bio-energetically, and I still chair a nonprofit that turns web-based special-occasion gifts into the deep satisfaction of charitable caring (*ChangingThePresent.org*—it's the thought that counts).

Wellness was the thread that connected each of these career experiences together. This was true too in my role as a senior executive of the *ToughLove*® behavioral health-care program for families of troubled teens, as the founder of an early Internet company that helped stressed-out people find getaway vacations for recreation and relaxation, and as an operator of a green transportation dealership with motor scooters that made people smile as they went *vrrrroooooooom!*

As a lawyer, I've been able to assist many more diverse clients involved with wellness. I've represented retailers selling organic fresh-juiced beverages and restaurants with vegetarian-focused fast food. I've advised remediators of environmental contamination and reclaimers of once-polluted brownfield lands. I've counseled celebrity makeup artists who empower women and men by making them feel more beautiful and branded cosmetics formulators who understood that true beauty was more than skin-deep.

Sometimes my legal client was Earth itself and all those affected by environmental degradation. I've litigated the destruction of an endangered species and its habitat all the way up to the US Supreme Court, and helped stop a state's nuclear waste dumpsite by bringing about federal judicial intervention. When I take on such cases, lines often blur, making it difficult to see who is the real client because so many are affected by the outcomes and so much is at stake.

Lines always seem to blur when it comes to wellness. In my career, I've seen how the cleanup of plastic waste can be viewed as harvesting a new green fuel stock and how a good craft beer can become a natural medicine. I've watched how business investments can be measured in both monetary and karmic returns.

Through all these diverse career ventures and pursuits, what I began to see were patterns and similarities common to wellness. I came to understand how a basic human desire for wellness—defined by a few core aspects of what it truly means to be well—connected together diverse expressions of what is now popularly called *the wellness movement*.

———

The more I examined the meaning and contexts of the wellness movement, the more I came to believe that the desire for wellness motivates and drives an even wider range of current trends, events, causes, and activities. I began to realize how *the worldwide movement toward wellness is one of the great evolutionary changes of human history, ushering in a new Age of Awareness.*

This evolutionary change is moving us past a long historical period of exploitation, brutal conflicts, and zero-sum games, where humanity had little or no regard for the impact and consequences of our individual and collective actions. It moves us toward a more harmonious, collaborative, and self-aware relationship with one another and Earth. That change has not happened overnight, and it is still happening, for evolution can take time.

The man who actually coined the word "wellness"—a man whose unusual story is told later in this book—described how the experience of the Second World War became the driving impetus toward wellness as the nations of the world joined together to adopt the constitution of the World Health Organization. Like all great historical movements, the movement toward wellness proceeds in fits and starts, zigging and zagging, with challenges and setbacks and lessons that are still being painfully learned, but it moves inexorably forward over time.

In a big-picture sense, the desire for wellness has also fostered and empowered numerous other movements, all of which also accelerated after World War II. Civil rights, human rights, animal rights, environmentalism, ecology, sustainability, spirituality, transparency, empathy, and even rock and roll, hip-hop, and other forms of postwar music are all movements that spring from the heart of wellness.

At first glance that statement may seem like hyperbole or overly broad exaggeration, but in truth each of these other movements is really just a different face of the same simple desire for human wellness—to proactively seek health, happiness, harmony, and love; to feel well and to be well. Wellness is a movement that leads us to the inevitable conclusion that we are all in this human experience together, interdependent and connected in ways we barely understand. It is a movement that reconciles and reconnects sides of ourselves that we had falsely separated, to restore our wholeness and the good health that comes with that.

———

Though I have been involved with many varied wellness enterprises, I'm not even sure how I found these eclectic projects—or more accurately, how they found me.

There is a spiritual *law of attraction* that says that we manifest into our lives what we think about and what we seek for ourselves, so perhaps that explains my career path. I think that's the same principle as, or at least closely related to, the biblical proverb that *"we reap what we sow."* So I guess I've been seeking and sowing wellness in my own life for quite some time now.

Perhaps that is what really qualifies me to write this book.

Looking back with the clarity of hindsight, my own personal search for wellness accelerated at moments of my greatest personal challenges. I've survived lung cancer and other frightening diseases; suffered business failures and financial setbacks; and experienced severe family relationship strife, including teenage intervention and rehabilitation. Those adult challenges and crises each taught me things about wellness in ways that my business and legal ventures could not possibly have taught me.

While these life challenges are meaningful to me, I don't believe my own adult hardships are all that remarkable. Sooner or later, to greater or lesser degrees, we all experience pain, suffering, and death in our lives. *All of us!* To borrow an old joke, *no one gets out of this life alive!* That is part of our common human experience, which we all understand on some level.

For us all, what truly matters is not the story of our suffering, but how we grow from those experiences. For me, each of my own life struggles made me think deeply about finding wellness. Each experience created an urgency to find peace and well-being in the midst of personal crisis. Though gripping and formidable, each crisis helped center and balance me, teaching me transformative lessons about what was important in my life. Each suffering was a disguised opportunity to discover how to become better from within, no matter what the circumstances, what the prognosis, or what the outcome. In so doing, each struggle increased my own true capacity to be well.

That's not to minimize the aching sadness and wretched pain that accompanied each crisis—for me as for most people—but finding meaning through the ordeal was part of their value. Really, if you think about it, finding a way to be well is the *only* positive choice you can make during these most trying of times. We have no other choice except to find some *calm inside* during the storm—even as the *storm outside* rages on. That simple truth has been said before many times and in many ways. The philosopher Friedrich Nietzsche, for example, famously said, *"That which does not kill us makes us stronger."*

My grandfather Moe Roth, my mother's father, who lived gratefully through all sorts of illnesses, infirmities, and medical procedures to the age of ninety-six, said it a different way. Lying in a hospital bed, then in his eighties, unable to return to his home and his daily routines, he told me with a smile that being in the hospital was just part of his growing *up*—not his growing *old*, as others might say. I still marvel today at his wellness even in the midst of a medical crisis.

Living as long as my grandfather Moe, you can see recurring patterns in your life by looking back. Memoir and history are a lot alike that way. Historians warn that by failing to understand the patterns of history, we are doomed to repeat them. Look back in memory, and you can also see the patterns that give your own life meaning and direction, which you can learn from and which can help move you forward.

———

Looking back, long before my own adult life challenges, I realize now that I was seeking wellness even as a child. At the age of thirteen, I picked up a guitar for the very first time and can still vividly remember the wonderful way it made me feel, despite the awkwardness of my early teens—creative and inspired, peaceful and yet vibrantly alive.

From that moment on, I vowed never to give up musical expression and the feelings of deep therapeutic wellness it gave me. I still play guitar and many other musical instruments, having kept that promise to myself forty years later and still counting. Keeping that promise to myself hasn't always been easy, especially since I eventually chose to make my living as a practicing lawyer, not a working musician. Some people reflexively believe that inspiration and artistry, traits typically associated with musicians, should not apply to lawyers.

But I think they're wrong, misguided and misdirected, foolishly following *"the hobgoblin of little minds"*—to borrow a phrase from Ralph Waldo Emerson, mentor to one of my personal heroes, Henry David Thoreau. Exercising my inner musician still makes me feel well, and feeling creative and inspired allows me to perform legal jobs at levels of excellence and intuition that I believe my clients have come to expect of me.

Looking back still further to when I was ten years old, I remember reading an unusual article on the front page of the *New York Times*. The story was written by an American journalist named James "Scotty" Reston during his visit to China in 1971, and it made me think about health and wellness in my own life in previously unimaginable new ways.

In 1971 the Cold War between democracy and communism raged on, with entire blocs of nations still hidden behind iron curtains. Communist China was then isolated from the United States of America, and formal diplomatic recognition of the Chinese mainland, apart from the island of Taiwan, was many years away. Richard Nixon was the US president, and working with his national security advisor, Henry Kissinger, American relations with mainland China were just beginning to thaw.

As part of this gradual restoration in diplomatic relations, James Scotty Reston was part of an elite group of journalists allowed by the American government to visit China for the first time in decades. What happened to him next on that historic trip was completely unexpected, and his story captivated the American public in a way he could never have imagined when he left his office in New York City. During his visit, Reston needed an emergency appendectomy operation and Chinese doctors in Beijing successfully treated his postsurgical pain with acupuncture needles and herbal medicines.

Back then, these therapies were strange and scientifically inexplicable to most Western physicians and most Americans, but Scotty Reston said the needles and herbs worked—at least for him. To address the skeptics, cynics, and resulting medical controversy of his account, he wrote: "There are many things I will do for a good story, but getting slit open in the night or offering myself as an experimental porcupine is not among them."[1]

Reston's story helped open my eyes and my mind, even as a young boy. For me, his article was not a lesson about Chinese medicine, acupuncture, or herbalism, although I developed a lifelong fascination with those modalities and other "alternative" therapies. Rather, Reston's story taught me the possibility of many paths to good health, including ways that were neither accepted by conventional wisdom nor understood by mainstream medicine.

Even as a ten-year-old boy, this lesson was very meaningful to me, because American medical doctors seemed unable to diagnose or treat my own agonizing childhood stomachaches. I still remember the awful feeling of being bent over in pain, clutching at my gut; and remember realizing that these childhood physicians might be the same doubters and medical cynics Scotty Reston described in his news story. He helped me understand that sometimes even so-called experts don't know what they don't know.

Reston taught me a joyous lesson that we all ought to humbly admit our own ignorance, so we can then begin to graciously learn from it.

———

In some ways, this book is a lot like James "Scotty" Reston's front-page story in the *New York Times*.

Like Reston's readers, readers of this book may come to discover mysterious medicines and exciting new therapies, but that was neither Reston's purpose nor this book's intent. To borrow Scotty Reston's own words, readers may learn about alternative ways to good health and then speculate about their value as "great new medical breakthroughs" for themselves, but "I do not know whether this speculation is justified, and I am not qualified to judge."[2] I have no medical degree; the only doctorate I have is in law.

To be clear, this book does not advocate any modalities for wellness nor demand adherence to any dogmatic doctrines of health. It won't tell you to avoid a certain kind of food or take a certain kind of drug, and it does not insist you live a certain kind of life. However, like Reston's story did for me as a ten-year-old boy all those years ago, maybe this book can help open your eyes and your mind and provide you with an underlying approach to wellness.

If "an underlying approach to wellness" sounds too enigmatic, think of the parable about teaching a hungry man how to fish, instead of giving the man a fish to eat. Giving the man a fish allows him to eat for a day, but teaching him how to fish allows him to eat for a lifetime. That parable holds true for those seeking wellness. If you are seeking wellness in your life, whatever your path and circumstances, whatever your needs and desires, learning first *how to approach wellness* will ultimately be of greatest value to you.

To be sure, the most valuable skill we can learn, adaptable for nearly any circumstance, is to *learn how to learn*. I read a quote recently

by the futurist Alvin Toffler that summed up the paramount importance of this skill. Toffler is considered among the most influential
and prescient thinkers of his time, and the author of the international
bestseller *Future Shock* and its sequels, who predicted that "Tomorrow's
illiterate will not be the man who can't read; he will be the man who has
not learned how to learn." [3]

I found that advice true in my own career. When I went to law school,
truly the least valuable part of my vocational education was the actual
laws I studied. That type of rote learning is easily forgotten, and besides,
laws change constantly and need to be rechecked and re-researched.
What was really valuable was learning a new way to *approach problems*, what
some of my law professors at Columbia University in New York City
described as "thinking like a lawyer." Learning a new way of thinking was
like acquiring a new set of tools that could be applied to new facts, new
circumstances, and new areas of law, and indeed, to help solve problems
well beyond the law.

Neuroplasticity is how my scientist friends describe the brain's ability
to learn entirely new ways of thinking, as if our minds were given a
new set of tools. Interestingly and historically speaking, the institutions of science and medicine had for generations mistakenly rejected
the very concept of neuroplasticity, falsely believing that the brain and
nerve cells do not grow and develop in adulthood, that they were fixed
and unchanging. That gross scientific error is a cautionary tale repeated
again and again throughout history.

Science and medicine have wonderful tools to offer, but wellness
requires tools of its own. Indeed, the tools of wellness are best used
by *you* for *yourself*. Science and medicine may not yet understand nor
appreciate these tools—which include your mind, heart, and spirit
beyond your physical body—but that should not stop you from using
these tools to benefit your own health and wellness. These tools are
capable of healing and transforming you, and healing and transforming others too.

We all have these tools to use, but not all of us have the *willingness to learn* how to use them. Like all good tools, these tools of wellness must be sharpened and honed for use. The more we use them, the better we become at using them. Sometimes they get rusty, but they just need to be polished and used again.

Truly, these tools are within us all, as great *truths* that are waiting to be revealed. This is not about religious faith or belief, although most religions and faiths say similar things. Although deeply buried in some people, nonetheless these tools and truths are inside all, available to be actualized and waiting to be used.

———

To make these wellness tools more accessible, this book weaves together true stories across diverse experiences.

As an old Native American proverb goes, *"Tell me a fact, and I'll learn; tell me a truth, and I'll believe; but tell me a story, and it will live in my heart forever."* As the picture on the cover suggests, this book is about the heart. To get to the heart and essence of the story, historically accurate words are quoted whenever possible. Sometimes, they are italicized or underscored too, to emphasize their meaning.

Some of the stories told are sad and preventable, like infant teething medicines that killed babies for more than a hundred years. Other stories in this book are happy and uplifting, like the story of an unreachable wild child condemned to an asylum who had a miraculous awakening that inspired millions. Stories of medicine merge with memoir, stories of science blend into philosophy, and stories of business converge with art and comedy. Some may call this approach *interdisciplinary* or *integrative*—while others unaccustomed to *big-picture thinking* may call it *chaotic*—but the truth is that *truth* cannot be narrowly separated into separate dominions of knowledge. That is surely true when it comes to something as important as your own wellness.

It may seem incredible that so much can be connected together, but truly, there are core commonalities. Those connections drive the stories of this book forward and inevitably lead to recognition how so much that we separate is already joined together in wholeness and unity, like *truth* itself.

That may sound complex, but one of this book's basic premises is that this *truth* is really simple and obvious. In a game show broadcast on television at the turn of a new millennium, comedian Jeff Foxworthy challenged Americans to be *smarter than a fifth grader*. The funny premise of the show was a reminder how often adults fail to think as clearly as a child—we make things far more difficult than they need to be.

To make it simpler and more accessible still, I tried to distill the heart and essence of what I've learned. In other words, I tried to keep this book short—or more accurately, as short as I could without losing the richness of true meaning. The great American humorist Mark Twain, another of my personal heroes, is said to have said *that he didn't have time to write a short letter, so he wrote a long one instead.* He was right about that, and it took me longer to make this book shorter, to get to the heart of the matter.

This book consists of thirteen chapters—a baker's dozen, or twelve with an extra for good measure (or "beyond measure" as the last chapter is titled). After this introduction, the chapters divide into two parts; how wellness can bring "better health" (part A) and how it can restore "wholeness" (part B). For further ease of reading, each chapter is divided into shorter and more manageable sections, each a pause to refresh.

Some may read the book rapidly in days, while others may prefer to linger slowly over months or longer, but whatever way you read this book is the best way for you. My own suggestion is to read the chapters in order, to build on intertwined stories and sequentially gain insights about wellness, learning about better health to gain a deeper appreciation of wholeness. If you disregard that suggestion, and find yourself jumping to favorite stories, looking for memorable quotations, or skipping directly to the paradigm-shifting conclusions of part B, well then I suppose your non-sequential approach has value too, especially for a non-fiction book like this one, which seeks the facts and truths at the heart of wellness and its new Age.

Perhaps this book could have been shorter still, and it may sometimes seem I'm meandering or that a certain message or lesson has already been said before. But those detours and redundancy are intentional, used to further develop an idea or expose the implications of a concept. Or perhaps its just my writing style, a reflection of my own personality and essence, for which I am unapologetic. Indeed, another lesson of wellness is never to apologize for who you truly are, to acknowledge and accept the beautiful differences and imperfections inside you as inside all, while you strive to become a better you.

Discovering and cultivating your best and truest self while accepting your differences and imperfections is a delightfully lifelong pursuit. It can surprise you and come at the expense of painful realizations about yourself—all of that has certainly been true in my own life—but that helps you grow. It is this self-discovery that nourishes your spirit, transforms your mind, and increases your capacity for wellness. But maybe I'm just meandering again...

It is my sincere hope that this book helps you find wellness in your own life in small or large measure. I am deeply humbled and grateful for that opportunity, and I wish you well.

S. J. (*"Steve"*) Spiegel

Part A

BETTER HEALTH

Chapter 1

START WITH SIMPLICITY

If you're searching for something, often the first step is knowing what you're looking for. *"What am I trying to find?"* you might ask yourself.

It may sound like a simple first step, but simple is not always easy. Especially when the thing you're seeking is difficult to define, when it's elusive and enigmatic, like *wellness*.

Like many powerful words, *wellness* means different things to different people. Some of these meanings were mentioned in the introduction, but bear repeating. For instance, to some people wellness means preventing disease and maintaining the body's good health; for others, it is a blissful state of mind and being. Some see wellness as a popular movement or a cultural phenomenon, while others disdainfully say it is unscientific quack nonsense. Adding further to its complexities and mysteries, many paths abound, with some insisting their way to wellness is the best way or the only way.

Despite all these definitional difficulties, few people would say finding *wellness* is not worth the effort. Wellness represents some of mankind's deepest hopes and aspirations for our selves, for others, and for the world. Across cultures and languages, humans use common expressions like *"I wish you well"* and *"I want to feel well"* and tell others *"Get well soon"* and *"Hope all is well."* These expressions evoke deep sentiments, thoughts, beliefs, and desires that are part of the universal human condition.

Wellness is a lot like love in that regard. Few would say that searching for love is not worth the effort, even though when it comes to true love, we don't quite know what we're looking for from the start.

Love can seem complex and irrational, yet some deep innate urge drives us to search for this elusive and enigmatic thing we call *love*—sometimes in unlikely places and at great personal sacrifice, though truly, love desires mercy but not sacrifice. Despite all its complexities, once love finally is found, it becomes intuitively obvious, as if we knew it was there all along, just waiting to be discovered. Once we are able to bask in its warm glow, love's beautiful simplicity seems self-evident.

How can something so seemingly complicated be so simple and true in its essence? Perhaps, like the heart of true love, the heart of wellness is astonishingly simple.

"If you can't explain it simply," Albert Einstein is said to have said, *"then you don't understand it well enough."*

Einstein should know. His theory of special relativity, which brought him into world prominence, was proven based on its *simplicity*. Call it the scientific law of parsimony or the heuristic principle of Ockham's Razor, but whatever the terminology, Einstein's understanding was so clear that it seemed to be simple common sense—at least in hindsight. His explanations of complex scientific problems seemed so obvious that Einstein's scientific peers eventually had to ask themselves, *"Why didn't someone think of that sooner?"*—even though Einstein had shattered their paradigms of physics, forever changing their old ways of looking at things.

———

Getting to the simple heart of the matter, like Einstein did, can be like finally seeing a forest through the trees. It can be like seeing an image in a Rorschach inkblot that we couldn't see before. It was there in the picture all along, plain as could be, but most didn't see it until someone else said, *"Look this way,"* and then it became easy to see—*if you were willing to look!*

Nicolaus Copernicus, and then Galileo Galilei, saw how Earth revolved around the sun, instead of the other way around, as was taught at the time. They offered a telescope so people could see for themselves, but at first, few were willing to look. Eventually the simple observations of Copernicus and Galileo changed how we look at the sun, Earth, the planets, and ourselves.

This may sound complex, but it's really simple. It's like the story of the tall truck that ignored the height-restricted warning signs at the entrance to a highway tunnel and got stuck, unable to move forward or backward in the tunnel. With traffic snarled and clogged up for miles behind the stuck truck, the police, the fire department, the highway engineers, and even the mayor all gathered at the entrance to the tunnel, scratching their heads in disbelief and trying desperately to devise a solution. They were stumped!

It took a little girl, waiting in one of the automobiles stuck in traffic, to make a simple suggestion, asking the mayor: "Why can't the truck just let the air out of its tires?"

Simply explained insights can change our perspective of the world and our own lives, opening entirely new vistas of understanding in great exponential leaps forward. So it is worth striving for these simplicities.

I once heard that there are three levels of understanding. The first and most basic level is simple; it is what we know on the surface of things, the common sense that anyone can understand. The second and deeper level contains the facts, figures, studies, and examinations, all of the intricacies and contexts and complexities beneath the surface, observations zoomed into reveal incredible detail, discovered and discussed by academics, professionals, researchers, and experts in the subject. This second level often uses convoluted abstractions and scholarly jargon and is obtained only after years of committed study, education, and research.

Finally, though, after all that study and all that detail comes the third level, with understanding greater than the intricate complexities of the second level. At this third and greatest level of understanding, things once again become simple, as the big picture with all its details is seen for what it is. The simplicity makes the complexities of the second level now easy to understand, obvious to those with common sense and willing to look.

Realizing the earth revolves around the sun finally explains the seasons and the movement of planets in the night sky. Understanding you can let the air out of a stuck truck's tire can suddenly set you free from traffic. Previously unexplained physics problems of space and time are solved instantly with Einstein's simple principles of relativity.

You *can* solve complex problems with simplicity; indeed, simplicity is often the *only* solution for complex problems.

———

If that sounds confusing, the real point is this: When it comes to something as fundamental for you as your own wellness, you don't need to be an Einstein to seek simplicity for yourself.

You may already know the obvious answers amid all the complexities of your life. It may just take a reminder, a lesson, a story, or someone to say, "*Look this way.*"

To those who think that it's too late in their life or too late in their own struggles to remember what makes them well, it's never too late to start! We are all on a life's journey—a journey that has its beginning and its end. Even at the end of a journey, we can desire wellness, to be at peace. If your own journey toward wellness seems overwhelming and insurmountable amid struggles for good health or happiness, try to remember that every journey begins with a single step—even a thousand mile one, as a Tao Te Ching proverb goes.[1] As your own journey of life continues, there are steps you can take towards wellness.

So take heart! Even prisoners in Nazi death camps somehow found wellness through their ordeals, a story told later in this book. So take your first step toward wellness, and continue your journey, even if *wellness* seems an unlikely place to go.

This book—*HEART* of *WELLNESS*—had its beginnings in an unlikely place too.

Most people think about wellness during life's most joyous moments but especially during their most troubled times. That was true for me too. Wonderful occasions like my marriage and the births of my three children brought me deep feelings of wellness, and I can still bask in the warm glow of those moments. The most terrifying times of my life, like the health ordeals of my lung cancer, the intervention for my teenage son, or the financial failure of my first major business venture, made me desperate for wellness, forcing me to search for wellness and appreciate how important it was for me and my family.

Though these troubled periods of my life were profoundly painful and unwanted, I am now deeply grateful for the valuable lessons they taught me. My lung cancer, for example, seems like a great blessing in hindsight. Like a strong and sometimes violent wind, the disease propelled me forward, helping me realize what was important to me, who I want to be, and who I am. I realized how I was but a sailboat on the water, for I could not control the wind, though I could hold on to the rudder to help steer myself in a direction, with faith in a higher power and purpose. Truly, I learned a lot from my lung cancer, but this book's beginning—its search for the heart of wellness—had nothing to do with that disease or with any other crisis in my life, or with any joyous moment either.

Instead, this book began with some business research and writing for career and financial purposes. That may seem an unlikely place to begin a search for wellness, but my topic was the commercial aspects of the wellness movement. As I researched and wrote about that topic, I began to realize something far bigger and more meaningful than the business subject where I started, something about the very nature of wellness itself. It was the unlikely seed from which this book grew—and where the next chapter begins.

———

Before proceeding to the next chapter, you may be asking where this is all leading, or perhaps you may be thinking I'm just meandering again. You may be wondering where the supposed simplicity of wellness is to be found and why I haven't explained it already if it's that simple to explain.

If you're looking for a brief explanation in numeric bullet points, as many books on wellness seem to offer, I'd say that these short lists may be concise, but they don't often convey *true meaning*. If you still emphatically insist on a numbered list, here's what I'd offer at this early stage of the book:

(1) *What we think we understand about wellness is like the exposed tip of an enormous hidden iceberg.*

(2) *As more and more people throughout the world openly seek wellness for themselves and Earth, the iceberg hidden below the water's surface will finally be exposed, revealing false assumptions about ourselves and our planet—false assumptions that have been accepted dogmatically and without question, except by a few, for many hundreds of years.*

(3) *Understanding the real meaning of wellness will enable us to better understand ourselves and seek better health, quality of life, and personal fulfillment. It will also change the dynamics of relationships among people and the dynamics of our relationship with Earth and its other inhabitants.*

(4) *These changes and new understandings are inevitable, unless our growing concern with wellness fades away, perhaps as a result of some cataclysmic*

8

event that forces us to struggle for survival—instead of strive for wellness. Indeed, the worldwide movement toward wellness can help avoid such a catastrophic event by correcting the false assumptions and mistaken separations that lead us in the wrong direction, away from wellness. Besides, for those struggling to survive, as we all do at some point in our finite lives, the true meaning of wellness helps uplift us through the struggle.

Lists like these—lists that offer readers *four simple steps to wellness!*— are more blunt than simple. The heart of wellness is simple, but it is not blunt. Wellness is not best explained with bullet points of proof, any more than it can be understood by sharp lines presented on compelling charts and measured graphs. As will be seen, the geometry of points, lines, charts, and graphs cannot capture the simple heart of wellness. Wellness has geometry of its own.

Maybe you're the type of person who looks for the lines or who needs mathematical proofs presented on scientific charts or logical graphs. Or maybe you're the type of person who believes you need to be an Einstein to find transcendent simplicity. If that's you, perhaps you can *think of wellness as existing in three dimensions*—like three dimensions of space. All three dimensions of wellness—you can call them three *keys* to understanding wellness, if you're still looking for bullet points—are discussed in this book, but over time.

Time may be the fourth dimension of wellness, but that time is up to *you*. Ultimately, this book is about *you* and the choices *you* can make about your own wellness. If you are reading these words, you're already moving in the direction of wellness and can get there in time.

As time moves forward unconsciously during our lives, there are still conscious choices we all make about time. Being well can be a conscious choice you make how to spend your time here on Earth.

Confused? This may not sound simple—at least not yet! Discovering the simple meaning of wellness for your self should make it so.

Chapter 2

FUZZY FORMALITIES FIRST

The thesis of this book grew from a formal and analytical white paper that I researched and wrote a few years ago on the topic of wellness.

This may be surprising to a great many readers, accustomed to warm and fuzzy musings on wellness. Indeed, most of the wellness books I've read are oriented toward being inspirational, heartfelt, and healing, with teachings and advice on how to achieve healthy and positive states of being. That was true too for a wellness book I wrote a few years back, while I was struggling to help my troubled teenage son and to find peace for my family and myself. It was a novel entitled *(((Tuning Jack FM)))*, written in the Chautauqua storytelling tradition, and it explored wellness practices like "self-tuning" and "mindfulness" of everyday routines.

These types of wellness books are often *qualitatively fuzzy* and philosophically nuanced. Those characteristics give the books their authenticity; it is what makes them deeply meaningful to their growing audience of readers.

By contrast, the white paper I wrote was *quantitatively formal* and factually authoritative. As customary for the white paper genre, it used logical precision and the techniques of detailed dissertation to convince its readers of its credibility and believability. Like most white papers, mine was written for formal presentation to an audience assembled in person to critically evaluate and review the paper's merits.

What may be surprising is the type of audience to which my white paper on the topic of wellness was formally presented. It was not delivered to spa seekers wrapped in terrycloth, nor spiritual sojourners clad in monks' robes. It was not even presented to academic audiences clothed in caps and gowns. Rather, it was given to Wall Street private equity investment banking professionals—those sophisticated elite of the financial world—dressed in formal suits and ties, many elegantly tailored with starched collars and monogrammed French cuffs.

Along with my business partner Antonio (*"Tony"*) Varano della Vergiliana and our own team of financial professionals, I presented the white paper to about two dozen groups of these private equity firms, mostly as we all sat across from one another at ceremonious conference room tables in architecturally elegant Manhattan skyscrapers dozens of floors above the avenues and streets of New York City below.

To many of my legal and business colleagues, a formal dissertation on the fuzzy topic of wellness may seem like an oxymoron, but these Wall Street private equity firms were considering investing many tens or hundreds of *millions* of dollars in the acquisition of companies that sold wellness-related products and services. These savvy financiers shrewdly recognized that the growing demand for *wellness*—whatever that word meant—was driving an expanding worldwide consumer market, presenting a unique investment opportunity.

The numbers told the story, and those numbers were measured in simple dollars and common cents. Wellness had become big business internationally, even though there was no consensus on how wellness was defined, then or now. What was clear was that new business categories were emerging to satisfy the growing consumer demand for wellness—like fitness clubs and health spas, vitamins and supplements, alternative medicines and therapies. Together, these types of easily identifiable wellness businesses collectively accounted for hundreds of *billions* of dollars in revenues.

What was even more financially significant to these investors was that traditional old-line industries, comprising many more *trillions* of dollars in revenues, were rapidly transforming themselves to accommodate the steadily growing consumer desire and demand for wellness. Among the giant industries adapting themselves to satisfy this growing consumer appetite for wellness were foods, beverages, cosmetics, pharmaceuticals, hospitality, health care, consumer goods, and household furnishings.

Some of the giant multinational conglomerates in these established industries had even created special wellness groups and divisions and were reorienting their business mission statements around wellness goals and platitudes. Many of these industry giants were acquiring smaller wellness-oriented brands and companies to gain a foothold in the changing consumer market dynamic—and helping create financial exit opportunities for enterprising entrepreneurs and investors.

There was a growing sense among these private equity firms that a train was leaving the station and that businesses that did not board this train toward wellness would be left stranded at the station's platform. In analyzing the data, the robust growth in wellness-related products and services across multiple industries did not have the usual trappings of a fad. Unlike fad-type revenues, there were no sales spikes that rose and then predictably fell again. The demand appeared to be slow and steady over many decades, with all indications of a long-term business trend, increasingly embraced by popular culture and in everyday life, with broad influence across diverse consumer markets and across international border lines. In other words, wellness appeared to be a worldwide business phenomenon, a movement worthy of the attention of savvy professional Wall Street private equity investors.

These investors wanted the pertinent facts and the numerical figures, the type of essential data and due diligence that provides important clues as to the direction and trajectory of a business trend like wellness. The white paper I wrote had this formal information, along with the whys and wherefores, so that these investors could better manage the risks of knowing where to put their money and how to place their bets.

And so, gathered together in conference rooms high above the streets of New York City, my business partner and I and other members of our team presented this crucial information to these Wall Street investors. They were all well-educated and well-trained financial professionals, so we knew their follow-up questions about the white paper and its conclusions would be analytically precise and logically spot-on, and we did our best to answer their questions.

My business partner, Antonio Varano della Vergiliana, and I were well-suited for such formal investment analysis with our respective educations and experiences. Tony was a gifted business operator, adept at managing the nuts and bolts of running businesses in a wide swath of industries, from agriculture to entertainment, construction to cosmetics, mining to manufacturing. A serial entrepreneur since his teens, with a talent for branding and positioning companies, he finally obtained an MBA in Finance, going "back to school" à la comedian Rodney Dangerfield when his grown children began attending college themselves. Antonio also had international business experience that ranged from his native Rome, Italy, to his adopted home of Perth, Australia, and many other places in between, including Orange County, New York, a rural enclave outside Manhattan, where the two of us first met.

Antonio Varano was a businessman to his core, with no special affinity for the wellness movement, although he was a natural—intuitively and reflexively—at understanding the importance of wellness in a balanced life, always seeming to enjoy diverse aspects of his life's experience with vigor and vitality. Tony would probably tell you that his interest in wellness was its ability to make money, and on one level that was true, but the truth was also that his vibrant and beautiful American wife, Andrea, had sparked his sincere interest in the topic through her own deep and abiding belief in wellness—not to mention her spending patterns on wellness, Tony would probably add with a playful loving chuckle.

By formal education and career, Andrea was an electrical engineer, demonstrably capable of scientific rigor and logical analysis, yet she regularly attended New Age yogic retreats and sought out the latest wellness supplements and healing regimens. For Andrea, *fuzzy* and *formal* were not mutually inconsistent; they were part of the same indivisible, multifaceted person—a seeming contradiction that was equally true for myself and perhaps for us all, part of the paradox of our basic human nature.

Maybe it was the *yin*-meets-*yang* connected duality that I've found unified at the heart of so many things, or so it seemed to me, then and now. Even back when I wrote the white paper, it occurred to me that these fuzzy Zen-like understandings helped to explain the direction of the consumer wellness movement and its future impact on business as much as any hard facts or figures, as much as any formal charts or graphs.

Our own team of investment banking professionals, however, properly reminded us not to engage in such fuzzy musings on wellness and the holistic unity of things. Our team included Clayton Jones, an elite West Point graduate and highly disciplined army captain, who had worked at such prestigious financial institutions as GE, and Michael Mendelson, a former Ernst & Young "Entrepreneur of the Year," who had astutely raised several billions of dollars for his investment banking clients on the London AIM's stock exchange. They had orchestrated the private equity presentations for Antonio and me and our company, Lotus Energetics Management. Though both Mike and Clayton had open minds and warm hearts, they were dutifully mindful of proper business decorum and the formal, polished ethos of Wall Street, and both knew—as did Tony and I too—that fuzzy conversations could be every bit as inappropriate as improper clothing attire.

So when Antonio and I met with these private equity firms to discuss the white paper, I happily donned a fashionably conservative business suit and tie, along with a politely formal attitude and demeanor, and gladly presented the logical analytical side of myself. This side of myself was sincere and genuine, in no way phony nor pretentious. It was a bona fide aspect of self that was entirely credible and consistent with my credentials and career as an Ivy League-pedigreed attorney, a Harlan Fiske Stone scholar rigorously trained in business transactions at the international Wall Street law firm of Skadden, Arps, Slate, Meagher & Flom—although this was but one single separate and isolated aspect of self out of many diverse and interwoven parts of me.

Some parts fuzzy, and some parts formal, all somehow inextricably connected and coexisting.

Chapter 3

BLURRING THE LINES

Beneath their formal attire and demeanor, I'd bet that these Wall Street private equity investors and investment bankers had some fuzziness in their own lives.

Perhaps they comfortably expressed their fuzziness within their families or with lovers and friends they cared about. Maybe they yearned for this fuzziness as a way of finding balance in their lives or to cope with despair at times of great personal crisis, reminded how vulnerably soft and fuzzily human they were beneath their suit-and-tie formal facades. For some this fuzziness was seldom revealed, like a skeleton kept in the closet. It may have been a side of self they didn't know they could share with others, or perhaps a side of self they didn't quite understand.

Indeed, finding and nurturing your truest self is a fundamental part of wellness. It is a way to bring light to the darkness, a way to heal your self. But that's just more fuzzy wellness speak, I reminded myself again, not appropriate for the white paper presentations; surely, I thought, there are lines of formality that should not be crossed.

And yet, reminiscing all these years later about my experience of presenting a white paper on wellness to professional investors, what left the most lasting memory for me was the presentation where the line between formal and fuzzy blurred, and then—in a brief but magical moment—seemed erased altogether.

It was late December, and the meeting was held in a building on Park Avenue in the New York City offices of one of the world's largest private equity investors, a London-based group. The team that assembled to evaluate the white paper was astute and inquisitive, and we had engaging and far-ranging discussions through the afternoon about the business of wellness, well past the time allotted. There was passion and imagination in the room, and it seemed as if no one really wanted the meeting to end. As night fell, we broke into smaller groups, still chatting about wellness and then about our plans for the evening. I was looking forward to holiday cocktails afterward with Tony and our management team, my festive red-and-green-striped tie giving away my Christmas spirit.

Though the meeting was interesting, what I remember most was how it ended. Moving with a group of private equity professionals from the conference room table toward the picturesque windows overlooking Park Avenue, we sat down and stared together at the snowflakes gently falling outside onto the boulevard below, the colorfully lit evergreen trees in the garden median shimmering with tinseled trimmings like a Thomas Kinkade painting. In that shared moment—that wonderful moment as we quietly gazed outside at a snowy scene—the line between formal and fuzzy disappeared for me.

It was a moment of good will and great warmth, *making spirits bright* in the words of a seasonal song. It was as if jingling bells could ring in joy and goodwill, palpably joining people's hearts together in peace. It was a shining instant, a moment of transcendence that could move people to share something more meaningful than the formal lines and labels of an analytical business presentation.

Some dismiss this invisible fuzzy feeling as mere *imagination*. You might call it the type of Christmas magic that delights children of all ages, yet others insist it is real—as real as anything can be! Whatever your opinion, these magical moments can linger in memory for a lifetime for reasons we don't quite understand. We might not be able to express nor explain such transcendent moments, especially not without poetry or song, yet their fuzzy feeling is common, part of our universal human experience.

———

The ability to transcend lines and limitations may seem implausible, something that we confine with formal lines of social acceptability. We may limit the feeling to religion or myth or artistic creation, but perhaps these lines and limitations were never there in the first place. Perhaps these lines are artificial separations, fictitious boundaries that were created for the sake of convenience or convention.

Lines may serve important purposes, which is why we initially draw them, but we can forget those purposes and become mistakenly attached to the lines themselves. One of the recurring themes of this book is that too-rigid attachment to these lines is at the peril of our own wellness.

Eventually events or insights can blur the lines we create for ourselves, forcing us to see beyond these lines, forcing us to recognize they were imaginary all along. We draw lines in the sand that are erased by the winds and the tides. Boundary lines separating nations disappear with wars and political bargains and have no meaning when it comes to natural movements like weather, species, and ideas. Color lines subjugating people into slavery or subservience are erased by the insight that people should be judged by the content of their character, not their surface skin appearances. Lines separating music into specific genres disappear with greater appreciation of the commonalities of musical expression, just as lines separating knowledge into separate fields of academic study disappear with the type of interdisciplinary thought that allows great leaps forward of understanding.

In a sudden, instantaneous moment of clarity and perception, we can understand that the lines we create for ourselves and our world, and the limitations and separations that come with line-drawing, were never really real. Realizing the lines are illusory, we can forever change how we view the world and how we see our place in that world.

Looking back, it seems appropriate for me that the line between formal and fuzzy was erased in a business meeting on *wellness*. The search for wellness has that effect on lines—it blurs the lines we've falsely assumed for ourselves. Lines are always blurred in the search for wellness, for wellness forces us to connect to the deeper humanity within us all, exposing the false separations we place upon ourselves. At the heart of wellness are unity and connectedness, which extend to our relationships with the world and with one another and to the many aspects of self within each of us.

The line-blurring effect of wellness is not limited to fuzzily sublime topics, like the multifaceted nature of self. As my white paper explained, wellness has the same line-blurring effect on mundane topics like the formalities of business.

———

Business surely has its own lines of separation, the type of lines upon which investors routinely base their financial decisions. Business people draw lines to separate consumers by market types and national borders. Lines are drawn to separate businesses themselves by industrial classifications and categorizations. There are lines of legal definition and terminology that separate an industry's regulation and its governmental oversight.

The wellness movement blurred each of these business lines. Even for readers uninterested in business, seeing lines of business blur in this short section of the book shows how other lines can blur too.

Like dinosaurs, those companies rigidly adhering to the old assumed lines of business in a changing wellness market saw market share erode and revenue base disappear, while agile entrepreneurs and open-minded companies of the wellness movement purposefully blurred lines of business to score big with breakthrough wellness products and services, growing new revenues and opening new markets.

Business line-blurring created both *disruption* and *opportunity*—yet another example of the type of fuzzily connected Zen duality where seeming opposites holistically contained the seeds of the other. Consider the beverage industry, for example. The beverage industry was built on the assumption that consumers buy drinks to quench their thirst. With the growing consumer market demand for wellness, resourceful beverage manufacturers began adding nutritional benefits or pharmaceutical impacts to their products, moving the beverage industry into new markets that overlapped with other industries. Beverage entrepreneurs created energy-enhancing drinks to stimulate well-being and vitamin-laden waters to improve health, innovating huge new product categories. As lines blurred between industries, a wellness-oriented consumer could now buy a beverage to boost their immune system or to provide mental clarity, not just to quench thirst. Similarly, wellness-oriented consumers began avoiding thirst-quenching beverages that was seen as too sugary or corrosive and that might lead to illness.

The beverage industry was not unique in its metamorphosis as a result of the consumer wellness movement. The line-blurring effect of wellness, and the business disruption and opportunity that followed, was felt across an improbably wide swath of other industries.

Food companies began to tout some of their products as "functional" foods, for their medicinal-like abilities to lower cholesterol, regulate digestion, or improve moods. Hotels began to offer spa treatments and fitness centers as essential to the wellness of their guests. Hospitals began to offer yoga and massage for patients and change the drab color of patient rooms to improve patient attitudes and well-being. Even furniture makers added ergonomic features as a therapeutic remedy for common public health and wellness issues, like bad backs and insomnia. As these examples each suggest, the search for wellness did not just create new products and services—it forced industries to reexamine *just what type of business* they were operating.

Businesses have historically been categorized into specific industry groups, so once a business is categorized, it is expected to behave a certain way. It's a lot like putting a square peg in only a square hole, and the round peg in only the round hole. Each separate industry group has different distribution channels, different points of sale, different industry associations, different marketing messages, even different legal rules and regulations. There is a beverage industry and a food industry, a pharmaceutical industry and a cosmetic industry, a hospitality industry and a home products industry, each conforming to the customs and practices of its respective industry.

As markets moved toward consumer wellness, all of these industrial lines—their classifications, characteristics, and categorizations—began to blur. As a result, the pegs and the holes seemed to lose their rigid shape, and the industries themselves began to look and act profoundly differently. It was as if these businesses were behaving like humans, suddenly learning the holistic nature of themselves in their own personal search for wellness.

The cosmetic industry is another good example of the profound changes that occurred as wellness blurred industrial lines. The modern cosmetics business began with industry pioneers like Max Factor, who developed face greasepaints to make up the faces of actors and actresses, changing their appearance for the stage and screen. This approach became the hallmark for the industry for a century; cosmetics focused on trademarked brands, with celebrity endorsements, that offered glamour and beauty by temporarily changing a person's appearance.

The wellness movement encouraged cosmetic entrepreneurs to move beyond surface appearances. Cosmetics industry innovators began adding botanical ingredients to their paints and powders and lotions and began making health and wellness claims for these new ingredients. They might add a botanical like calendula, a flowering plant known for its ability to soothe the skin, or an extract of a rare melon believed to have anti-aging properties. Then they made drug-like claims of therapeutic value or medical cures, since the supposed effects of these new botanical ingredients went beyond changing surface appearances.

Industry insiders called these new product formulations "cosme-ceuticals," combining aspects of cosmetics and pharmaceuticals. By the time I wrote the white paper, the new category of cosmeceuti-cals—which didn't even exist a few years earlier—was already calcu-lated to constitute the *majority* of all cosmetic products sold. The white paper offered case studies of the seismic changes that cosmeceuticals brought to the cosmetic industry, but what was really exciting was the way that it blurred the lines of industry, creating new opportunities for entrepreneurs.

Like a conventional cosmetic, cosmeceuticals could still be trade-marked, branded, and marketed with celebrity endorsement. But now, like a pharmaceutical, these innovative new wellness products could also be patented, with clinical trials proving their efficacy, and then endorsed by doctors and medical professionals. There were no more lines to dic-tate how the product was positioned in the market, and entrepreneurs could pick and choose their approach depending on their strategies for the product itself.

And when it came to the channels for distributing and selling the new cosmeceuticals, the line was again blurred; indeed, the line may have been erased altogether. One highly respected business research group, Packaged Facts, called the phenomenon the "Big Blur of Channel Overlap." The product might still be distributed in a drug-store aisle or sold at a department store counter, the way cosmetics had been sold and distributed for generations. Alternatively, the cosmeceu-tical might now be sold by prescription or through a doctor's office, the way drugs were conventionally distributed and sold.

Innovative marketers soon realized that they were no longer confined by the old lines of either the cosmetic or the pharmaceutical industries, and they ventured into entirely new channels and sales outlets, like television infomercials, health and beauty spas, direct response and multilevel marketers, wellness service providers, natural food stores, and many others. There seemed to be no lines and limitations anymore on cosmetic products; indeed, many were forced to ask what was a "cosmetic" anyhow?

Government regulators, accustomed to rigid definitions to enforce their industry laws and rules, were especially perplexed by the blurring of the lines. In the United States, the Food, Drug and Cosmetic Act of 1938 created laws, with rules and regulations to be enacted by a federal agency known as the FDA. The FDA was given broad powers of oversight and enforcement depending on whether a product was classified as a "food," a "drug," or a "cosmetic." Given the blurred lines of wellness products, with their benefits and attributes that spanned across multiple industries, how would the FDA apply and enforce its legal rules, with their rigid lines of definition and categorization?

This was not just a regulatory question for products like "cosmeceuticals."

One of the first questions for government regulators was the legal classification of the fast-growing market of dietary and nutritional supplements, which were specifically sold to provide health and wellness benefits to consumers. Should these supplements be regulated as a "food additive" or as a "drug"? As both or neither or something else? In 1994, as the FDA was considering regulating these nutritional and dietary supplements, the US Congress was said to have received more complaints from its constituents against these proposed regulations than against any other proposed legislation that year by far.

Wellness consumers would not stand for regulation and enforcement of definitional lines that they knew no longer existed. Congress bowed to this overwhelming public pressure by passing the landmark Dietary Supplements and Health and Education Act, which explicitly barred the FDA from regulating the fast-growing body of wellness supplements (with some limited exceptions focused on fraud and misrepresentation).

As the lines blurred, broader questions were raised. Is marijuana, a plant that grows naturally with pharmaceutical-type effects, a "drug" that should be regulated? What about gluten, which is a "drug" found in naturally growing wheat and other grains, or lactose, a "drug" found in naturally produced milk and dairy products? How about coffee or chocolate and other "beverages" and "foods" that act as "drugs" to regulate mood?

All drugs have the potential for harm as well as good. For those who are allergic to tree nuts, for example, an everyday food with nutritional benefits for some can create medical emergencies. Where are the lines, and why should they be applied to some substances, but not others? As lines get blurred, with substances producing different effects for different people, should we force definitions that don't really exist? Or is self-education and self-responsibility the only way to prevent harms that differ dramatically for different people?

These deep but practical questions may go far beyond the scope of this book, but the first step is to begin to recognize that wellness has blurred certain lines that we had accepted without question—and that these lines may have been convenient, but they never truly existed in the first place.

They were fictions, illusory separations and limitations that sometimes came at a steep price for our own wellness. This applies to formal lines, like definitions of drugs and foods and cosmetics, as well as to fuzzy lines, like aspects of our selves.

———

Learning to blur lines and limitations—or erase them altogether—is just another way of thinking and understanding. It is an underlying approach, an essential tool for our toolbox that we can utilize to approach our own wellness.

Mostly we don't even recognize that lines are placed upon us or that these lines create limitations upon us. We take these lines for granted in our lives and for our world, believing them to be real and undeniable, perhaps because everyone else we know believes they exist too. So an essential step toward wellness is to see those lines and limitations for the fictions they are and to work toward blurring or erasing those lines as appropriate for your own wellness.

Surely some lines and limitations may be helpful for your individual wellness. If you're gluten-intolerant or lactose-intolerant, for example, you may need to draw lines against eating a plate of pasta or a scoop of ice cream—even as your family and friends enjoy these same foods, promoting their happiness and well-being with something that makes you feel ill. That's not dissimilar to a drug like alcohol, which is toxic and dangerous to some, yet wellness-enhancing to others.

Similarly, if a situation calls for formality in behavior, then it is up to us to draw that line for ourselves and use it as a limitation to act appropriately. Yet it is also up to us to erase those fictitious lines of formality when we are ready to achieve the type of fuzzy human connection that is essential for meaningful personal relationships, so important to our wellness.

Others can offer suggestions and guidance and advice about where or when to draw the lines or to erase the lines altogether. But in the final analysis, it is *your* responsibility and obligation to draw lines that promote *your* wellness and to erase lines that detract from *your* wellness.

And it is our responsibility and obligation to respect and appreciate that others may draw those imaginary lines differently for themselves and for their own wellness.

Chapter 4

THE MEANING OF A WORD

If you were asked to guess who had the first recorded use of the word *wellness*—at least the first time it appeared in print—you might guess the person was a health guru or a spiritual sage. The person who coined the word *wellness* had neither of those career descriptions.

Maybe you'd next guess it was a songwriter singing of hope or a poet contemplating tranquility, or speculate it was a mystic talking of a "New Age" of human awareness or a researcher rediscovering ancient healing wisdom. The person who first talked of *wellness* held none of those jobs either.

If you asked for a clue, I'd give you a time frame in history, as historians do, and tell you that the person who first used the word *wellness* and sought to give that word meaning predated the idealism and romanticism of both hipsters and hippies. His visionary insights into *wellness* predated even the aspirational hopes of a return to an enlightened Camelot under John F. Kennedy, who was elected president of the United States in 1960.

Surprised? The man who introduced the word *wellness* into the English language was a senior government bureaucrat in the Eisenhower administration. He first spoke on the topic of wellness in the late 1950s, eventually writing a short paper entitled "High-Level Wellness for Man and Society," published in the American Journal of

Public Health.[1] Halbert L. Dunn, MD, PhD, was chief of the Office of Vital Statistics, an agency then within the US Department of Health, Education and Welfare, and it was Dr. Dunn's job to statistically analyze the demographic data that the American government collects about the health and welfare of its citizens.

Some might consider that job description to be the epitome of dull and tedious employment, but Dr. Dunn knew he had important work to do—the vitality, health, and well-being of America were at stake!

On the surface, all seemed well in America during the presidency of Dwight D. (*"Ike"*) Eisenhower, the administration in which Dr. Dunn served. The 1950s were can-do years that followed America's victory in World War II. As the supreme allied commander of Europe, General Eisenhower had triumphed over Nazi tyranny, and he was celebrated not just as a military victor but as a liberator of subjugated peoples and nations. It was a time of peace and prosperity, and the general was president, winning landslide elections with his slogan of "I like Ike." Business was booming, and in the field of health, America was scoring victories over dread diseases like polio. It seemed like happy days in America.

Yet with all America's obvious successes in the 1950s, there was something amiss. You could see it in America's artistic expression by reading Beat-generation classics like Jack Kerouac's *On the Road* and J. D. Salinger's *Catcher in the Rye*, which spoke to growing disillusionment and alienation. It was echoed in the emergence of rock-and-roll music and a growing countercultural movement. You didn't need to be a Beat poet or a rock star, though, to see that something was ailing the American public. If you only knew where to look, you could see it in some disturbing public health statistics.

Dr. Halbert Dunn had access to a treasure trove of public health data in his job as chief of the Office of Vital Statistics (he was eventually promoted to assistant surgeon general at the end of Ike's administration). Of course, data is only as useful as one's ability to interpret the information, but Halbert Dunn was particularly adept at data analysis. He was a pioneering visionary in the application of bio-statistics to public health and a founder of the National Association for Public Health Statistics and Information Systems.

In a sense, Dr. Dunn proceeded like any good physician diagnosing the health of his patient—which for him was the American public. He began his examination by measuring his patient's vital signs and by gathering his patient's medical data before asking probing questions about what was wrong with his patient's health.

Eventually the answer came to Dr. Dunn. Despite his biostatistical and scientific expertise, it did not come from quantitatively *formal* science and mathematics. According to Halbert Dunn himself, the answer came in the qualitatively *fuzzy* words of purpose and declaration adopted a decade earlier in the late 1940s of the constitution of the World Health Organization.

It is easy to understand why this constitution for the world's health was so important and inspirational for Dr. Dunn, as it was for so many leading doctors and health-care workers throughout the world in the 1940s and 1950s. More people died in the Second World War—*as many as eighty-five million estimated dead!*—than any other event in all of recorded history, and that includes humanity's many epidemics and famines, tragedies and catastrophes. For the world's medical and health-care community, World War II was a global health crisis of unprecedented scale and proportion. In the war's aftermath, the time was again ripe to restore good health throughout the world.

After deliberation and adoption by nation-states around the world, this new World Health Organization constitution *"declared"*—in the familiar pattern of America's own founding documents—that certain *"principles are basic to the happiness, harmonious relations and security of all peoples."* It was the very first of these fundamental constitutional principles that inspired Dr. Dunn to answer what was ailing the American public. Dunn quoted these words of declaratory purpose—the #1 basic principle for all the world's health—in the very first paragraph of his pioneering essay on high-level wellness:

> *"Health is a state of complete physical, mental and social well-being and not merely the absence of disease or infirmity."*[2]

The words may seem obvious, but it may be worthwhile to carefully reread these words again for yourself, to glean their profound meaning. Dr. Dunn himself acknowledged that it was difficult to truly understand these simple words of principle, even though Dunn knew that these words were frequently quoted by the health-care community of the 1950s. Even simple, commonly quoted words are often misunderstood, in the same way that simple is not always easy.

"Our eyes have been so long turned in a different direction," Dunn lamented to his fellow physicians and health-care workers, that "most of us" did not understand the meaning of these powerful words of constitutional declaration. As Dunn explained, it was like water "seen through a glass darkly"—for how do we know if the glass is half-full or half-empty if we can't even see the water through the darkness? Metaphors and similes, like Dunn's comparison of water seen in the glass, are fuzzy ways to impart true meaning when precise words of formal explanation are still not being understood.

Even today, "most of us" still misunderstand the meaning of these words, though we can read and recite them and though they seem simple and obvious. We still call in sick with fake coughs and imagined sniffles to justify a much-needed day off from work. We still require proof of illness, like a doctor's note, to excuse our children from school attendance. We still need the name of a disease to justify to our friends or to ourselves why we're not feeling well. If we aren't diagnosed with a sickness that can be identified in the medical literature, most physicians still believe that we are healthy, and most medical insurance companies will not pay for our treatments.

Think about that! These words of constitutional principle were declared "basic" to our health, happiness, harmonious relations, and security in the aftermath of the deadliest event the world has ever known, after discussion and deliberation by the leading doctors and nations of the world. And yet, when all is said and done, most of us still define health as "merely the absence of disease and infirmity."

———

"Health is a state of complete physical, mental and social well-being" is just an empty platitude until we give it meaning.

Only after we give it meaning can we see what a powerful concept it is and how it gives us tools for our own wellness. Only after we give it meaning can we see how it leads to deeper insights and how those new insights lead to still more tools for promoting our wellness, as it did for Dr. Dunn.

Words are empty until we understand and honor their meaning. And then, once we understand and empower their meaning, it's as though we suddenly see a forest through the trees. Their meaning was there all along, like an image in a Rorschach inkblot that we couldn't see, just waiting for us to change our viewpoint and perspective or waiting for us to change our attitude—or *altitude*, as Dr. Dunn might joke, wellness being in his words a "high-level" concept.

Indeed, changing our level of sight can change our level of insight. It is said that the very first picture of the planet Earth taken from outer space—dubbed the "Blue Marble"—did more to change our view of ourselves and how we share this world together than any other photograph in history. Wanting to further change humankind's view of its place in the cosmos, the visionary astronomer Carl Sagan encouraged a picture of Earth from even farther away in space, as the NASA spacecraft *Voyager 1* was leaving the solar system in its mission to explore the universe. This photograph of Earth, taken from the edge of our solar system, was named the "Pale Blue Dot" and has similarly altered our understanding of what it means to live together on planet Earth.

Changing your viewpoint isn't limited to dramatic photographs from faraway space. I've searched for my own eyeglasses—*silly me!*—when they're already sitting on the nose of my face. The eyeglasses are plainly there on my face, yet they're unseen and waiting for a change of perception. As Dr. Dunn suggested, sometimes we have to look at things from a different vantage point.

———

It's up to us to change our perception, to change our approach, so we can see what was there all along.

You may know that health is more than the mere absence of disease and infirmity, yet what meaning do you give to those words when it comes to your own health? Sometimes, as Mark Twain quipped, we can "know merely things" without being "familiar with the meanings of them."

Mark Twain was the pen name for author Samuel Clemens, one of America's greatest humorists and sometimes described as the father of American literature. In writing those words about *knowing the meanings of things,* Twain was speaking of his friend Helen Keller, whom he helped launched to worldwide fame. Helen Keller was known for her brilliant mind—despite her not being able to see, not being able to hear, and some thought not being able to think either. Here's how Twain told the story:

> Helen Keller has been dumb, stone deaf, and stone blind, ever since she was a little baby...and now at sixteen years of age this miraculous creature, this wonder of all the ages, passes the Harvard University examination...and does it brilliantly, too, not in a commonplace fashion. She doesn't know merely things, she is splendidly familiar with the meanings of them. [3]

Twain was an admirer of the type of education you could get at places like Harvard, but mostly he was a big fan of the type of learning that required self-education and self-knowledge. Dr. Halbert Dunn could not have agreed more with Mark Twain. Elaborating on the core principle of high-level wellness, Dr. Dunn explained in his seminal essay *"that the central bastion to be conquered involves teaching people how to 'know themselves.'"*[4]

"Know thyself!" has always been a cornerstone commandment of common wisdom. It may sound simple, but it is not easily applied. It is well worth the effort, though, for self-knowledge can lead to great personal awakenings. Self-knowledge can bring profound wellness to yourself and to others. Indeed, you cannot really understand the meanings of *things* if you do not first understand the meanings of your *self*.

It may seem obvious too, but self-knowledge cannot be accomplished by others, only by you for yourself. Each of us must do this for ourselves—though good teachers can help!

———

Helen Keller's remarkable teacher was Anne Sullivan. She was portrayed in Hollywood movies as *"The Miracle Worker"*—the name that Mark Twain first gave her.

Miss Sullivan enabled a miracle to unfold because she would not give up on young Helen, even when the educational system itself banished the child to life in an asylum. It was the belief of these educational institutions that Helen was an unruly wild child who needed to be maintained and restrained beyond the lines and boundaries of civilized society.

Anne Sullivan's breakthrough was running Helen's hand under cool water while motioning the word for water in Helen's other hand. The deaf, dumb, and blind child could not see, nor hear, nor some say think—but she could still feel in the palm of her hand. Helen

32

Keller described that breakthrough experience with her teacher Miss Sullivan in her best-selling autobiographical book *The Story of My Life*, which she wrote in 1903 while a student at Harvard's Radcliffe College. In a beautiful passage from Helen Keller's autobiography, she wrote how the meaning of a word can suddenly come alive; how discovering meaning for ourselves can finally awaken us, allowing the light of understanding to shine:

> As the cool stream gushed over one hand she [Miss Sullivan] spelled into the other the word water, first slowly, then rapidly. I stood still, my whole attention fixed upon the motions of her fingers. Suddenly I felt a misty consciousness as of something forgotten—a thrill of returning thought; and somehow the mystery of language was revealed to me. I knew then that "w-a-t-e-r" meant the wonderful cool something that was flowing over my hand. That living word awakened my soul, gave it light, hope, joy, set it free! There were barriers still, it is true, but barriers that could in time be swept away. [5]

Miss Sullivan also described the experience from her vantage as the teacher, recording an entry in her own diary, on March 20, 1887, following her student Helen's miraculous breakthrough:

> My heart is singing for joy this morning. A miracle has happened! The light of understanding has shone upon my little pupil's mind and behold, all things are changed! The wild little creature of two weeks ago has been transformed into a gentle child. [6]

One of the great appeals of Helen Keller's story—that led to books, movies, fortune, and fame—is how transformation is truly possible. Helen's transformation began from "wild little creature" to "gentle child," but it did not end there. Her miraculous transformation continued the more this "light of understanding" continued to shine.

According to another of Miss Sullivan's journal entries, just two and a half years after Helen's initial breakthrough, Helen's curriculum included "arithmetic, geography, zoology, botany and reading." [7] The demands of Helen's academic curriculum nearly exhausted her teacher, but Miss Sullivan said that was the easy part of her job:

> It must have been evident to those who watched the rapid unfolding of Helen's faculties that it would not be possible to keep her inquisitive spirit for any length of time from reaching out toward the unfathomable mysteries of life. But great care has been taken not to lead her thoughts prematurely to the consideration of subjects which perplex and confuse all minds. Children ask profound questions, but they often receive shallow answers, or, to speak more correctly, they are quieted by such answers. [8]

In so many ways, Helen was no different than any other child, each asking "profound questions" to parents, teachers, and other adults in their lives, each trying to learn true meaning and understanding, each an "inquisitive spirit" in his or her own way. Thankfully, there are amazing teachers like Miss Sullivan who take "great care" not to give "shallow answers" that quiet these questions and silence the spirit.

———

At the heart of the story about Helen Keller is a lesson about how we learn and how we discover meaning. It is a hugely important lesson that is at the heart of wellness.

It is also a hugely important lesson for the institutions and systems that we entrust with our children's education. This lesson helps answer questions about what makes a teacher or a school effective. It helps answer questions about what makes teachers and schools good—or even great, like teacher Miss Anne Sullivan.

The first thing to realize is that teacher and student may have different perspectives of these questions and their answers, because they have different vantage points. As a teacher, Miss Sullivan wanted what she called "the light of understanding" to shine upon her student Helen. Helen reminds us, however, that the light was never gone. It was always there—"a misty consciousness as of something forgotten—a thrill of returning thought"[9] in Helen Keller' own words—just waiting to reappear.

Great teachers are those who kindle the light of understanding that is already inside the student. When that happens, it results in miracles—little miracles of childhood learning and big miracles of awakening like Helen Keller, but all miracles just the same—which may be why Mark Twain described Miss Sullivan as a "miracle worker." If miracles occur when "the light of understanding" shines brightest, then perhaps what makes for a great school is supporting more miracles. Imagine how many more miracles of learning there would be if institutions and systems of education encouraged and facilitated teachers and courses that kindled these miracles![10]

Surely a teacher and a school can instruct and lecture and test, but for the student, the light first needs to *shine from within*. Fortunately, all children are naturally inquisitive, and each asks "profound questions" in his or her own search for understanding. The light is already there inside of each child, even in infancy; to know that is true, just spend some time with a toddler and his or her unceasing questions of *"Why?"* and *"What?"* and *"How?"* A teacher or a school, in haste to instruct and lecture and test children, can quiet their questions and silence their spirit. Indeed, it is far too easy for a teacher or a school (or the bureaucratic systems and institutions that seek to control teachers and schools!) to squander the opportunity for more miracles of learning by discouraging a student's own natural search for understanding and meaning.

We ought to remember that "the light of understanding" shines brightest when the light of teacher and student come together. Each light needs to join with the other in unity. When the light of teacher and student converge, both learn from each other and become more brilliant in their own way, as the story of Anne Sullivan and Helen Keller teaches.

Teacher and student may seem like opposites, separate and apart from each other, but this is just another example of a seeming duality that is fuzzily connected at its heart and in its essence. It is the same unity at the heart of so many things that really matter. In *truth*, there are no lines between teacher and student, for they are inextricably connected to each other; truly, if the "light of understanding" does not shine between them, then the teacher is not teaching, and the student cannot be learning.

Helen Keller reminds us that this proverbial light is already there inside each of us. Indeed, it is everywhere, already connecting us all, but waiting for the understanding and meaning that make the light bright. That too is a fundamental lesson of wellness.

———

One of many things I like so much about Mark Twain is that he could never resist a joke to remind us of what's obviously true, even when others ignored the simple *truth*.

"I have never let my schooling get in the way of my education," Twain quipped. I liked that witty remark and quoted it in the dedication to my book *(((Tuning Jack FM)))* because it reminds us to proactively take charge of our own education, no matter how we are schooled. It reminds us too to vigilantly guard and kindle the light of understanding from within as part of a lifelong search for self-knowledge. We learn more from schooling that way besides.

It is a huge mistake to let schooling get in the way of our education, for the two are not the same. The price to our learning is costly, yet we pay again and again, repeating the same patterns of mistake.

When Mark Twain saw this mistake in the story of his friend Helen Keller, his humor grew sarcastic and biting, understanding how the same mistakes kept recurring in the educational systems of East and West and everywhere the Twain met. In his book *Following the Equator*, Twain explained:

> Has Miss Sullivan taught her [Helen] by the methods of India and the American public school? No, oh, no; for then she would be deafer and dumber and blinder than she was before. It is a pity that we can't educate all the children in the asylum.[11]

Then, as now, it was easier for school systems to give up on children like Helen Keller. By labeling Helen Keller as incapable of learning—as an untreatably insane and enraged "wild little creature"—there was no need to discover the engaging and precious "gentle child" that was always inside her. Cast aside by a system interested more in schooling than education, Helen Keller could be sent to an asylum, where she would be physically shackled and restrained, or in a later era, electroshocked and lobotomized, or in a still later era, pharmaceutically sedated and stigmatized.

There is a lesson for the health-care system here too, but the lesson is much broader than health care, for it applies to each of us and to the way we see one another. It is usually easier to see someone as an *object* than as a *person*, but a simple change in perspective makes all the difference.

Mark Twain did not intend to disparage an entire institution—*no, oh, no!*—and neither do I. Institutions and systems, like teachers, schools, doctors, and hospitals, can do good—*yes, wonderfully good!*—but sadly they can also hold us down and keep us out, preventing us from finding meaning and understanding by enforcing imaginary lines that were never really there in the first place. As Helen Keller discovered for herself, there were no lines or barriers—or at least, only lines or "barriers that could in time be swept away."

When systems and institutions fail us, as they do from time to time, we must take charge! Taking charge to find the answers we are looking for is our prerogative. It is not just our choice; it is our responsibility and duty to ourselves, for when it comes to the things that really matter to us—vital things like wellness—only we can find meaning for ourselves.

Even if you have been quieted by the system's shallow answers to your profound questions, your questions of meaning and understanding patiently await better answers.

It is up to you to use the quiet and the silent stillness of this quiet as an opportunity to listen closely. It is up to you to hear the part of you still asking those profound questions. It's the part of you that wants to know your self and to honor who you are—it's the part in you, as in each of us, that seeks wellness.

Maybe that part of you is buried deeply, its voice now just a barely audible whisper, forced into quiet submission or quiet desperation by the routines and demands of adulthood or by the shallow answers you were given as a child. Or maybe that part of you is now screaming for attention, the result of years of ignoring its voice, or the result of a health crisis that forces you to confront your inevitable mortality, demanding you answer these long-forgotten questions. But surely, either way, the profound questions are still there, waiting and wanting to be answered.

Take a moment to listen to yourself in perfect silence and stillness, and you'll know that's true.

Chapter 5

WHO'S IN CHARGE OF CHANGE?

What happens when we desire meaningful change—like a positive change toward good health and wellness in our lives—but the institutions that regulate and control these areas of activity do not support our personal desires? Indeed, what happens when the institutional systems actively *oppose* our desire for positive change in our lives?

By turning its focus away from the student, an educational system can banish Helen Keller to an asylum. It's not that systems and institutions are inherently bad or have bad intentions —*no, oh, no,* it's not like that at all. An educational system can begin by truly helping literacy and learning, but then turn itself toward rigidity and rote repetition. Focus can shift from learning to testing, from literacy to homogenized instruction. The institutional motive may have been innocent enough, like economy or convenience or administration, and yet the educational system nonetheless condemned Helen Keller, and countless others like her, to ignorance and failure.

It's not just Helen. It happens with systems and institutions throughout history, and it is happening today. It happens around the world, and it happens in our backyards. It may happen unknowingly and unthinkingly, but it still happens.

Governments that once protected its citizens and secured their freedom turn toward tyranny and repression, warring against their own people and denying them their liberty. Churches that once provided beacons to follow toward morality and spirituality turn toward dogma and depravity, corrupting and stealing from their own worshipers. Financial institutions that once enabled personal savings and business growth turn toward predatory avarice and greed, cheating and bankrupting their own customers and communities.

All systems can become entrenched and self-perpetuating. They can aggressively resist reform and deny meaningful change.

When these breakdowns happen and the system no longer functions as it should or could, trying to change the system can be especially difficult. Ask someone who has tried—like a whistleblower, reformer, protester, pioneer, maverick, statesman, rebel, entrepreneur, misfit, visionary; ask them if change comes easy? They might shake their head in disbelief at the naive innocence of the question and talk frankly about the slim chances of changing City Hall. I've fought City Hall as a lawyer and activist many, many times, and I can confirm that's true.

———

It was against these long odds that Halbert L. Dunn, MD, PhD, with his keen understanding of statistical probabilities, tried to change the medical and health-care system to reorient it toward "high-level wellness."

Dr. Dunn may have thought that changing the system was within his power, that he could beat the odds. As a senior government public health official, with a distinguished career beginning at New York Presbyterian Hospital and the Mayo Clinic, he was the type of "system insider" that is supposed to have access to the levers of power and influence.

He knew he was delivering a simple but profound message about *good health being more than the mere absence of disease.* He knew this message was not a radical proposition, for it was embodied in the first and most fundamental principle of the constitution of the World Health Organization, a foundational document cherished by the medical and health-care system itself. It seemed such a simple idea—such an easy way to promote public health—to begin focusing attention on the wellness of patients, instead of merely treating their diseases.

All he needed to do was to convince his peers of the need to change the system from within. Dunn selected the perfect platform to deliver his message of change—the prestigious and peer-reviewed *American Journal of Public Health*. It was read and discussed by those policy makers, thought leaders, physicians, and health-care workers who Dunn believed could *"activate"* a system-wide change in perception.

Dr. Dunn was a frequent contributor to this journal, having already envisioned the power of biostatistics and computer automation systems for advancing public health. His articles were widely read, forever changing medicine through application of better mathematics, record keeping, and information databases to public health practices. Now he was ready to change the system once again.

So, from his pulpit in the *American Journal of Public Health*, Dunn preached change to the system, urging his colleagues to move medicine toward the positive health of wellness, instead of merely treating disease:

> Without prejudice to the importance or the continuation and support of existing medical and health programs...it seems clear that many of today's and tomorrow's problems call for the stimulation and development of a new major axis of interest directed toward positive health—one strong enough to activate physicians, health workers, and others in devoting a substantial segment of their time, resources, and creative energies toward understanding and culturing good health in a positive sense.[1]

Armed with a mountain of facts, figures, signs, and statistics, Dr. Dunn explained how the change toward wellness was urgently needed to combat a menacing new public health crisis in America. In the copious data, which he assembled as the chief of the National Office of Vital Statistics, a position he held for a quarter century, Dunn saw chronic new epidemics and unclassified new illnesses. He understood these new problems demanded a reorientation of the health-care and medical system itself, a change toward wellness:

> [T]he problems which face the medical and public health professions have changed character drastically in the last few decades. Chronic illness and mental disease are far more prevalent. A great range of neurotic and functional illnesses, which seldom destroy life but which interfere with living a productive and full life, are on the increase.
>
> The preventive path of the future, both for medicine and public health, inevitably lies largely in reorienting a substantial amount of interest and energy toward raising the general levels of wellness among all peoples. [2]

The medical and health-care system, said Dunn, was ignoring the *root causes* of these new diseases, treating only their *symptoms*. Treating the symptoms on the surface was like playing a cruel game of "Whack-A-Mole" with public health. Each time a new symptom was diagnosed and treated, another ailment would pop up with increasing frequency and take its place. To Dunn's way of thinking, the system itself now needed to look deeper, to understand and then address the underlying causes of the problem.

This was classic wisdom that still applies to today's problems. Aristotle taught, *"If you would understand anything, observe its beginning and its development."* Aristotle himself was the wise product of a celebrated ancient educational system, an institution that passed down its methods and teachings from Socrates to Plato to Aristotle to Alexander the Great, where true *understanding* was the system's objective—a marked contrast from an educational objective like standardized examination competency.

Seeking to understand the underlying causes, Dunn discovered that these drastic new public health problems were *"rooted in the changing demographic, social, economic, and political character of civilization."* Although these changes to civilization *"are well known,"* Dunn said, *"their significance is usually not fully appreciated."*[3] His insight was reminiscent of Mark Twain's quip about how we can *"know merely things"* without being *"splendidly familiar with the meanings of them,"* and truly, Dr. Halbert Dunn was no casual observer of things. He sought to understand their *meanings*.

In his pioneering paper on wellness—aimed at convincing the health-care and medical system to change itself—Dunn summarized four of the root causes of the recurring public health problems:

> *"It is a shrinking world,"* where *"communication time has shrunk to the vanishing point."*
> *"It is a crowded world,"* with *"population pressures and scarcities of materials and living space."*
> *"It is an older world"* in the age of its *"people, productivity, and resources."*

And lastly, perhaps scariest in its potential impact on public health, Dunn foretold: *"It is a world of mounting tensions,"* where *"the tempo of modern life and its demands on the human being and his society are steadily increasing with no corresponding readjustment and strengthening of the inner man and the fabric of his social organizations."*[4]

Dunn's insights now seem prescient, the words of a wise but nearly forgotten visionary who used biostatistical skills to connect disparate dots in public health data long before others could appreciate their significance.

But the year was 1959, and in that year and in the decades to follow, the medical and health-care system and its institutions ignored Dr. Dunn's words and their meaning. Dunn's peers and colleagues within the system, whom he hoped to "activate" to change the system from within, turned a deaf ear and a blind eye, and just plain acted dumb, in a way that Helen Keller never *could*—and in a way that Helen Keller, always eager to understand the true meanings of things, never *would*.

It would take a long, long time for bright new minds to come along and reveal for the rest of us what Dunn saw in the late 1950s. Someday the information systems that Dunn pioneered would evolve and develop into the computers and communications of today, stretching Dunn's notion of a *"vanishing point"* in a *"shrinking world"* still further. Someday there would be new social networks via mobile smartphones and worldwide Internet access that allowed ordinary people to directly strengthen the *"fabric of their social organizations,"* bypassing the institutional systems that ignored the exigencies of *"the tempo of modern life and its demands on the human being and his society."* Someday critical best-selling thinkers like Thomas L. Friedman would write paradigm-shifting bestsellers like *The World Is Flat* and *Hot, Flat and Crowded*, explaining and further expounding on many of these same causes and their effects, but that was a half century later.

Simple truths that were obvious in hindsight were not yet understood by the systems and institutions of 1959. Halbert L. Dunn, MD, PhD, the first man to write of wellness and the father of modern public health information systems, died in 1975, never really seeing the changes to the system that he hoped to bring about.

Perhaps, as someone skilled at finding needles in a haystack of data, Dr. Dunn took comfort in the signs of the coming changes, scattered bits of information that portended seismic changes. These signs of change included the story told by James "Scotty" Reston of the *New York Times* in 1971—just four years before Dunn's death. His tale of acupuncture needles and Chinese herbal medicines seemed to captivate and intrigue the American public, hungry for alternative possibilities for wellness.

James Reston's strange and mysterious story awakened many ordinary people to these possibilities for wellness, among them a ten-year-old boy suffering painful stomachaches. Reston's story suggested the possibilities for good health and wellness in ways that American medical institutions and health-care systems didn't understand and would scarcely acknowledge. His story offered hope that people could somehow proactively improve their own health and wellness for themselves in ways that the medical and health-care systems couldn't dictate or control.

In other words, positive change could come, whether these institutions liked it or not.

———

One of the defining characteristics of the wellness movement is that it grew from the *bottom up*. Instead of the health-care policy makers and medical thought leaders changing the system from the top down, as Dr. Dunn had hoped his peers and colleagues would do, change came from *people themselves*. Ordinary people sought and demanded positive health and wellness for themselves, for their families, and for their world.

Economists sometimes describe this as a demand-side model because consumer demand triggered market response. For instance, bottom-up demand created an opportunity for entrepreneurs to develop and innovate new wellness products and services. From fitness centers to health spas, nutrition bars to energy drinks, holistic foods to natural medicines, wellness entrepreneurs looked for new ways to serve an evolving wellness market and to supply the growing consumer demand for good health and wellness. New markets were created and older markets were changed as wellness products and services clamored to gain the public's attention and become the next hot wellness trend.

But the bottom-up change affected much more than just market economics. As people sought wellness outside the system, they changed the community's attitudes about good health. They changed values and beliefs about health priorities and about life purposes, about our relationships with one another, and about how we share Earth together.

These cultural changes began slowly and proceeded gradually, almost imperceptibly, permeating society from bottom to top until one day it became obvious that something truly fundamental had changed.

In retrospect, it is remarkable that ordinary people brought about these changes in values and beliefs and began to change the very systems that would not change themselves. These changes are ongoing; the wellness movement is like a swift ship on the water, still changing society and its institutions in new ways, moving forward not only by the winds of change and the engines of progress, but by its very own momentum. It is sometimes difficult to see that momentum when you're on board the ship, in the same way that we forget how fast Earth itself is moving through space even as seasons change and day changes into night over and over again.

It may seem abstract and exaggerated to say that people changed themselves and then changed the system because of their own quest for wellness. But consider a wellness basic, like yoga or meditation. These approaches to good health were virtually unknown in America in the 1950s, when Dr. Dunn first wrote of wellness. Initially the practices were ridiculed and seen as the fringe behavior of a few freaks; they were sharply criticized by health-care systems and institutions as being without any medical benefits.

Today, though, the practices of yoga and meditation have permeated society, with instruction and guidance commonplace in nearly every large city and small town in America. Remarkably too medical institutions have finally, albeit grudgingly, acknowledged and accepted their value in the prevention and treatment of a wide variety of chronic illnesses and functional ailments. Clinical studies and brain imaging scans have now scientifically substantiated what yoga and meditation enthusiasts have known all along: that these practices can make people feel well—calmer, healthier, and at peace—in a crowded, shrinking, hectic world.

That example may seem too simple, as yoga and meditation are no longer divisive wellness practices. But the public's search for wellness has changed society and institutions and continues to do so in profound ways that may not be as obvious.

Two of the most controversial issues of the present day, as I wrote this book, are both news stories about people changing the system simply because of their own personal quest for wellness—gay marriage rights and marijuana legalization. These seemingly unrelated topics also illustrate the system's sad and misguided resistance to cede control to people over their own personal wellness choices.

When Dunn wrote his paper on wellness in 1959, homosexuality was seen by the health-care system as a deviant psychiatric disorder and treated by the legal system as a serious criminal offense. For fear of the system's widespread condemnation and its penalties, gay people attempted to repress their homosexuality; or alternatively, if an individual was willing to acknowledge his or her homosexuality as an aspect of self that could not be and should not be repressed, homosexuality was mostly secreted away in the closet or within isolated communities for fear of humiliation and retaliation.

Denial of an essential part of one's own self is antithetical to good health and wellness. True health and wellness requires *"a state of complete physical, mental and social well-being"* that comes from acceptance of who we are. As Dr. Dunn explained in his seminal journal article on "High-Level Wellness for Man and Society", good health and wellness requires that people seek self-knowledge, so that people can learn *"to know themselves and thus become better balanced and able to meet their daily problems more adequately."*[5] Dunn even posed a rhetorical question about the problems created by misunderstanding of one's self:

> "How much of the demand for sleeping pills, alcohol, and tranquilizers is due to this deep-felt need? It will not be easy to help some adults achieve a better understanding of self. In fact, it is quite likely that the majority of people are fleeing from a deeper knowledge of themselves."[6]

Good health and wellness happen when a person feels love and acceptance for who he or she is. The Gay Pride movement, beginning with the marches and rallies that followed the Stonewall Riots of 1969, finally allowed homosexual people in America to celebrate this aspect of themselves without the self-loathing and sickness that accompany shame and fear and denial. It was a bottom-up movement by ordinary people that demanded that the systems and institutions that condemned, persecuted, and denied civil and human rights to people because of their sexual orientation be changed.

The gay marriage debate was yet another chapter in the gay community's search for understanding and institutional acceptance. Gay marriage symbolized, among other things, the hopes and desires of an estimated 4 percent of the American population who are homosexual to be happily who they are, to love one another without societal condemnation or institutional retaliation, to be loved within their families, and to be part of an extended family of humankind that offers acceptance of who we are to all of us. In 2015, the US Supreme Court narrowly decided to affirm these rights of gay marriage, but it was apparent that change came first in popular attitudes, and that change was driven from the bottom up.

Four percent may not seem like a lot of people, but that number represents many tens of millions of people in the United States and many hundreds of millions more worldwide. More importantly, whatever the actual number of gays or whatever their percentage of the population, good health and harmonious relations *for all people* is measured by the tolerance and humanity shown *to each and every person.*

Acceptance of one another is about healing and not hurting, helping and not hating. It is about embracing fundamental World Health Organization constitutional principles that are *"basic to the happiness, harmonious relations and security of all peoples."*

———

The number of marijuana users is estimated to be much higher than the figure for gays, with approximately 7 percent of the American population admitting to regular use, and more than half of the total US population admitting to having inhaled or ingested parts of the cannabis plant at some point in their lives. Despite this widespread usage by tens or even hundreds of millions of people in the United States alone, marijuana remains an illegal drug, scorned by the health-care and medical systems, still currently subject in many states to severe criminal and legal penalties imposed for its use.

Like the debate over gay marriage, the debate over marijuana legalization is about the system's attempts to repress and control individual wellness choices, and it is about the hard-fought and limited successes of people to change the system from the bottom up.

Unlike the debate over gay marriage, however, the movement in favor of marijuana legalization has been directly framed as a health and wellness issue, with much of the current argument focused on the medical uses of cannabis. Opponents, especially those in the system whose livelihood benefits from criminalization of usage, argue that marijuana is not a medicine.

Understanding the meaning of the word *medicine* is a worthwhile exploration for a book on wellness. The current debate over marijuana's legalization is a window through which we can better understand the word's meaning—the hidden assumptions and implications of the word *medicine*—and just how medicines benefit our health and well-being.

Historically, we know that what is considered a medicine changes over time. Indeed, the health-care system itself classified marijuana as a medicine from 1850 to 1941, listing cannabis as a drug in the *United States Pharmacopeia*, the official standard of the medical system. During this time, large American pharmaceutical companies like Parke-Davis, Eli Lilly, and Squibb marketed and sold marijuana as a medicinal drug.

Cannabis usage gradually began to be banned in the 1910s in a historical wave of antidrug temperance that also resulted in fifteen states banning tobacco cigarettes, with twenty-two others considering such anti-tobacco legislation. This same societal wave of antidrug moral idealism culminated in the legal prohibition of alcohol from 1919 to 1933 by adoption of the Eighteenth Amendment to the US Constitution.

Even during alcohol's infamous Prohibition, though, there was still a legal exemption to buy alcohol for medicinal purposes through a physician's prescription. Doctors of this era objected to restrictions on their medical authority to treat patients with any drugs, including alcohol, they saw fit to prescribe.

It may seem funny today, but in a nearly forgotten chapter of history, medicinal beer became a divisive-wedge issue of the day, taken all the way to the US Supreme Court in 1924. As one prominent physician told the *New York Times* during Prohibition's vigorous national debate over the definition of a medicine, "I have always maintained that every family ought to have an alcoholic stimulant in the house all the time. There is nothing more valuable in emergency." This doctor often prescribed it for patients stricken with "nerves" and admitted that he himself always took an alcoholic drink at the end of the day, explaining "It braces me up." [7]

As that Prohibition-era doctor suggests, perhaps the medical benefits provided by marijuana should not be defined narrowly just in terms of curing illnesses, but must be seen in terms of providing wellness for the whole person. In the words of the World Health Organization Constitution, perhaps alcohol and marijuana promote a sense of *"mental and social well-being"* for the user, steadying nerves, dulling life's pains and pressures, or facilitating social interaction. During the height of Prohibition, illegal speakeasy saloons and home-distilling equipment proliferated beyond the system's control as tens or hundreds of millions of people demanded alcohol for their mental and social well-being. From the bottom up, consumer demand led to the legal repeal of Prohibition, with the eventual adoption of the Twenty-First

Amendment. It was the end of a failed social engineering experiment for alcohol that we seem to have repeated for marijuana.

Even if good health is seen as *"merely the absence of disease or infirmity"*—contrary to the principles of this book and the World Health Organization Constitution—marijuana may be good medicine. Cannabis has been used successfully to treat debilitating diseases and infirmities that include seizures, multiple sclerosis, nervous system disorders, pain, nausea, migraines, loss of appetite, the effects of chemotherapy, and of course—the classic punch line of many stoner justification jokes—glaucoma! For those afflicted with these and other illnesses, the health-care system's so-called medicines are often far less effective than marijuana; pharmaceutically manufactured drugs for treatment of these diseases often have harsh and undesirable side effects.

What is a *medicine* supposed to be, then, if not something that gently and effectively provides cures for disease or symptomatic relief for illness or infirmity?

There is rising cultural acceptance of marijuana's medical value, both in the broader sense of its ability to promote individual wellness and the narrower sense of its ability to treat diseases. Change appears to be coming from the bottom up, as voters in a growing number of states where referendums have been put on the ballot have demanded tolerance for marijuana. Local communities and their local police forces are increasingly turning the other cheek toward users and lowering legal penalties for use. Even a few high-profile physicians are bravely advocating for this change, even as most of the health-care and medical system still deny marijuana's status as a medicine.

We often draw arbitrary lines and give things judgmental labels. Lines and labels may serve important purposes, which is why we initially created them, but—to paraphrase an earlier chapter of this book—we can forget those purposes and become mistakenly attached to the lines and labels themselves. One of this book's recurring themes, which bears repeating, is that too-rigid attachment to these lines and labels is at the peril of our own wellness.

We call some things medicines though they induce horrid side effects and though they may be proven years later to be downright dangerous to public health (like thalidomide and Vioxx, which were later found to cause birth defects and heart attacks, respectively), yet we refuse such status for other substances that help and that heal. There are real human consequences to these illusory lines in shifting sands; try telling a parent of a child suffering chronic crippling seizures or a cancer patient coping with the debilitating side effects of chemotherapy that marijuana cannot be a medicine.

The health-care system has other arguments too why marijuana should not be considered a medicine, but when examined closely, these arguments are self-serving. For example, one argument is that marijuana is also used—or misused—for purposes besides the treatment of disease, including profit, addiction, recreation, religion, experimentation, creativity, discovery, boredom, stress relief, and social coping. But the same multiplicity of uses applies to many other pharmaceutically produced drugs, sold by large conglomerates and often resold illegally by dealers on the street, as well as for alcohol, tobacco, caffeine, sugar, and other substances tolerated or regulated by the system. Nearly all substances—including "medicines" and "drugs"—have alternative uses and unintended consequences, and nearly all can be misused too.

Another argument given by the health-care system is that marijuana has not been studied enough, so there is not enough evidence-based data of effectiveness and no known mechanism of action. The mechanism of action argument is certainly false, since marijuana's pharmaceutically identified active components act through cell membrane receptors in the brain, now known as cannabinoid receptors. The lack of studies may be a function of the stigma associated with research and the absence of funding for such research, but it is a conclusory argument besides—since studies often prove what they set out to prove.

Studies by pharmaceutical companies seeking approval for new drugs as medicines, for example, often ignore conflicting data and conflicting inferences and routinely overlook horrid side effects of usage.

Even without studies, other substances have been accepted as medicines—aspirin, for example. Aspirin was originally derived from willow bark, its therapeutic properties known since antiquity. Though similar to marijuana in its natural derivation and its ancient recognition, aspirin somehow historically managed to earn recognition as a medicine. Yet in the often haphazard way in which we draw lines and apply labels, other naturally occurring substances with therapeutic properties, like marijuana, are not called medicines.

———

I myself enjoy a hot cup of ginger tea for an upset stomach or nausea. It gently soothes my digestive system, and like aspirin and marijuana, ginger is an ancient natural remedy that comes from a naturally occurring plant. But ginger, which comes from the underground rhizome root stem of the *Zingiber* plant, is generally denied recognition as a medicine. *And why?*

Some cynics would say that medicines are limited to drugs that can be patented and sold for profit by a pharmaceutical company, but cynicism aside, many doctors and health-care authorities would insist that medicines are limited to drugs that are chemically identified, synthesized, homogenized, and standardized. This is an especially troubling argument because it means that a naturally occurring plant cannot be a medicine—by definition—because the plant contains numerous components that have not been scientifically identified, or that work in combinations that are not scientifically understood, or that are not uniform from one plant specimen to another. In other words, awe-inspiring nature has wonderful cures, but since our still-crude scientific knowledge cannot duplicate their compositions and combinations, ipso facto they are invalidated as medicine.

There is certainly merit in providing effective dosages, and the best part of the argument against naturally occurring medicines may be that physicians are unable to prescribe precise amounts because of the lack of pharmaceutically processed uniformity and standardization. All once-living plants, including ginger and marijuana, are disqualified from use as medicine by this argument since they all have individual compositions and potencies, differences and distinctions, as is characteristic of all living things.

But this ignores that even standardized medicines—with the same administered dose—will affect different people differently. We humans are naturally occurring living things ourselves, and we each have our own differences and distinctions. That's why individual side effects will vary, and it is impossible for any medicine to operate with the degree of specificity and precision sometimes claimed by the medical system. *We humans are not standardized either!* Part of the wellness movement is an acknowledgment—*indeed, a celebration!*—of our individual uniqueness and imperfections, even as we learn how similar we all are inside.

The argument for synthesized sameness is insidious because it eliminates the best solutions nature offers for our health and wellness. There is an old saying that *"an apple a day keeps the doctor away,"* and modern science continues to discover new medical benefits of the ancient wisdom about eating apples and other fruits, especially those high in antioxidants. But apples will vary, not just based on their particular variety, but upon their freshness, the orchard where they were grown, the tree that produced them, the season picked, the weather and climate, the fertilizers used, the pesticides applied, the soil conditions, and so forth. There are even studies, though widely ignored by scientific institutions, that suggest variations in fruit yields based on the love and caring attention paid to the fruit-bearing plant!

In other words, apples have *qualitative* differences that cannot be measured with the tools of *quantitative* standardization. Perhaps some apples will keep doctors away better than other apples, but the health and wellness benefits of an apple are not diminished by the apple's lack of pharmaceutical standardization. Indeed, do we really benefit from standardizing and homogenizing apples? Do we really want to strip apples of their varieties and variations?

Some ginger tea merchants, knowing the therapeutic value of ginger and the opposition of the medical establishment to its status as a medicine, are now claiming to manufacture their teas using "pharamaceutical-like" standardization and quality assurance processes. Perhaps such standardization will someday make a qualitative difference to the medical system, which largely ignores these attempts to reconcile natural goodness with medicinal standards. Despite the resistance of the system, I personally know and admire some open-minded physicians and surgeons who recommend naturally occurring herbal teas like ginger as helpful and effective adjuncts to their own medical practices.

Denying a naturally occurring substance the label of medicine— even though it is relatively safe and therapeutically effective—has important consequences for our health and wellness. For instance, consider the complicated questions raised by denying ginger tea's medicinal value:

- Should the health-care and medical system *prevent* me from utilizing ginger tea, offering me only a pharmaceutically synthesized and standardized chemical pill to calm my stomachache?
- Does it matter to these medical doctors that the pharmaceutical pill they recommend, unlike the ginger tea, may cause some other unintended side effect, like kidney disease? [8]
- Will doctors who recommend ginger tea instead of the synthesized pill be ostracized from the medical community and prevented from practicing medicine in the way that they want?
- Even if the medical system does not mandate that I take the synthesized pill for my stomachache, will my government-regulated and government-mandated health insurance cover

only the cost of the patent-protected expensive pill and not the commonly available cost-effective ginger herbal tea?

————

These questions may seem complex, whether for controversial substances like marijuana or noncontentious stuff like ginger tea, but there is a very simple question hidden inside, at the heart of all the seeming complexity: *Who's in charge of your health and wellness?*

The answer may depend on your point of view. Do you support an individual's liberty to freely make his or her own choices? Or do you favor an institutional system's sovereign prerogative to make choices for people and then support those choices with financial support and legal penalties? Maybe you believe that the answer is different based on the type of choice being made? Perhaps you believe that choices involving health and well-being are especially personal and should be reserved to individuals to make for themselves.

This is not a question about who makes better choices, since both people and institutions often make very bad decisions, even about questions of health and wellness. There are no guarantees, despite all the assurances to the contrary. Oftentimes, as history teaches, what seems to be a good decision can turn out to be a very bad one; other times, what seems to be a bad decision can turn out to be a very good one.

Being in charge of decision-making, by its very nature, can be a humbling experience, and choice implies the right to get it wrong.

Chapter 6

TAKING CHARGE OF YOUR HEALTH

My grandfather William Spiegel—my father's father—bravely fled Russia as a young teen during the Bolshevik Revolution of 1917. A bullet was said to have pierced his large Cossack hat, grazing his skull, although other members of his immediate family were not so lucky, and they were killed by flying bullets of the Russian Bolsheviks.

Never having experienced such horrors in my own life, I can only imagine the pain of that event in his young life. But my grandfather was a tough man, with a gentle soul, and was determined to live up to his name, *"Will."* Though he seldom talked about his experiences in Russia, he took time to remind me when I was a child of the power that a strong will can exert on our destiny. To him, a strong will was never an excuse to be inconsiderate or impolite or unkind.

As a young man forced to grow up very fast, William Spiegel left his homeland for America, speaking Russian and Yiddish, eager to learn English. He went on to learn a trade as a plumber and raise a family. He was a resourceful self-starter, who ingeniously kept old cars running with plumbing pipes and fittings, and he helped his son, my father Albert, attend dental school and start a family of his own. In short, William was an American through and through, adopting its culture gladly and gratefully. I was his first grandchild.

I can vividly remember him beaming with pride at my graduations from high school and college. He was quiet and reserved, as usual for him, but I can still *feel* his joy at these graduation ceremonies. I have precious few other memories of those graduation events many decades ago, but that warm feeling of my grandfather's joy—his pride in me—I can remember like yesterday. Some of life's best moments are emotional remembrances like that, and I cherish that I still have such wonderful memories.

My strong-willed, self-starting grandfather survived civil insurrections and persecution, bullets flying through his hat and one-way steamboat trips to a new world, but he was eventually taken down—too early—by a simple bacteria, known as *H. pylori*. It was like the classic scene from *War of the Worlds*, the visionary H. G. Wells's book turned into blockbuster mass media entertainment, where the all-powerful Martian invaders are ultimately destroyed by tiny microbes. The Martians underestimated what they did not see, although if only they'd looked—if only they'd asked the right questions—what was unseen was there all along.

My grandfather William Spiegel died during my first year of law school. He was the one who suggested that I go to law school in the first place, to become a real estate lawyer, like some of the suit-and-tie men with white hard-hat helmets who walked around on big construction jobsites that my grandfather observed as he helped install the plumbing. He never got to see me graduate law school and was too sick by then to even visit me at Columbia University, in Manhattan's Morningside Heights, a short hour's ride away from his home in suburban Long Island, New York. I am sure he would have liked to have visited me, very much so.

How could this health crisis have happened to someone so strong and so brave?

My grandfather had simple gastric distress—a bad stomachache—originally. The health-care system eventually diagnosed a peptic ulcer and surgically operated on him in 1961, based on then-prevailing medical wisdom that surgery was essential for his stomach condition. The year 1961 was the same year that Dr. Halbert Dunn brought his message that good health was more than the mere absence of disease to an even wider audience with publication of a book entitled *High Level Wellness*. Twenty-one years later, my grandfather died of stomach cancer, in some ways because the health-care system failed to heed Dunn's message.

The stomach cancer might have resulted from the scars and inflammations of the ulcer surgery, since inflammation is now believed to be a trigger for such cancers. Or it might have been the result of the bacterial infection in his stomach—but like Martians and microbes, this root cause of peptic ulcers was completely overlooked by the health-care system of the time. Either way, the health-care and medical system got it wrong. They ordered unnecessary surgery, with all its risks, and ignored the true bacterial nature of the problem, which they left untreated.

It took a couple of rogue Western Australian physicians and researchers, Barry Marshall and Robin Warren, to prove that nearly all peptic ulcers and certain stomach cancers are caused by a bacteria known as *H. pylori*. The two eventually won the Nobel Prize in medicine for their discovery in 2005, but when they announced their hypothesis in 1982, the medical establishment judged the two harshly. The year 1982 was the year my grandfather died, and back then, most doctors never suspected his stomach problems started with bacteria. Long after Marshall and Warren's landmark study was published in *The Medical Journal of Australia* in 1985, most physicians worldwide continued to dogmatically assert it was impossible for bacteria to live in conditions as harsh as the highly acidic stomach.

"It was a campaign and everyone was against me. But I knew I was right," [1] said the courageous doctor Barry Marshall. He was so committed to proving his hypothesis that Dr. Marshall infected himself with the *H. pylori* bacteria and induced his own painful peptic ulcer—just so he could cure himself!

The hypothesis should not have been that controversial for anyone willing to connect the dots. Bacteria had long been suspected as a root cause of stomach ulcers, and several German physicians prescribed anti-bacterial bismuth compounds as treatments in the 1860s and 70s. Even before Marshall and Warren made their hypothesis, autopsies revealed bacteria in the stomachs of the deceased, researchers discovered stomach ulcers could be caused by bacteria in animals, and some studies even suggested simple antibiotics could successfully treat peptic ulcers. One New York physician, Dr. A. Stone Freedberg, actually identified *H. pylori* in the human stomach but was then forced by his hospital research supervisor to abandon the research, as his findings were too controversial for the medical institution that employed them both. Indeed, 2005 Nobel Laureate Dr. Robin Warren speculated that Dr. Freedberg would have won the Nobel Prize way back in 1951—if only the medical system had allowed Dr. Freedberg to continue his *H. pylori* research. But it didn't, so my grandfather had surgery he didn't need for a stomach ulcer it couldn't help, which is why this medical history matters so much to me.

———

Knowledge evolves all the time, so it is not an indictment of the health-care and medical system to say they got it wrong about my grandfather, his diagnosis and treatment, and all those countless other patients with common stomach ulcers.

However, perhaps we ought to begin by admitting to ourselves, honestly and humbly, that none of us are infallible, that perhaps we may be wrong. It is often conceit and arrogance that blind us to the *truth*. Perhaps we ought to admit that others, the ones with crazy ideas—like those who said peptic ulcers were caused by an *H. pylori* bacterial infection—might be right after all.

Perhaps we ought to acknowledge that—even now, at this very moment—there are other surgeries and medicines, protocols and treatments that are falsely but dogmatically demanded by health-care systems and institutions. Perhaps we ought to admit that there are things that the medical system gets wrong and will likely fix someday.

Knowledge continues to evolve about common health conditions that we thought we fully understood, including stomach ulcers. After doctors stopped attacking the uncommon ideas of Marshall and Warren and finally accepted that these two rogue Australian physicians were correct, the medical system stopped surgically treating peptic ulcers like they did for my grandfather. Then they began using strong antibiotic drugs to kill the *H. pylori* bacteria, and that became their new medical protocol to treat stomach ulcers. It seemed a simple and obvious solution, consistent with a systemic view that saw bacteria as harmful "germs" to be exterminated, as if an enemy in a brutal war for good health.

That's not the end of the story, though, because knowledge continues to evolve even today and even for peptic ulcer protocols. Prompted by proactive patients who asked about the value of *probiotic* bacteria cultures (like the type found in foods like yogurt), some open-minded medical doctors began to understand how not all bacteria were *harmful* and how some bacteria were *helpful* for healthy digestion and stomach wellness. Some of these doctors began to realize how the strong antibiotics prescribed for stomach ulcers were also killing the helpful bacteria, creating unwanted side effects, and how *H. pylori* was not always an enemy to be violently vanquished.

In an article published in April 2006 in the journal of *Alimentary Pharmacology & Therapeutics*, researchers M. Gotteland, O. Brunser, and S. Cruchet reviewed clinical studies worldwide on the use of probiotic bacteria for good digestive health and concluded that "probiotic micro-organisms may be used as a 'possible' tool for the management of *H. pylori* infection and its associated gastric inflammation."[2] They summarized that these helpful probiotic bacteria cultures "are able to inhibit *H. pylori* growth" and "maintain lower levels of this pathogen in the stomach."[3] These studies showed how probiotics played a major role in "stabilization of the gastric…function" and "decrease of… inflammation" and, more generally, "healing" of stomach ulcers. [4]

Interestingly too their systematic survey of clinical studies from around the world suggested "similar effects on *H. pylori* by food-stuffs," including berry juices and garlic, red wine and fermented milk products, and that "regular intake of these and other dietary products might constitute a low-cost, large-scale alternative solution applicable for populations at-risk for *H. pylori*…" [5]

Dr. Dunn would surely have enjoyed that common sense approach, to eat common foods that lead to stomach wellness for you.

——

While my grandfather was ill, I recommended to him certain herbal teas to help soothe his fragile stomach, and I fondly remember enjoying a hot cup of chamomile tea together with him during that time. My grand-father liked that particular tea, and I knew it made him feel well, even if just for a moment. I was not yet steeped in the study of medicinal teas back then, so I did not yet know about ginger tea, which—as explained earlier—I have found to be marvelously useful in treating my own stom-ach distress in the many years since my grandfather passed away.

Genetics plays a part in many disease states that recur over genera-tions, including peptic ulcers. Back when my grandfather was ill, and for many years before that, I myself had frequent painful stomach-aches. That family history concerned me, in the way that most people are concerned for themselves about diseases that afflict their own families. It was my own proactive health and wellness research that eventually led me to ginger tea, which has been a safe and effective staple "medicine" of mine for many decades now.

I found other "medicines" that worked well for me too. Back when my grandfather was still alive, suffering from his own severe stomach maladies, I'd often have stomach distress after eating meals. The painful distress came from so many different types of foods that it seemed impossible to draw any conclusions. Some well-intentioned doctors and other concerned people told me it was because I enjoyed spicy peppery foods, which seemed to be the common sense wisdom of the time. I later discovered that this "common sense" was false—for me at least—but even at the time I wasn't willing to give up the spicy tastes that I enjoyed and the peppery foods that my body craved; I wanted to continue to live my life with gusto.

It was a college girlfriend's father—a nice, down-to-earth man who immediately asked me to call him "Dan"—who first recommended a commonly available remedy called Pepto-Bismol® to me to calm my aching stomach. Its only apparent side effect, as Dan told me to expect, was a strangely blackened tongue the morning after. "It's made with bismuth, Steve," he told me with kindness and patience, "and bismuth is an ancient remedy for the stomach."

Pepto-Bismol for an upset stomach seems obvious today, but this was 1981, a year before Barry Marshall and Robin Warren hypothesized about a bacterial root cause of peptic ulcers and stomach cancers; it was also the year before my grandfather died. Pink bismuth medicines may have been available in 1981, yet no doctor had ever recommended I try them—no doctor, that is, until Dan, who happened to be an endocrinologist and dean of Boston University Medical School. I tried the medicine he recommended, and it soothed my aching stomach. *Relief at last!*

Why was this common medicine not seen as a commonsense prescription for stomachaches like mine then? Back in 1981, pink bismuth compounds were not in vogue within the medical community. They had fallen out of fashion, like polka dots or flower prints can do. Most doctors had told me—each in their own "medical opinion"—that too much stomach acid was the root of my stomach distress. They would recommend strong antacids, telling me to lay off the spicy food and to reduce my stresses. Often these doctors would judgmentally label me a type A personality, jumping on an "excess stomach acid caused by personality type" bandwagon that the medical system was then driving. Back in 1981, the medical system did not believe in a bacterial basis for stomachaches like mine, so until Doctor Dan, no doctors would think outside those sharp lines and tidy boxes to prescribe a mild antibacterial containing bismuth, even though it was an ancient remedy for the stomach.

But Dr. Daniel S. Bernstein certainly possessed an open mind.

In long, animated conversations we had together over red wine—which Dan informed me was an ancient digestive aid too, many years before studies would later confirm red wine's many "medical" benefits—I remember talking about the controversial health theories of Dr. Linus Pauling. Doctor Dan showed enthusiasm for Pauling's radical theories of intensive vitamin C therapy as a cure for both the common cold and cancer. "Don't just write off Linus Pauling," Dan told me; "he's a winner of two Nobel Prizes and has pioneered our understanding of the nature of chemical bonding and structure of DNA." Dan knew too that many doctors in the medical system were disparagingly saying that Linus Pauling was a medical quack—some foolishly still believe so today—but Dan would have none of that. He insisted that Pauling's great innovative mind, already proven to be well ahead of his time, deserved our own open-minded consideration.

Doctor Dan's own open mind was the very reason he gave me such good "medical" advice, like telling me to try a pink bismuth concoction for my stomachaches. He was well read too, so perhaps Dan knew of the innovative German physician Dr. Adolph Kussmaul, who was successfully treating peptic ulcers with antibacterial bismuth compounds back in the 1860s.

Thinking about wise old Doctor Dan all these many years later, what I find most amazing is that Daniel S. Bernstein, dean of the Boston University Medical School, made his recommendation of a bismuth compound for my stomach, even though he watched me voraciously eat spicy foods. Even though he knew my family history, having recommended a surgeon for my grandfather's stomach cancer and having reviewed my grandfather's history of peptic ulcers. What was he thinking? That maybe—just maybe—an antibacterial bismuth compound would do the trick for his daughter's boyfriend's health? Maybe he even knew that the peppery food he watched me eat had antibacterial properties too, so he assumed my body was craving something it needed?

Truly I don't know why he made his recommendation to me, because he never articulated his thought processes, other than bismuth's history as an ancient stomach remedy, but I do recall Dan joking about people's opinions. *"Opinions are much like assholes, Steve,"* he once laughed in amusement, *"because everyone's got one."* He had opinions too, but my stomach and I greatly appreciated his opinions.

In 1981 and in the years to follow, I regularly consumed Pepto-Bismol® whenever my stomach was in distress. Today, many decades later, I still do occasionally, though in the years to follow, I would proactively learn better ways to manage my digestive health to prevent my stomach from aching in the first place. Now the pink concoction is just another "medicine" I can decide to take, when I need it, where I need it, how I need it.

It's just another arrow in my own personal health quiver, a tool in my wellness toolbox.

———

There are *three keys* to understanding the wellness movement—that's what I would tell the Wall Street private equity investors when presenting my white paper on the subject of wellness. They are better described and understood as three *dimensions* of wellness, but that sounds fuzzy and the word *keys* was more appropriate for formal private equity presentations, more reminiscent of bullet points in a chart or variables in a graph.

The *first* of these three keys, I would explain, was that people were becoming increasingly *proactive* about their wellness. In other words, growing numbers of people were taking charge of their own health and well-being, no longer content to unquestioningly "do what the doctor ordered." They were no longer willing to let physicians, systems, institutions, and industries decide what medicines they should take, what foods they should eat, what therapies they should use, and how they should make themselves feel well.

By 1998 according to a study[6] published in the *Journal of the American Medical Association*, more people in the United States were visiting so-called alternative medicine practitioners—squarely outside the mainstream of the medical system—than primary care physicians, the medical system's gatekeepers. As Dr. David M. Eisenberg, who authored the study with several of his colleagues for the prestigious Harvard Medical School, concluded: *"The market for alternative medicine is vast and growing."*[7]

The numbers weren't even close. By 1997 Americans made 629 million visits to alternative medicine practitioners, compared to just 386 million visits to primary care doctors. The study noted that the visits to these alternative health-care providers had risen by 47 percent in just seven years.

It wasn't that these alternative practitioners were preying on the uneducated or the poor, who didn't know better or who didn't have access to conventional medicine. Quite the contrary, the study found the use of alternative therapies was greater among *college-educated and higher-income people,* than among those with less education and lower incomes. These were capable consumers, proactively making their own wellness choices in a marketplace that was beginning to give them these choices.

They were willing to spend their own money to make these alternative health-care choices. Among the most surprising statistic to Eisenberg and his Harvard colleagues was that the growth in alternatives occurred "despite the low rates of insurance coverage for these services."[8] In other words, they were ignoring the strong economic incentives the system had in place to perpetuate itself and to ward off challengers.

It was as if people were refusing the synthesized pill that doctors had prescribed for their stomachaches and were willing to pay for natural ginger tea alternatives out of their own pockets. Not surprisingly, it wasn't just stomachaches. As the study revealed, the most sought-after alternative health-care treatments were for chronic and nervous conditions, the types of ailments that Dr. Halbert Dunn had described forty years earlier as a *"great range of neurotic and functional illnesses, which seldom destroy life but which interfere with living a productive and full life."*[9]

If the medical system was not going to address their headaches, backaches, arthritis, anxiety, and depression, all of which interfered with everyday wellness, then people were going to go outside the system and find solutions for themselves. According to the study, the alternative medicines and therapies that people were trying included herbal remedies, relaxation therapies, massage, chiropractic, hypnotism, acupuncture, homeopathy, self-help behavioral modification, spiritual and energy healing, nutritional counseling, and high-dose vitamin regimens like Linus Pauling advocated, among many other modalities.

In 1998 when Eisenberg published his study in the American Medical Association's journal, the institutions of health care and medicine stridently voiced their disapproval of these alternative medicines and therapies. Institutional attitudes had not changed much since 1959, when Dunn first wrote about wellness in the *American Journal of Public Health*. Most of the medical system still dismissively said these alternatives were not *"scientifically proven"* or *"evidence-based"* approaches to health care.

Their stern rebuke came with the same self-assured tone of conviction and conceit with which most doctors said, in 1981, that antibacterial medicines could not treat a peptic ulcer. Their negative opinions about alternatives were not stopping the American public, though. Increasingly people were making their own health and wellness decisions, regardless of what the doctor ordered.

Knowing that their doctors disapproved, however, the American public avoided the confrontation. As the study revealed, less than half of all patients told their primary care medical physicians about their use of alternative medicines and treatments.

What the study also revealed, but did not say explicitly, was how disconnected many of these physicians had become from their own patients. These doctors were bothered by their patients' wellness choices and their infidelities in straying outside the medical system. These patients were bothered by their doctors' contemptuous disapproval and their close-minded refusal to acknowledge what they didn't understand.

It was not a productive relationship. A disconnect between physician and patient did not lead toward the goal of good health, any more than the goal of true education would be furthered if student and teacher no longer communicated.

A moment of simple insight can change everything. Almost immediately following publication of Dr. David Eisenberg's landmark study in the widely read and widely quoted *Journal of the American Medical Association*, the systems and institutions of medicine and health care began to change themselves. They began to accommodate the alternative choices of their patients, even embracing these alternatives.

"Alternative Medicine Goes Mainstream" declared the headline in *Psychology Today* in 2000.[10] This was less than two years after the publication of Eisenberg's study in 1998. What "was once considered the domain of snake oil charlatans and gullible consumers," the magazine article explained, was now being recognized by "more and more traditional physicians and major federal organizations…as a potentially valid form of treatment."

Some doubters, those skeptics and cynics who ask tough questions and demand precise answers, might say that medicine was just following the money. A headline in the *Harvard University Gazette* read, *"Americans Spend $27 Billion a Year on Herbs, Massages, and Other Elective Treatments"*[11]—and that was in 1997 dollars. An estimated $12.2 billion of that number was spent without health insurance reimbursement, perhaps the best proof that medicine was leaving a lot of money on the table, as a Wall Street shark might opportunistically say.

It is not easy to overcome doubt and to embrace change. The *Psychology Today* article reminded its readers, many of whom were psychiatrists, therapists, and psychological treatment centers, of the perceived dangers of allowing patients to run amok. *"As people learn to take health into their own hands, however,"* they cautioned, *"they still need guidance from science."*[12] In other words, conventional institutional medicine needed to take charge of these new alternatives to once again direct their patients' health care.

The first step by *conventional* medicine was a new name for *alternative* medicine. You can't reconcile with outsiders if you are still calling them infidels or quacks. What was once dismissively labeled *"alternative"* was quickly renamed *"complementary"* or *"integrative"* medicine. Oh, what a difference a new name can make! Change a word, and our understanding can change too. It's all about how we draw the lines of our own perception and about the meanings we give to the words we use.

In 1999, just a year after the Eisenberg study was published in the AMA journal, the Memorial Sloan-Kettering Hospital in New York City formally established its Integrative Medicine Service. It proclaimed its mission to *"complement mainstream medical care and address the emotional, social, and spiritual needs of patients and families,"* to *"focus on quality of life,"* and *"to increase self-awareness, enhance well-being, and help prevent health-related problems."* Their Integrative Medicine Service has since grown and evolved and has become a model copied by hospitals and clinics worldwide.

To some, the Memorial Sloan-Kettering Hospital may seem an unlikely place where alternative health care and wellness would be tolerated, much less welcomed. The physicians and health-care professionals of Memorial Sloan-Kettering are internationally renowned medical experts on the front lines of the war against cancer, not "snake oil charlatans" peddling alternative wellness wares to "gullible consumers."

Doubters might say that this is all just window dressing, empty platitudes to appease patients. These cynics might say that this "integrative" and "complementary" approach has no real benefit to medical outcomes. These skeptics might argue that wellness has no real place in real medicine, certainly not when it comes to something as lethal as cancer at a serious scientific institution like Memorial Sloan-Kettering Hospital.

Four years after the founding of Memorial Sloan-Kettering's Integrative Medicine Service, just five years after the publication of the Eisenberg study, I had the opportunity to see for myself, more up close and personally than I could have ever imagined.

———

In 2003 I was admitted to Memorial Sloan-Kettering Hospital to surgically remove an entire lobe of my lung. My lung was diseased with an adenocarcinoma, sometimes known as the nonsmoker's lung cancer.

What I found in my own firsthand experience as a lung cancer patient at the hospital was that wellness at Memorial Sloan-Kettering was not some opportunistic embrace of the Eisenberg study. The hospital seemed to understand that wellness has an essential place in even the most serious of medical sciences. Its embrace of wellness did not seem limited to alternative medicines or complementary therapies either.

It seemed to me, as a patient, that wellness was intentionally woven into the very fabric of health care at the Memorial Sloan-Kettering Hospital. The hospital seemed to grasp the deeper meaning of the World Health Organization's constitutional principle that *"Health is a state of complete physical, mental and social well-being and not merely the absence of disease or infirmity."*

As Dr. Dunn taught so many decades earlier, a health-care system should treat the whole patient—not just the disease. Treating patients like a whole person may not be *quantitatively measurable*, yet such treatment is *qualitatively discernible* to a patient. On some deep and intuitive level, we all know when we are being treated like *objects*, not as *people* with feelings and thoughts, hopes and fears.

Treating the whole person promotes well-being and aids in patient recovery, even when a patient's health is severely compromised by disease. This has been statistically shown time and again through what some call the placebo effect—the powerful healing ability of mere belief in administered care. *Truly caring for a patient is often the best medicine of all.* As Dr. Dunn suggested, in an increasingly fast-paced high-tech mechanized world, slow-paced high-touch personal caring becomes more important to good health than ever before.

Though my prognosis was far from certain in 2003, I was made to feel like a whole person as a patient at Memorial Sloan-Kettering Hospital. Although I did not take advantage of a single class or treatment through the hospital's Integrative Medicine Service program, the hospital did its very best to address my "emotional, social, and spiritual needs"—to borrow the words of their own mission statement.

All of the hospital's doctors, nurses, technicians, orderlies, and administrative staff, every single person, treated me with warm regard and with genuine concern. This seemed the real essence of everyone's job, and it also seemed to me that this caring was not random or accidental, that such caring had been formally established and enforced by hospital policy and protocols. They helped me to feel well in ways that are hard to explain but that really mattered to my health and healing.

There were practical consequences to this caring too. When I reacted adversely, allergically, to the high-dose morphine drips for my postsurgical pain, for example, my medicines were quickly changed. When the substitute pain relief medicines proved insufficient, my painful agony in the middle of the night was promptly and compassionately addressed. I also appreciated the special wellness attention paid to the foods I was eating; caring sensitivity was paid to my dietary needs, restrictions, and tastes, and I was given a choice of well-prepared ingredients and options, instead of being forced to eat stereotypically drab hospital food.

The hospital encouraged my wellness in other fuzzy but therapeutically significant ways. My wise and wonderful surgeon, Dr. Manjit S. Bains—to whom I am deeply grateful not only for saving my life but for being part of it—encouraged me to gradually restore my lung function by walking a little bit at a time, so I would stroll the hospital's corridors, trying to balance and catch each shallow and difficult breath.

During these short rehabilitative walks, I immediately noticed how the hospital walls were brightly and artistically decorated, and I would absorb their colorful cheerfulness. The art helped me feel well! That may sound vague, but I've long known how art and creative expression provide me with feelings of deep therapeutic wellness and peace. As I mentioned in the introduction, I learned about that aspect of myself the moment I picked up a guitar at the age of thirteen.

Some readers of my book *(((Tuning Jack FM)))* have asked me whether the story told about the character Jack playing piano in a hospital waiting room, dressed only in a hospital gown and recovering from cancer surgery, was autobiographical. Yes, that story was true, though many others in that book were fictional. The story is a wonderful illustration of the true wellness that Memorial Sloan-Kettering Hospital helped me to feel as a patient in its care:

Perhaps my favorite remembrance of my time in the cancer ward was when I strolled down to the hospital's waiting room, with its beautiful baby grand Steinway® piano. I remember the odd feeling of sitting down on the piano's bench, wearing only my hospital gown, neatly tucking aside the tubes and bags attached to my frail body, pushing these tethers gently out of the way of the keyboard, with its glistening ivory and ebony. I remember the feeling of gratitude and good fortune at being able to play this magnificent instrument, so much lovelier than the beat-up and slightly out-of-tune piano I sometimes play at home.

And then I began to play. The music that day was spontaneous improvisations and remembered muses, and it flowed in inspired musical waterfalls. Out came cascading songs of hope and melancholy, of beauty and grace, like a river from someplace both deep inside me and yet far, far beyond me, through my fingers, onto the black and white keys. It came in musical waves, ebbing and flowing and ebbing and flowing, before ceasing.

An audience of patients and visitors and some hospital staff gathered to share the experience, some were already seated in the large hospital waiting room before I sat down at the piano, some strolled in and sat down and politely listened. I'm not sure whether they were drawn to the sad and sweet musical compositions themselves, or just to the unusual sight of a cancerous hospital-gowned Piano Man, his wounded lung draining into a mobile surgical bag, pouring his aching heart out through the piano's keys, but, either way, I felt warm and appreciated and loved during the shared experience.

73

I remember too catching glimpses of the faces of the audience. Some had anguish visible on their own faces, with painful stories of their loved ones right at the surface of their being. But even these troubled souls seemed to pause for a while, listening and even quietly praying to themselves, as they became part of the rhythmic flow of the music. I noticed how the music leapt from my heart to theirs, for an instant, before they moved on with their own journeys and their own busy lives. On their way out of the hospital waiting room, when the music ceased, some thanked me and some blessed me...

Some even told me that I was inspiring and that I gave them hope. That got me thinking. Was I inspiring to them because I was a cancer patient myself, or was it the music itself which spoke to them?...I'm not sure, but I do know that I did not sit down at the piano to play with the intention of inspiring a hospital waiting room, or with the intention of inspiring anyone else for that matter.

I played because the music was a release for me. The music helped me to reach deep down to the very core of my being, the music helped me reach that same spirit that I sensed intuitively was the very best part of me. At that moment, weakened by surgery that removed a cancerous lung, I did not know how my body would heal, but somehow I knew that my spirit was all that ultimately mattered. I might not be able to measure that spirit scientifically, or even explain it religiously, but somehow I knew that I needed to connect to my spirit, to find the deep peace that I craved. I sensed that my spirit could be found deep in my heart, and yet someplace far beyond my body.

As I shared the music of my soul with that hospital waiting room audience, I interacted with that audience in a way that I'll never forget. I felt like I was sharing much more than music with the people in that waiting room. I felt like I was sharing my spirit, and, even more surprising to me, I felt the audience sharing their spirits with me. As our spirits mingled and danced together in the music, I felt incredibly light and yet awesomely strong. At that magical moment, I realized that I was not merely a body sickened by cancer and surgery, I was *in spirit*. And I felt *in-spired*. [13]

———

In looking back at this experience at Memorial Sloan-Kettering Hospital, I am grateful there was no myopic close-minded health-care system, led by some unthinking and unfeeling hospital administrator, to say, "No! You may not play the piano; you are merely a patient with a disease, so go back to your bed, lie down, and take your meds!" Instead, this hospital was an enlightened institution, providing a gorgeous piano in a waiting lounge that could be played by patients like me—how many hospitals would have even thought to do that?

I am grateful too that Memorial Sloan-Kettering Hospital was sensitive to the "emotional, social, and spiritual needs" of patients like me, wholeheartedly embracing their mission statement, and that they encouraged their patients to be proactive in their own health and wellness. For me as a patient, proactivity was through music and creative release. The piano helped me to heal in ways that were meaningful and real, though perhaps scientifically inexplicable. If asked to explain, I'd guess that the experience helped me to heal because I was able to express and share my spirit.

In sharp contrast to my experience at Memorial Sloan-Kettering Hospital, I've stayed at other hospitals, where I felt like a mere object for medical treatment of a disease, not a whole person in need of genuine wellness. At some of these other hospitals, I felt as if I was nothing more than a quantitatively precise chart of numbers hanging by the side of my hospital bed, next to a metaphorically drab gray wall, for a qualitatively uncaring health-"care" staff to examine.

Sadly, all these many years after Eisenberg's study and Dunn's thesis, that uncaring *"you-are-your-disease"* attitude is still far too prevalent in the health-care system, strongly encouraged by insurance payment systems that mandate quantitatively calculable hurried speed of treatment over qualitatively intangible empathy. Why government enables and enforces such "check-the-box" insurance protocols in a "health-care" system—where the Hippocratic oath once demanded *humanity* from its physicians above all else—is deeply disturbing to me, although a full discussion of insurance's role in health care is beyond the scope of this book.

Suffice it to say that government, health-care insurers, and health-care institutions all must be reminded, again and again, that treating mere diseases—instead of treating the whole person—is the antithesis of good health and wellness. To borrow an old expression, no one cares how much you know until they know how much you care.

Chapter 7

WHAT MAKES YOU FEEL WELL?

Ask people a simple question—*What makes you feel well?*—and you'll get a lot of different answers.

If you asked me in that hospital waiting lounge, recovering from lung cancer surgery, playing piano made me feel well. At other times in my life, if you asked me this same simple question, it might be sharing a good meal and good conversation with friends or family. Or a saunter in the woods on a crisp, sunny day with my dogs. I can feel well when engaged in meaningful work on the job with interesting people, giving generously to a cause where I know I'm helping others, or by comforting a friend who's feeling down. Swimming on a hot day, strumming a well-tuned guitar, and sipping black coffee as I ease into a new morning. These are but a few more ways I can feel well.

If I'm aching or itching, twitching or sneezing, feeling ill or infirm in any way, I have many other ways to feel well as well. Sometimes, it's an acupuncturist or masseuse, doctor or clinic. Other times, it's as simple as a pill, spray, ointment, cream, tonic, tablet, tincture, or tea. I've felt well by burying myself under blankets in my cozy bed to rest and sleep, by reading a good book in a bathtub of warm water and Epsom salts, by holding hands or making love with my wife, by quietly praying to God and meditating, or with an alcoholic cocktail at happy hour. And that's just me, and that's just for starters...

Continue to ask the same simple question to different people, and the number of answers will increase dramatically.

Each and every person brings uniqueness and individuality to the question, so the answers will vary wildly. The answers will vary even from the same person, depending on when he or she is asked. The answers will vary at different times of the day or on different days during a lifetime. They will change with the point of view of the person or based on the particulars of the situation. The path to feeling well is not a "one size fits all" pursuit.

It seems that there are so many different answers to this one simple question.

Think of it from this perspective: With all these many answers, there are so many opportunities to try to feel well, even when you're feeling ill. So many options and choices! It could be a medicine or a therapy, a type of food or fitness regimen. It could be a product, service, program, or technique.

Thanks to the innovators and entrepreneurs of the wellness movement, there are many new options for wellness. Thanks to the burgeoning interest in wellness, some of the ancient ways to wellness, once nearly forgotten, have once again become accessible too. All of these choices have the potential to invigorate, uplift, relieve, relax, restore, remedy, pamper, beautify, heal, entertain, calm, care, comfort, and connect. There are more wellness options to help you grow, give, gratify, laugh, learn, and love.

Some people—perhaps who mostly see a glass as half-full—may rejoice in all this choice. Indeed, if the first key to understanding the wellness movement is that people are becoming more and more proactive about taking charge of their health, then there are surely a lot of varied ways we can become proactive for ourselves!

To other people—perhaps who mostly see a glass as half-empty—all these choices may be overwhelming or discouraging. Finding wellness, especially when it is desperately needed most, may seem a bit like searching for a needle in a huge haystack of other people's answers. Options and choices only have value if they can be applied to the situation at hand; otherwise, all these answers become useless muddled overload.

The diversity of these answers may be seen as a good thing or a bad thing; but really, it is neither. Like so many things in life, it is what *you* make of it.

———

At the outset of this book, I suggested that there may be three levels of understanding. First, on the surface of things, there is simplicity, which everyone can understand. Then, probing deeper, on the second level of understanding, there is the realization of complexity, which requires expertise. Finally, on the third level, comes true insight, when understanding evolves past complexity and becomes simple once again—often elegantly simple.

If this is true, then what appears to be complexity in the answers to the question of *What makes you feel well?*—answers that initially seem diverse and individualized—can ultimately reveal simple, common truths. How, then, can you find these simple truths about wellness for yourself?

Many researchers have waded through the complex answers, trying to extract useful information and uncover the simple truths at the heart of well-being. Physicians, public health officials, and wellness gurus have all followed this process, hoping to find a fountain of health in a mountain of data. Looking for commonality in the diversity, these researchers—like Dr. Dunn, who was privy to mountains of data in his perennial position as chief of the National Office of Vital Statistics—all try to distill the complexities into practical advice and helpful wisdom.

As these researchers have discovered, the complexities compound the more you search the data. Each answer has different forms and dimensions, adding to the complexity. Probing deeper into the answers, questions of *"what?"* lead to questions of *"why?"* Understanding *why* some things make you feel well adds layers of additional inquiry and analysis, bringing subtlety and nuance, like *why* you make certain choices for wellness and *why* you avoid other wellness options. With all these many complexities, answering the question *What makes you feel well?* can seem overwhelming, as if you are stuck at the second level of understanding.

Searching is well worth the effort, though, because the question is so very important to ask. You don't need to be a physician, public health official, or wellness guru just to *ask the question!* It is a question that we can all ask ourselves, and a question that we must all ask ourselves.

What makes you feel well? Even if you are accustomed to letting others answer the question for you, even if you are accustomed to obediently following the advice and guidance of others as to what would make you feel well, wellness requires that *you* ask the question. That bears repeating, partly because it is so obvious, yet so often overlooked— only *you* know whether or not *you* feel well, so only *you* can answer the question. The question is directed at *you*. It's that simple.

In the way that simple is not always easy, answering can seem difficult, but that does not prevent you from asking the question. No matter how complex or how far away the answer may seem, you must remember that *by asking the question, you begin the process of answering.* So— what makes you feel well?

Outcomes are often about the questions you ask. Ask the right question, and you can get the right answer. Ask the wrong question, and you will never get the right answer. *"Garbage in, garbage out"* is an old adage of the computer software industry, and it applies to wellness because our questions dictate and limit our answers.

If you ask for wellness, you're more likely to find it.

———

I learned that lesson—to take time to *ask* for wellness—the hard way when I arranged an intervention for my teenage son. It was the most difficult decision I had ever made.

I knew that the teenage years can be a frenetic rite of passage from childhood to adulthood, fraught with tension and drama for teens and their worried parents. Of course, long ago, I had been a teenager myself, struggling with my own parents over independence and what it means to be an adult. I now regret some of the aggravation I caused my parents back then, but time passed, and our adult relationship emerged stronger than ever.

I had also experienced the teenage stage as a parent before. With my other children, though, I somehow managed to muddle through until the teen years thankfully passed. *"I know you'll love me again by the time you're twenty-five!"* I once teased my then seventeen-year-old daughter, Melissa, at a time of great strife in our personal relationship. Judging from my daughter's behavior, and perhaps my own, when she was seventeen, I would never have imagined that in just a few short years, our relationship would evolve to the point that she would be adapting her artwork for this book's cover. She now teases me that she didn't need to wait until twenty-five to love me; she says she always did. Relationships can grow and evolve wonderfully that way, even after periods of struggle.

With this teenage son, though, I sensed that muddling through was not an option. The teenage phase for Nicholas seemed qualitatively different, and I was worried as he approached seventeen that something unthinkable might happen long before the age of twenty-five. In just a few months, Nick transformed from a light and happy spirit, whom I could spend hours happily chatting with, to someone dark and difficult to communicate with, whom I hardly recognized. *Who was this person who replaced my son?* I asked out loud as he failed high school classes, destroyed family cars, and ran away from home, all in rapid succession. During his downward spiral, he came and went with abandon, and troubles fell like rain.

It was a turbulent period, when wellness sometimes seemed like a luxury that I couldn't afford. My own emotions grew from concern, to worry, to terror for the health and safety of my son and of others whom my son's behavior may have threatened. All of my prior experiences and my preconceptions about the teenage years somehow seemed irrelevant. Our lives, and the peace we hoped for in life, seemed shattered and gone. I had a lot to learn about what would make me and my family feel well again.

Ironically, before my own children were teenagers, I had already seen up-close the devastation that out-of-control teenagers can wreak on themselves and their families. One of my wellness business ventures involved the celebrated ToughLove® parenting support program and my close involvement with its founders, therapists David and Phyllis York. Syndicated advice columnist and cultural icon Ann Landers popularized the Yorks' approach when she recommended their program to a mother seeking help with a troubled teenager. The response to the Ann Landers column was overwhelming, as if a social epidemic suddenly came out of the closet, leading to movies, television shows, and magazine stories about the program and the problems of the teenage years.

From a parent support group that began in Doylestown, Pennsylvania, in the late 1970s, the Yorks rapidly grew their ToughLove®

program to more than fifteen hundred chapters across America and internationally to places as far away as New Zealand. Phyllis and David touched many lives in their journey—sometimes in unexpected ways. For instance, the Yorks introduced me to Alice Gosfield, their health-care lawyer, who for many years since has been sending me e-mails of awful—sometimes awfully good—jokes that have kept me laughing, contributing to my wellness and many others' in meaningful ways.

All jokes aside, the Yorks helped countless families feel well through their understanding and support of how *behavior* is an important *health* issue for many families with teens. Though my own children were still young back then, I learned many things from the Yorks, their pro-grams, legalities, finances, organizational structures, and management, but all I learned could not prepare me for the firsthand emotional experience of a teenage crisis happening in my own family.

As mentioned, the intervention for my son Nicholas was perhaps the most difficult decision of my life, but it was a decision to proac-tively feel well again. I wanted this wellness not just for my son, but for myself and our whole family. It took commitment and courage to simply *ask* what might make us feel well, and at first it was not easy for me to muster that level of commitment or courage. What seems so simple in hindsight was so difficult then.

Asking the question for my son, myself, and my family—*what would make each of us feel well?*—I realized that none of us were feeling well. The situation didn't look like it was improving on its own. Perhaps, I thought, something needed to change, and the intervention would be a good fresh start over for us all. One part of my mind hoped the intervention might be like the "reset" button on a machine that breaks down.

Then another part of my mind would push back, causing me to reconsider the idea to intervene. I imagined how my son might feel angry and betrayed and how that feeling might scar our father-son relationship for a lifetime. That type of pain would never make me feel well or help my son feel well either. I did not want to make a wrong decision, knowing that fools can rush in where angels fear to tread. So indecision paralyzed me, and it held my family hostage from a chance at wellness.

Eventually I realized—in my own heart—that the decision to intervene was an act of love and kindness, and I hoped that my son would someday see that *truth* too. I was determined to tell him that, if he would ever listen to me again.

The intervention took place in the stillness of the night, and it awakened my son from a deep sleep. It was nonviolent, which was very important to me and my inner Thoreau, but the final result was that my son would leave our home, taken away from all that was familiar. After first introducing my son to the two large men who would be escorting him from our house, my wife and I left the premises, which we were told would help facilitate the intervention. Driving a few blocks away from our home, my wife and I cried together in each other's arms. That remains one of the most vivid and painful memories of my life.

At that moment, we had no idea the direction our son and our family would take or whether we'd ever feel well again. At least I knew that we asked the right question.

———

Extensive family therapy followed the intervention. It was during these family therapy sessions that I was required to truly ask the question of *What makes you feel well?* and also ask the underlying *Why?* questions. In therapy there were many forms of the same basic question, but each variation forced us to look closely at our own wellness. For me and my family, asking these questions and grappling with the answers was insightful and transformative, and it slowly helped us regain our family's wellness.

There were one-on-one therapy sessions and group discussions with members of my own family, as well as get-togethers with many other families. The therapies could take many forms, to help us better look at what made us well and what made us feel unhappy and ill too. Professional therapists and trained facilitators guided us through these questions. They used role-playing games, storytelling techniques, and soul-searching discussions. We were encouraged to be supportive and understanding of one another, yet not hold back on critical analysis and truthful revelations.

These therapeutic approaches were often uncomfortable, especially for families like mine that valued their privacy. Some methods seemed strange at first, yet resulted in great insightful leaps forward, like using emotionally sensitive horses and dogs to help connect to the wellness of family dynamics. Throughout the process we were urged to embrace the unusual and confront our discomfort.

It took real commitment to continue, and setbacks were an essential part of the process that taught lessons of their own. Yet for each of the many families I met, just asking these questions and committing to answer them was highly impactful and wonderfully healing.

What the questions revealed was often surprising. Although all of the families were experiencing similar teenage problems, which seemed the same on the surface, the underlying causes could be quite different, very specific to the dynamics of the family in therapy. Each family had their own painful and unique stories to tell. Each family came from different places, with different backgrounds, different financial means, and different cultural attitudes. For each, these questions of *what* and *why* needed to be asked and then answered as best they could.

On the surface, the problems appeared to be substance abuse, trouble in school or with the law, communication breakdowns, disrespect in relationships, and all sorts and manners of rebellious and self-destructive behaviors. We learned how these behaviors were really not the "problems"; they were always *symptoms* on the surface of something far deeper and more revealing.

These symptoms were like the visible froth spilling over the sides of a boiling teenage cauldron. A teenage girl intentionally cutting herself, slicing her own skin till it bleeds, may tell you she feels a moment of wellness in her release of pain, and a teenage boy binge-drinking, oblivious to all life's pressures and unfairness, may say he feels a moment of wellness in his stupor. For both, it is the complicated *whys* beneath the surface that help explain their self-destructive choices. These *whys* varied widely for each teen and their families, but understanding these *whys* offered hope of a way back toward good health and higher-level wellness.

There were *whys* like anxiety, depression, resentment, addiction, bereavement, absence, abuse, alienation, attachment, self-image, self-esteem, expectation, exhaustion, dependence, obsession, imbalance, fear, inadequacy, bullying, belittlement, boredom, numbness, disconnect, and separation. Indeed, even these supposed underlying causes were *mere words!* We needed to resist using these words as bland psychological jargon with clinically sterile meanings. These *why* words rarely, if ever, captured the devil in the details of each family's story. These *why* words did not settle or substitute for each family's own individualized search for answers.

Indeed, in many ways the real hard work of therapy was getting people *just to ask the questions.* Just asking these questions, honestly and sincerely, was an essential step forward for all of the teenagers in therapy. For my son Nick, it enabled him to confront his fears and insecurities and imagine a bright new future with new meaning and new purpose in his life. That made all the difference to him—it was *transformational!*—and I saw too how it made all the difference to the other teenagers I encountered.

At the start of the process, I thought that it was only my son and the other teenagers who needed to ask these questions. But I was wrong!

I needed to ask these same wellness questions for *myself*; indeed, my entire family and all the other families needed to ask these questions for *themselves* too. Each and every member of an extended family suffers in a family crisis, so each family member needs to seek wellness for himself or herself.

Sometimes the questions also revealed how family members could fall into unhealthy patterns of seeing one another as *objects*, not as *people* with their own hopes, fears, and needs for love and wellness. In the midst of a crisis—this is true in any crisis—it is far too easy to objectify people, to forget our common humanity and connection.

As family members suddenly realized how their actions were hurtful or uncaring to one another, families achieved breakthrough insights in their relationships. This clarity, though sometimes painful, was an essential first step for the healing that comes from acceptance, reconciliation, and forgiveness.

During the experience of teenage intervention and family therapy, asking these questions of wellness for myself, I wrote the book *(((Tuning Jack FM)))*. Although the book is not about the intervention or its aftermath, writing was a way of asking questions about wellness for myself, and it helped me find answers of deeper meaning and purpose. One of the important lessons of wellness is how finding meaning and purpose in your life promotes healing and wellness during even the most troubling of times.

By asking what makes you feel well, you are forced to confront yourself, to ask core questions like *Who are you?* and *What are you doing with your life?* No one has all the answers, but we can all ask these simple questions. *Each and every time you ask these questions, you get to know yourself a little bit better.*

This search for self-knowledge is essential for wellness, and it begins the process of proactivity for your own health. This is the same lesson about wellness that Dr. Halbert Dunn understood so long ago, when he declared *"the central bastion to be conquered involves teaching people how to 'know themselves.'"*

There are many ways to say the same thing. The protagonist of my earlier book, Jack F. M. Hernandez, would say that wellness begins by *(((tuning in)))* to your self.

I like to say that *self-discovery is essential for self-recovery.*

———

We take much about our own lives for granted. You can live unconsciously, as if you were sleeping, scarcely acknowledging your own routines and habits, not knowing what you do and never thinking about why you do it.

Consider your breathing. It may be obvious, but mostly you are unconscious of its movement; at other times, you can consciously observe, change, and control your breath. If you're asking *what makes you feel well,* breathing is a very good answer! Not only because consciousness of your breath can be a simple way to maintain good health, but because *"don't stop breathing"* is good medical advice too.

Health-care lawyers would smartly advise me to emphasize that *I am not giving medical advice.* Indeed, I am not a physician—just a lawyer, and then only in certain jurisdictions and certain practice areas. My comic side thinks it is funny, though, that our systems and institutions require formal medical education and licensure to make statements about what is good for our health, perhaps even the obvious need to keep breathing.

It is easy to lose sight of simple things in life that are essential to good health. Simple things like your breathing or what goes into, onto, and out of your body. Simple things like how your body moves through its environment and how you interact with all that surrounds you—people, animals, plants, technologies, transportation, buildings, landscapes, air, and water. Asking questions about these simple everyday things in your life is good for your health.

You don't need to be a medical doctor to know that, but some doctors do. For example, Dr. Kenneth H. Cooper, a physician whose work became celebrated for the well-being it promoted—and whose story will be briefly told in the next section—said it another way: *"It is easier to maintain good health through proper exercise, diet and emotional balance than it is to regain it once it is lost."*[1]

Through the intervention and the therapy that followed, my son Nicholas learned the importance of these three simple common denominators for his health and well-being, in ways that most of us—myself included—have never had the opportunity to experience. Perhaps the most transformative part of the entire therapeutic experience for him, or so Nick tells me, was wandering for months through the wilderness with only food, water, and some other essentials carried on his back. In this stark environment, with the complexities and technologies of contemporary society removed, and only sky and stars above, good health is stripped to its bare essentials.

As he spent each day hiking miles and miles with a heavy physical load to carry, Nick became acutely aware of his body's movements, and his muscles turned taut, strong, and lean. Water and food in this environment were never taken for granted, for both the nourishment they provided and the camaraderie they created with those who shared their sustenance together. Alone with his thoughts and feelings for hours or days at a time, he discovered more about himself, what was bothering him, and what kept him from peace.

He realized how you can feel like a tightrope walker sometimes with all the pressures and demands of modern life, but even way up on the high wire, you still need to keep balance just the same. He realized how you need to find healthy, productive, and fulfilling ways to make yourself feel well.

Preparing meals in this wilderness environment, Nicholas rediscovered a childhood dream—a passion that he had almost forsaken in the midst of his teenage crisis. His renewed inspiration reset the purpose and meaning of his life, and in the years to come, he would graduate from the renowned Culinary Institute of America in Hyde Park, New York (the hometown of President Franklin D. Roosevelt, who of course also understood how important *purpose and meaning* was for world peace—as well as everyday life—as his American nation fought to end a world's war).

Today, Nick seems to take life in stride, brightening the day for everyone he meets with his laughter and easygoing nature. I know that he is a source of balance, inspiration, and wellness for me personally now. As a bonus, I get to enjoy good food and drink with him, some of which he calmly and lovingly prepared or selected and which he helps me appreciate even more. Nicholas may have found meaning at mealtimes, but he also found purpose in painting, *prolifically so,* I might add; I've already picked one of his paintings for the cover of my next book, if the fates allow.

Nick would probably tell you that Dr. Cooper's prescription for *"proper exercise, diet and emotional balance"* remain core objectives for his own personal health and wellness, and it's why he gravitated to fields like foods and beverages to comfort and nourish people—it is an expression of a desire to care for other people and help them feel well. He'd probably say that many top chefs today would agree with that assessment, which is why they gravitated to their careers too.

Most public health officials, physicians, and wellness gurus today would also agree that *"proper exercise, diet and emotional balance"* are basic to maintaining good health. However, when Dr. Cooper first uttered these words in 1968, most of his colleagues in mainstream medicine refused to believe that these three aspects of daily life had much connection to health or could prevent disease and infirmity.

It may now seem current medical wisdom, but its insight is not new. Hippocrates, called the father of Western medicine, recommended much the same basic formula for good health thousands of years earlier. We sometimes forget what we knew all along—the way most physicians forgot about ancient bismuth stomach remedies for my grandfather and me—so Cooper's common sense is a welcome reminder and helpful encouragement.

There still may not be any medical consensus on the *meaning* of these simple things. What is proper exercise or a healthful diet? What is emotional balance, and how do you get there? Once more, regardless of the answers to these questions, there is no substitute for simply *asking* the questions for yourself.

———

Consider "proper exercise"—the first of Dr. Cooper's three common denominators for maintaining good health.

Exercise was a topic near and dear to Kenneth Cooper's heart. As a colonel and physician in the US Air Force, he developed a cardiovascular fitness and exercise program (along with his colleague Pauline Potts, a physical therapist and colonel herself) that was good enough to train astronauts. Dr. Cooper eventually started a national exercise craze with his famous book *Aerobics*, first published in 1968.

Aerobics may be a wonderful exercise for wellness, but Dr. Cooper would surely agree that there are many other forms of "proper" exercise. When it comes to exercise, there are also dancing and frolicking, sports and recreation, the hikes I like, farming and gardening, hunting and foraging, yoga and stretching, body sculpting and boogie boarding. The list goes on and on, and depending on your individual exercise preferences, you may choose to run, jog, jump, walk, trek, cycle, climb, crawl, meander, race, pace, push, spin, flip, twist, twirl, lift, surf, ski, curl, carry, skip, swim, saunter, or swing. What is "proper" for one person is not "proper" for all people. A recurring theme of this book is that we need to embrace our individuality and uniqueness, instead of blandly insisting on our sameness. *One size does not fit all.*

Even for the same person, what is "proper" exercise during one phase of life will not remain so during the course of an entire lifetime. For example, the exercise regimen for a top professional athlete is not appropriate for that same athlete as a small child, nor is it appropriate when the athlete becomes old, ill, or infirm. What is proper exercise for you will be different too, based on your stage of life or the stage of your day. Life changes things, bringing new phases and new circumstances, even changing the physical shape, condition, and metabolism of our bodies.

Life is always changing—that's one of the beautiful things about life. Look at a sunset, the waves on a beach, the flowering landscape of a meadow, the thoughts and emotions in your mind. These scenes all change—from season to season, from day to day, from moment to moment—countless times in the course of a lifetime. We may hope for a life on Earth that is fixed and unchanging, but even what seems like forever cannot be, for change and death and renewal are part of life's inevitable cycle. We may not enjoy or value change, but life's changes will happen regardless; acceptance of that simple fact goes a long way toward our own wellness.

As appropriate for these life changes, the way we exercise will change, and we need to proactively know our bodies and our individual capacity for exercise as part of our own proactive approach to fitness. This may mean testing yourself, and it may mean proceeding slowly until you find comfortable levels of exercise for you. You may want to consult with experts, like physicians, coaches, and trainers, but— even with their guidance and advice—*you* still need to be vigilant about knowing what exercise makes *you* feel well. Whatever these physicians, coaches, and trainers may recommend, you have many choices.

With the growth of the wellness movement, your options for proper exercise continue to multiply and expand. Consider Dr. Cooper's aerobics exercise regimen as an example. Today you can seek the companionship of others and take an aerobics class at a local health and fitness center, or you can exercise alone in the comfort of your own home with an aerobics video. You can find aerobics exercises set to many different types of music and customized for many different cultural environments. In other words, even if you choose aerobics as a way to feel well, you still must find an aerobics program that's right for you.

It's worth remembering that aerobics instruction itself didn't exist when Dr. Halbert Dunn coined the term wellness while he was a senior public health official under President Dwight D. Eisenhower. Both Eisenhower and the next American president, John F. Kennedy, openly worried about the lack of exercise and fitness among American youth, creating federal task forces like the President's Council on Physical Fitness. Wellness entrepreneurs like Jack LaLanne and Vic Tanny began to provide community places to exercise in response to growing consumer demand. These pioneers and their peers vastly expanded the range of locations and changed the focus from body-building gyms for improving physique and appearance to fitness centers for good health and longevity.

Since those early days, wellness entrepreneurs have expanded aerobic workouts in the gym by developing new types of exercise equipment. They have brought new exercise equipment affordably into our homes to expand home aerobics options too. Wellness innovators have also created new types of aerobics fitness regimens for ever-widening audiences. They have provided technologies to monitor heart rates and other health and fitness indicators to improve aerobics' capacity to make us feel well.

This evolution of choices and options for Dr. Cooper's aerobics is reflected for many other forms of exercise. If proper exercise is a common denominator for wellness, there are more opportunities than ever before to *proactively decide for yourself* the type of exercise that might make you feel well.

———

The same pattern emerges with *diet*, the second item on Dr. Cooper's list for maintaining good health.

Like proper exercise, diet is a simple common denominator for good health and wellness, but what is *"proper"* and what does *"diet"* mean anyway? A diet is used to lose weight, and a diet is used to gain weight. It can be about calories, carbohydrates, or cholesterol and can be affected through nutrients, vitamins, and minerals—even molecules like free radicals and simple H_2O. Diet is about the foods we eat, the beverages we drink, and supplements and substances we introduce into our bodies. It is not only what we consume through our mouths, for diet includes anything we introduce into our bodies or absorb through skin and other bodily membranes.

There are many physicians, health gurus, nutritionists, and experts all ready to give advice on what is a "proper diet"—but like exercise, *one size does not fit all*. Though there may be commonalities in nutritional needs, what is "proper" will vary from person to person and will change based on stage of life and lifestyle. A competitive runner needs a diet to maintain the physical needs and energy-burning demands of an intensive lifestyle, and a baby barely able to crawl must have a diet that supports precious life functions and healthy childhood growth. Diets for the runner and the baby may be vastly different, but "proper diet" makes both feel well—requiring both the runner and the baby's caregiver to proactively take charge of diet.

It is worth taking charge of your diet too, because the many positive health effects of a proper diet are very broad. Diet can be used to heal you from diseases, purify and cleanse your body of toxins, and change your moods and mental state—among many other positive benefits.

There are negative effects of a poor diet, as well. Not meeting certain basic dietary requirements will result in disease and poor health. For example, the failure to consume vitamin C—commonly found in fresh citrus fruits—results in a dreadful disease known as scurvy, as early sailors learned at sea. The dietary deficiency made them feel awful, their gums bleeding and their spirits depressed, before progressing to more advanced stages, eventually death. Eating an orange or a lime suddenly made them feel well again.

British sailors were once ridiculed as *"Limeys"* because of the type of citrus they added to their alcoholic grog at sea. It's funny if you think about it—how a food chosen to prevent scurvy, by people making healthful dietary choices, made the British into objects of derogatory criticism. Another theme of this book is that if a lime makes you feel well and you're not hurting others by adding a lime to your diet, then by all means eat the lime—no matter society's ridicule or contempt for lime-eaters!

Being proactive and making informed choices about our diets should be simple. But it is not always easy when society belittles people for eating certain foods—like limes—and keeps limes away from those who want to eat them. It is common, historically speaking, for political, legal, economic, or health-care systems to unwittingly or wrongfully dictate dietary choices available, to the detriment of a community's health and well-being.

Consider the wretched disease of beriberi, once rampant throughout Asia. For those afflicted with this disease, speech slurs, walking becomes difficult, and mental confusion sets in. Eventually, the circulatory system and heart shut down, causing death. It turns out that beriberi—once a focus of international medical attention and health-care studies—was caused by bad food choices that society made for everyday people.

In the 1800s, industrial factories milled rice, a staple of most Asian diets. Unpolished brown rice degrades much more rapidly than polished white rice, so by removing the coatings on the outside of the rice grains, the rice could be stored longer for sale by these industrial enterprises. International politics, policies, and laws protected the economic trade in white rice. Cultural values further reinforced the consumption of white rice, demeaning brown rice as peasant food and otherwise strongly encouraging ordinary Asians to buy the industrially milled white rice. As brown rice disappeared from diets, the once-rare disease of beriberi became epidemic, although few saw a connection that seems obvious in hindsight.

The connection was discovered in the decade or so before 1900 by a Dutch physician named Christiaan Eijkman. In 1886 Dr. Eijkman set out to Indonesia, hoping to discover a treatment for beriberi, which had become rampant among the Indonesian people of what was then known as the Dutch East Indies. Upon his arrival Eijkman immediately began to conduct medical laboratory tests on rabbits, monkeys, and chickens, hoping to learn in animals how the disease of beriberi was contracted and how it could be cured. These scientific tests did not lead to any insights, but Dr. Eijkman's big breakthrough was when the caretaker of the laboratory chickens told Eijkman that the chickens all got sick from eating leftover white rice, but quickly recovered when fed unpolished brown rice. Eijkman then proceeded from one clinical trial to another in animals, confirming how the brown rice coatings successfully treated the disease. By 1895, he conducted tests among human populations and soon after confirmed that unpolished brown rice prevented and treated the disease of beriberi in humans.

You might think that if brown rice was a cure for beriberi, the medical system would flock to the solution. But medicine can be a lot like fashion, imitative and vainglorious alongside its great allure and appeal, and back then, in the late 1800s and early 1900s, the *germ theory* of disease was all the rage in the fashions of medicine. This theory that bacteria, microbes, and other germs were responsible for most diseases won German physician Dr. Robert Koch the Nobel Prize in Medicine in 1905. The germ theory became so popular that most doctors believed a germ must be responsible for beriberi too, ignoring the obvious solution that there was something vital for nutrition in the brown rice coatings.

The way we think—our underlying approach—can change what we see, so it may not be surprising to see the reluctance of the medical community to accept Eijkman's findings. Indeed, even Dr. Eijkman himself stubbornly insisted that beriberi must be caused by a germ, erroneously believing that the brown rice coatings contained an antibody against the bacteria causing the disease. The young Dutch Dr. Eijkman had studied under the famous German Dr. Koch in Berlin in 1885, before leaving for Indonesia in 1886, and became thoroughly indoctrinated into his mentor's germ theory of disease. His narrow-minded refusal to admit that beriberi could be a mere nutritional deficiency, even decades after discovering the link between the brown rice coatings and beriberi, earned Dr. Eijkman the nickname of the *"Unwilling Father of Vitamins"* at Utrecht University in the Netherlands, where he was a professor for the latter part of his distinguished career. [2]

It wasn't just Eijkman who mistakenly clung to this fashionable medical notion about a bacteria causing beriberi. As medical historian David Arnold wrote, describing another beriberi epidemic in the mid-1920s, decades after Eijkman's discovery: "But the principal reason for [this beriberi epidemic]…was that many influential figures in the medical establishment clung to the belief that beriberi was better explained by [bacterial] 'toxi-infection'…[because] this bacterial explanation, influenced by germ theory and the Pasteurian tradition, was widely held…"[3]

In other words, many leading scientists and physicians of the day erroneously supported the germ theory at the expense of simple common sense and a widely available nutritional treatment for beriberi—wholesome brown rice. The story reminds us that narrow-minded adherence to widespread but mistaken beliefs can have a major impact on our health and wellness, sometimes leaving populations of people to suffer or die from an entirely preventable disease. It reminds us how history can be cruel indeed.

———

It did not need to be that way. Hearing of Dr. Eijkman's discovery of the link between beriberi and the brown rice coatings, a bright open-minded young Polish chemist named Kazimierz Funk was inspired to discover how substances found in common foods like the brown rice coatings were essential to good health. By 1912, the brilliant twenty-eight-year-old Dr. Funk revealed that many vital nutrients shared a chemical structure called an *amine*—brown rice coatings had thiamine aka vitamin B1-so he coined the term *vitamin* for *vital* amine. Funk hypothesized that vitamin deficiencies caused a whole range of then-common illnesses, from beriberi to rickets, pellagra to celiac disease.

Yes, history can be cruel, but sometimes it can be funny too. *"Dr. Funk's vitamins"* might sound to you—as it did to me—like a catchy new wellness brand, telling the story of an early Doctor Feelgood who restored health with his magical new vital amines. Perhaps the Nobel Prize committee was not similarly amused, for they ignored Kazimierz Funk in their 1929 award for medicine, acknowledging the scientific discovery of *vitamins*, the very word to which Dr. Funk ironically gave meaning.

That year, the Nobel Prize in medicine was jointly awarded to Dutch Dr. Eijkman, who uncovered the hidden connection between the brown rice coatings and the prevention of beriberi, and Sir Frederick Hopkins of Britain, who found "accessory food factors" that prevented diseases in animals fed different diets. Vitamin pioneers like Poland's Dr. Funk and Japan's Dr. Umetaro Suzuki (the first person to succeed in isolating thiamine from the brown rice coatings) were snubbed by the Nobel committee in 1929. For that matter, also over-looked in the award was ancient Greece's Hippocrates, the so-called father of medicine who, thousands of years earlier, is said to have said, *"Let thy food be medicine, and thy medicine be food."*

This ancient wisdom seems both simple and obvious, embraced by people and cultures around the world, yet common sense can be far too uncommon in the systems and institutions that affect our health care. Knowledge may evolve, but it is difficult to advance true understanding if we stubbornly cling to definitional lines that really do not exist—and never did.

Even as the wellness movement forces us to acknowledge the fiction of these lines, health-care institutions continue to cling to these lines, and create illusory new ones too. For instance, as part of the US Food and Drug Administration's evolving response to the wellness movement, the FDA created a new hybrid check-the-box category called *"medical foods"*—extending their regulatory authority through erroneous new lines with new legal meanings. It makes me wonder what the FDA has in mind.

Does the FDA believe that a physician's signature is now necessary to purchase a lime to regain health for those afflicted by scurvy, or that a doctor should write a script for brown rice for a patient to get well from beriberi? Should nutritional remedies only be available through a doctor's prescription, in the same way that we limit the legal availability of medicines from people who need them the most? Is medical regulation really about protecting businesses and economics, much like the industrial trade in white rice was legally enforced in another era?

It also makes me wonder why the medical system has not fully embraced diet's obvious effect on health, requiring future physicians to study more dietary healing and nutrition courses in medical school to learn how to use foods to prevent and treat medical conditions. Most medical schools don't even offer such nutritional medicine courses, outside of the basics—at least as I'm writing this.

To date, the only medical doctors that I know who truly understand and appreciate the connectedness between food and health are those who have engaged in their own serious *self-study* of the topic. To borrow Mark Twain's quip, these physicians never let schooling get in the way of their education. Thank goodness that *true education* does not begin and does not end with formal schooling!

Thankfully too, ordinary people don't need a doctor's license or a doctor's prescription to use foods as medicine—at least not yet—and ordinary people don't need to be physicians to proactively take charge of their own diets.

Chapter 8

LEARNING WHAT MAKES YOU

FEEL WELL

The first step in proactively using diet for good health and wellness is *knowing* the foods you are eating and *knowing* the beverages, cosmetics, medicines, and other things that go into or onto our bodies too. How can you seek out foods that make you feel well or avoid foods that make you feel ill if you don't even know what you are eating?

The concept is truly simple—when it comes to your diet, the foods and substances you put into and onto your body, you need to know what you are consuming. The concept may be simple, but knowing the ingredients in our diets is not as easy as it might seem. In an age of industrialization, when consumables are often processed, prepared, and packaged for compelling reasons like economy, convenience, marketing, preservation, and standardization, the identity of ingredients in our foods, beverages, cosmetics, and medicines can be hidden and unexpected.

When Tony Varano and I were doing our presentation of the white paper, I would explain to the private equity firms that there was one obscure statistic that I thought emblematic of the wellness movement and its sales trends: *the growing numbers of "label readers."*

I reminded the private equity investors how few consumers were once willing to slow traffic in the grocery store or linger in supermarket aisles to learn more about what they were buying. As the wellness movement gained momentum, however, more and more people each year took the time to read the labels on the packages of their foods, beverages, cosmetics, and medicines.

These label-readers want to learn about the ingredients they are consuming into their bodies, but they want to learn so much more than a mere list of ingredients. As Mark Twain quipped, we can *"know merely things"* without being *"familiar with the meanings of them."* These label-readers wanted to understand the *meanings* of these ingredients, for themselves and their families.

Label-readers wanted to know the *quantities* of ingredients that were in their foods, medicines, beverages, and cosmetics, but they also wanted to know their *qualities*. They wanted to learn the ingredient's nutritional value. They wanted to understand its health risks and benefits and its proper uses and dosages. Label-readers wanted to know how the ingredient was sourced and the process for manufacturing. They wanted to learn how the ingredients were grown, where they were grown, and about the farmers who grew them. They wanted to know about the attitudes and ethics of those who made and sold the products and the economics of whether they were fairly traded.

With all of their questions and concerns and with the knowledge gained from their inquiries, a remarkable thing began to happen. These label-reading consumers actually *accelerated* the wellness movement, bringing meaningful change from the bottom up. They would spread the news of how an ingredient helped make them feel well, and as the news spread, that ingredient would suddenly get "hot" in the marketplace, increasing sales of all products with that ingredient.

The "hot" ingredient might be a type of oil for beautifying cosmetic use, like tea tree oil or Moroccan argan oil, or a type of oil for heart health, like omega-3 fish oil or olive oil. It might be a new superfruit with touted antioxidant health benefits, like an acaí berry that people would hear about but not even know how to pronounce, or it might be a common apple, with age-old health benefits that would be reconfirmed for a new audience. In what seemed like the blink of an eye, whole grains would get hot in the marketplace, rapidly replacing processed grains in cereals and breads on supermarket shelves, and new grains like quinoa would sprout on menus everywhere. None of this should be surprising. Brown rice sales undoubtedly surged too after the news of its health benefits in cultures sickened by beriberi.

Or it could go the other way, and products could go "cold" in what seemed an instant. Label-readers would spread the news of how certain ingredients made them unwell, and when people heard this news, sales of products with these ingredients would be ruined. For example, once-popular food products would be shunned by the market in an instant, even legally prohibited, because they contain trans fats and high-fructose syrups. It is worth noting that these types of fats and sugars are *qualitatively* different than the types of fats found in the heart-healthy oils and the types of sugars found in the oxidant-rich superfruits, so simple *quantitative* disclosures of "fats," "sugars," "proteins," and "carbohydrates"—like the basic nutritional breakdowns mandated by law on labels—are not sufficient for wellness consumers.

Antonio and I knew that the topic of driving sales would pique the interest of business investors, and that was certainly the case during our presentation of the white paper. Investors always want to understand the trends that affect business, its products and services, because being able to correctly forecast sales—predicting the future—is how investors make more money. In that sense, understanding how the wellness movement drove sales was a chance for rapid financial gain, motivating investors.

Fear of loss is also a powerful motivator in business. Business investments could be lost overnight as wellness consumers made certain ingredients obsolete, sometimes compelling retailers to remove products with shunned ingredients from their shelves. For those investors in tried-and-true industries like foods, beverages, pharma-ceuticals, and cosmetics, where consumer demand was once thought to be stable and recession-proof, ingredient trends could now happen so fast, so furiously, that forecasting sales figures might seem like a rough day on the ocean, in waves that rapidly rise and fall, surge and crash.

Take the example of aspirin and acetaminophen, seemingly simple medicines providing pain relief to many people. In one business cycle, aspirin sales would fall because label-readers learned of aspirin's link to stomach ulcers, as well as the rare but potentially fatal Reye's syn-drome; as inquiring consumers learned of acetaminophen's gentler nature for the stomach and hospitals touted the safety of Tylenol® and other generic versions, acetaminophen surged in popularity. Then, years later, in another dramatic business cycle, aspirin would once again be purchased in droves because of its newly discovered ability in low doses to prevent heart attacks, while acetaminophen would see its sales tumble, because label-readers learned of the link to potentially fatal acute liver damage from small overdoses. With these wild and unpredictable wellness waves, if you're a business investor focused on the medical category of pain relief, how could you even make a sound investment decision?

This is not a book on investing in wellness businesses, so the ques-tion is mostly rhetorical, but I'd say find something to invest in *that makes people feel well*. In this medical category, the product should provide effective pain relief to many people, like aspirin or acetaminophen, but should also be safe and free of side effects for most people. I wouldn't want to place my bet on products that can give people stomach ulcers or inflict potentially fatal illnesses and infirmities, which scare label-readers and lower sales.

Actually, I did make a bet in this investment category many years ago. It was then a struggling start-up, with a synergistic blend of natu-ral medicines applied topically to the skin on affected areas. In its early years, each time I heard a heartfelt story about how Topricin® eased someone's pain and improved his or her quality of life, I was able to *"make another deposit into the emotional bank"*—as Lou Paradise, the patented product's formulator and company founder, would say. Like most investors, I appreciate monetary deposits into the bank too, but financial investments always have risks and rewards, so I need to *feel good* about what my investments *do*, not just what they *earn*.

Knowing that my investment in a pain relief medicine company helps heal people without hurting them—well, that makes me feel well too. Topricin is free of any known side effects and safe to use, because of Lou's next-generation homeopathic approach, in which combinations of low dosage ingredients are serially diluted and succussed. Topricin's disclosure of its ingredients and their homeopathic safety on its label pleases me, as it pleases other label-readers, but today's label-reading wellness consumer wants to know much more about a product than just its ingredients, safety, and quantity. Label-readers also need to know that there's also a qualitative difference in the caring and concern of the people that make the product, which resonates beyond the label, encouraging the booming sales of "artisan" and "craft" products made with love to a growing audience of wellness consumers.

———

Once upon a time, not that long ago really, most consumer products in the United States and throughout the world did not reveal their ingredients.

Labels were seen by manufacturers as an advertising tool only, to tell stories that sold products, and there were no laws or regulations that required disclosure of ingredients. So most didn't tell, and the more unscrupulous manufacturers intentionally hid harmful ingredients from their customers—ingredients that they and their doctors might have been outraged and alarmed to find out about.

A movement began in the 1870s to awaken the public to the dangers of impure foods and drugs. Pure foods and drugs seemed like such a simple idea, a cause that everyone could rally around. But purity and simplicity were not easy then and are not easy still.

The *"pure food"* movement in America was led by activist crusaders like Dr. Harvey W. Wiley. In his role as the American government's chief chemist, Dr. Wiley tested the widespread use of food additives on a staff of civil service employee volunteers, who became known as the *"Poison Squad."*[1] These human guinea pigs consumed foods laced with then-common food additives like formaldehyde, borax, sulfuric acid, and copper sulfate. These additives helped preserve the shelf life of foods and gave foods the appearance of freshness by making their colors brighter. Red meats seemed redder and green vegetables seemed greener, while concealing the dangers of the hidden ingredient.

The exploits of the Poison Squad were glorified in song and celebrated by journalists, educating the public about how common food additives could make them sick, causing headaches and stomachaches and far worse. Still, Dr. Wiley and his Poison Squad could not effect legislative change. The pure food movement was heavily opposed by industrial food and drug manufacturers, who believed that disclosing ingredients would harm their businesses. These powerful and entrenched institutions—sellers of our foods and makers of our medicines—lobbied the US Congress year after year, preventing legislation. American consumers had no legal right to know what they were consuming.

When the Pure Food and Drug Act was finally adopted in 1906, it was not through the exploits of the Poison Squad. Nor was Dr. Wiley himself responsible for the law's adoption, although many historians still consider him to be the father of the Pure Food and Drug Act. It took a bestselling book, *The Jungle,* written by the muckraking journalist Upton Sinclair and published by Doubleday in 1906, to shock Congress into acting.

The public was horrified by Sinclair's undercover accounts of disgustingly unsanitary conditions at meatpacking plants in Chicago, and Congress had no choice but to act to calm the national hysteria over food. The Meat Inspection Act and the Pure Food and Drug Act were both adopted into law on the very same day in 1906, during Theodore Roosevelt's presidency. Finally there was some measure of transparency in our foods and our medicines. Consumable products—or at least a few of them—needed to be labeled. Historians would point out that the Pure Food and Drug Act legislation did not go very far, but it was a start.

Some readers may still ask: *Why do labels even matter?*

I would answer that what we don't know can hurt us. That our ignorance can even kill us.

One of my favorite labeling stories of this early 1906 Pure Food and Drug Act period is the tale of a medicinal infant remedy known as Mrs. Winslow's Soothing Syrup. It was brilliantly marketed, widely available, and trusted by mothers and their doctors. Growing in popularity sometime after 1844, millions of bottles were sold for babies who had *"teething"* pain or who had *"colic"*—and also to *"give rest to the mother."*

Mrs. Winslow's Soothing Syrup worked wonderfully, soothing the crying infant into restful sleep almost immediately. As far back as 1860, the *New York Times* had printed glowing endorsements about the safety and effectiveness of the medicine, helping build confidence over successive generations of mothers and grandmothers, all without ever disclosing its proprietary ingredients. [2] Well-intentioned parents trusted the label's claims that it was the *"oldest and safest remedy for children teething"* and believed its advertisements that it was *"perfectly harmless"* for a baby's teething pain. Many mothers took a soothing spoonful of Mrs. Winslow's Soothing Syrup for their own headaches too, as advertisements for the medicine encouraged them to do. [3]

The problem was that some infants never awoke from their restful sleep, because of the undisclosed qualities of the medicine. In 1910—four years after the passage of the 1906 Pure Food and Drug Act and fifty years after publishing praise for Mrs. Winslow's Soothing Syrup—a new *New York Times* exposé revealed the results of a US chemist's analysis, disclosing that Mrs. Winslow's Soothing Syrup contained high doses of morphine, a powerful narcotic. No wonder it stopped teething babies from crying and gave rest to mothers!

The 1910 newspaper exposé led to a popular outcry, which in 1911 goaded the American Medical Association to publish their own exposé, describing Mrs. Winslow's Soothing Syrup as a *"baby killer"* that was also addicting countless other children. [4] The American Medical Association's forceful condemnation led to a popular outcry and the product's rapid demise in the American and British consumer markets—after a *seventy-year period* of the medicine's big profits and widespread popularity.

———

Today's label-readers still need to pressure health-care leaders to force disclosures on labels. Although foods and medicines now need to be labeled because of continuing legislation and regulation dating to the 1906 Pure Food and Drug Act, it does not mean labels can be trusted. Wellness-oriented consumers know they must take charge of their health and wellness and cannot rely solely on systems and institutions to do it for them.

It took an outside muckraker's accounts about how meats are processed before the US Congress was shamed into passing its 1906 legislation, and it took a newspaper account of unwanted ingredients in an infant teething medicine before the American Medical Association finally spoke out against Mrs. Winslow's Soothing Syrup. The more things change, the more they stay the same, and these self-similar historical patterns still recur today.

Acetaminophen is a good example. [5] For many decades, beginning in the mid-1950s in the United States, the pain relief medicine's safety was loudly proclaimed by corporate manufacturers, government regulators, and the medical establishment. In the early 1970s, however, following reports and studies from rogue, ridiculed, and underfunded scientific researchers, word of mouth began to circulate among wellness-oriented consumers about the hidden dangers of acute liver failure from even slight and unintentional overdosages of acetaminophen.

Hearing of these bottom-up concerns, the FDA—the US agency responsible for the safety of foods and drugs—convened an expert panel to determine the safety of acetaminophen. This panel concluded in 1977 that acetaminophen can cause *"severe liver damage"* if overused even in small amounts and urged that this warning should be *"obligatory"* on all labels of acetaminophen products, like Tylenol®. Despite the unambiguous conclusions of its own expert panel, the FDA delayed implementing this obviously needed label warning until 2009—*a delay that lasted thirty-two years!*

We can endlessly debate whether such conscience-shocking delays by health-care institutions are benign or sinister, innocent or intentional. Some will argue that these delays are the direct result of corruption and greed, part of a system that protects entrenched financial interests ahead of people's health and wellness. Others will insist that these delays are just unfortunate by-products of process and procedure, necessary to gather scientific proof and slowly reach consensus. The real truth may be somewhere in between these two extremes—or the truth may be something else entirely—but in the final analysis, does the FDA's motive and explanation even matter?

During the thirty-two long years of the FDA's delay in warning the public of the dangers of liver damage from even small overdoses, thousands of people accidentally died from acetaminophen use. Each and every year during these thirty-two years, whatever the motive or explanation for the FDA delay, however understandable or reprehensible they may be, many tens of thousands more children and adults were hospitalized from accidental acetaminophen overdoses.

Sadly, we tend to objectify and depersonalize data and statistics, ignoring the immeasurable costs of damaged lives, ignoring the pain and suffering of victims and their families. Surely these victims and their families are the real human costs of the failure of our health-care systems and institutions to provide simple ingredient label information pertinent to health and wellness.

These were innocent people treating a baby's teething or a head-ache, a fever, or some other pain who believed the promise of the popular Tylenol® brand's label of *"safe, fast pain relief."* They believed that the product's safety and efficacy—even for small children—was the reason it was *"recommended by pediatricians"* and the *"brand hospitals use most."* In these popular advertisements by Johnson & Johnson's McNeil Healthcare Division, consumers were specifically asked to *"Trust Tylenol®,"* and these innocent people gave their trust—they trusted the pharmaceutical manufacturer, they trusted the hospital and its doctors, they trusted the medical associations, and they trusted the FDA's government regulators. And yet, for their misplaced trust, these innocents wound up in an emergency room, needed a liver transplant, or died.

It was all preventable. All that was required was disclosure of truthful information about the medicine's ingredient and its dangers of liver failure from small overdoses, which had been discussed and known by researchers since the early 1960s, but as any business-minded person knows, that type of disclosure would have jeopardized the brand's profits and its robust sales of more than a billion dollars per year. How many were killed or injured from the lack of disclosure from the introduction of Tylenol® by McNeil Laboratories in 1955 to the initial labeling of overdose warnings in 2009-after a *fifty-five-year period* of the medicine's big profits and widespread popularity?

———

Another good lesson of these stories—if you're trying to answer the simple question of *What makes you feel well?*—is that one person's medicine can be another person's poison.

Though Tylenol® and Mrs. Winslow's Soothing Syrup both proved harmful poison to some people, there is no doubt that these medicines soothed and helped many millions of others feel well, helping ease the pain of little babies teething and screaming and the headaches of their well-intentioned mothers. The line between medicines and poisons can blur, just as lines can blur between foods and medicines, or between drugs and cosmetics, or between so many other fictitious separations we create in our lives and in our laws. Imaginary lines often come at the peril of our wellness.

These are not isolated examples of a line blurring, some exception to a rule. One of the most popular and effective cosmeceutical products in America today is Botox®—which is derived from one of the most lethal toxins we know. Though it can cause the fatal illness of botulism, medical researchers are learning how the *botulinum toxin* can manage acute pain and spasms or smooth the wrinkled skin of aging. So, is it a wonderful medicine, a beautifying cosmetic, or a deadly poison? Is it all of these things, or none of these things? *You decide.*

You deciding is at the heart of wellness. The decision to proactively take care of ourselves and our loved ones—which as I've said is the *first of three dimensions* to understanding the wellness movement—requires good information and good support.

That's why the labeling lapses for Tylenol® and Mrs. Winslow's Soothing Syrup mattered for the health and well-being of so many. When information about quantities and qualities of ingredients is not disclosed, people lose the ability to make their own informed decisions about what they and their families consume.

I've heard heartbreaking stories of well-intentioned, loving parents giving their sickened child acetaminophen, trusting the medicine to help their son or daughter. Wanting to give their child a sufficient dosage to ease their disease but not knowing the acute danger of small overdoses, these parents unwittingly poisoned their child, causing a failure of their child's liver. They killed through misinformed caring, unaware that a trusted medicine could become a deadly poison, unaware that there were no bright lines of separation between what can heal and what can harm.

Some may have opinions—even strong opinions—about these lines of separation. They'll tell you what is a medicine and what is a poison; they'll tell you how a certain food will make you ill or how a certain diet will make you feel well. Their opinions may be well-intentioned and they may even be correct for you, but their self-assurance often masquerades as "irrefutable fact" or "rational science." Remember how wise old Doctor Dan joked about opinions being like assholes—everyone's got one.

People's opinions about the medicines we take and the foods we eat can be woefully wrong. That's another simple but important lesson of the Tylenol® and Mrs. Winslow's Soothing Syrup stories. Was Tylenol® any less dangerous before the FDA finally got around to mandating warnings about liver failure on its label? Was Mrs. Winslow's Soothing Syrup any less safe after the American Medical Association was finally shamed into calling it a baby killer? The products were the same—only the opinions changed. Both were wonderful medicines for many people and lethal for the wrong person in the wrong situation.

———

One more good lesson of these stories, then, is that people can't be put into neat and tidy little boxes, to be treated without regard to their individuality and uniqueness. When it comes to our medicines and ourselves—like our exercises, our diets, and what makes you feel well—one size does not fit all.

"No genuine cure," wrote Dr. Samuel Hahnemann in 1810, *"can take place without the strict individualized treatment of each case of disease."*[6] Dr. Hahnemann, considered the father of homeopathy, warned against *"useless and wrongful disease names"* that compel physicians to treat according to the commonalities of the disease, instead of individualized treatment based on *"the entire complex of all the signs of the individual state of each single patient."*[7] Samuel Hahnemann's patient-focused protocols were once so revered, his contribution to medical arts and healing so renowned, that in 1900 the US Congress erected a statue to him in Washington, DC—still the only monument ever erected to a physician in America's capital.

Some skeptical scientists and doubting physicians consider Hahnemann's homeopathy to be quack medicine today. Though they may not yet understand its "mechanism of action" (with homeopathy's serial dilution and succussion of its *"like cures like"* medicinal formulas), that is no reason to disregard Dr. Hahnemann's common sense wisdom about "individualized treatment." Sometimes our opinions can blind us to the truth, forcing us to accept what is otherwise false or to reject what is otherwise true. To borrow an old adage, we must remember not to throw out the baby with the bathwater.

Like fashion, ideas about medical care change over time, and Dr. Hahnemann's opinions fell out of favor with a medical system unable to explain homeopathy. We forget, though, that ideas and opinions are always changing, which is why homeopathy may be returning to public favor today, even in an era of *one-size-fits-all* "managed care."

Who manages your health care? The burgeoning concept of "managed care" in America can be traced to the administration of President Richard Nixon, with the adoption of the Health Maintenance Organization Act in 1973. Spurred by this legislation, medicine rapidly evolved from its charitable principles, to care for the sick and the infirm, to a system with specified managed care protocols. In other words, instead of individualizing treatments (as Dr. Hahnemann once admonished), insurance companies, government regulators, and medical institutions now compel physicians and health-care workers to treat patients in specified and inflexible ways, with standardized treatment mandates.

There are specified medicines and specified procedures for specified disease states to be completed within specified time allowances, with specified insurance codes, to which health caregivers must strictly conform—just to get paid! Doctors and nurses must fill in lines on their charts and check boxes on their forms as dictated by reimbursement requirements of the managed-care health-care system. Their busy routines are dictated by protocols, instead of patient needs. The best and brightest physicians are now forced to imaginatively bend the lines and stretch the boxes, pretending to conform to the inflexible managed-care protocols, all the while doing their best to treat the patient's individualized needs.

It may sound simple and obvious, but today's managed-care health-care system may have forgotten that the true role of a health caregiver is *to give care*. Caring is *qualitative*, which is why a *quantitatively* managed system cannot understand or account for caring's central importance for a patient's health. When a doctor or nurse finally puts down his or her charts and check-boxes and takes time to listen, sympathize, empathize, and comfort the patient, that is when true wellness happens. Those remembered moments of individualized caring are often cherished by a patient, moving him or her toward good health and wellness in ways that managed-care systems cannot—and never will.

Mark Twain told a tragically true story of how his younger brother Henry Clemens suffered a horrible steamship accident, a boiler explosion that killed and wounded many others on board a Mississippi riverboat. Henry was brought to a makeshift hospital in Memphis, and Twain, then a riverboat pilot, helped care for his ailing brother night and day. Henry's precarious health soon improved, thanks to "Doctor Peyton, a fine and large-hearted old physician of great reputation in the community," who gave Henry "his sympathy and took vigorous hold of the case and in about a week...had brought Henry around." [8]

But the story sadly did not end with wise old Doctor Peyton's devoted caring and brother Henry's improved health. One night, the wise old doctor warned Twain to guard Henry's restful sleep and told him to "ask the physicians on watch to give him an eighth of a grain of morphine" but cautioned that "this is not to be done unless Henry shows signs that he is being disturbed." The inexperienced young physician on duty overnight showed no such individualized care and gave Henry "a vast quantity" of morphine "heaped on the end of a knife blade, and the fatal effects were soon apparent." [9] Twain grieved his whole life from the loss of his brother, feeling he could have somehow prevented Henry from dying.

The story's fatal ending may seem extreme, but the truth is that a *one-size-fits-all* standardized approach to medicines and foods can make us feel ill even when it doesn't kill us. From time to time, we're all members of the Poison Squad, getting sick from something we consume, whether it is prescribed for us or otherwise. From time to time, we all have adverse reactions to foods, medicines, cosmetics, beverages, or even remedies that we thought would make us feel well but didn't.

Morphine was prescribed for me too, to treat the excruciating pain of open-lung cancer surgery. It worked in one sense, as it alleviated my surgical pain, but an allergic reaction to the medicine made me want to crawl out of my skin. It was a horrible feeling, and I begged the doctors and nurses to take me off the morphine. Thankfully they did, caring enough about my individualized well-being to find a new medicine to relieve my pain without the dreadful skin side effect of the medicine.

Health-care providers are at their very best when they care enough about patients to help them feel well, just as teachers are at their very best when they help students learn. They can become *miracle workers*—as

Mark Twain said of Helen Keller's teacher Anne Sullivan—when they *truly care*. Miracles can happen when teacher and student both care about the student's learning, and miracles can happen when a doctor and patient both care about the patient's wellness.

You can let others decide for you *what makes you feel well*. You can place your trust in the systems and institutions that sell, serve, administer, regulate, and police your medicines and foods. You can place your trust in your health caregivers—the doctors, nurses, therapists, technicians, chiropractors, acupuncturists, midwives, nutritionists, homeopaths, healers, orderlies, or others who take on that vital role. Just be aware that there are consequences to blind trust, to burying your head like an ostrich in the sand. Henry Clemens was on the path toward a miraculous recovery in the "vigorous" care of the "large-hearted" and "sympathetic" Doctor Peyton; tragically, disinterested one-size-fits-all treatment protocols were no substitute for individualized care.

Of course, there are times when you cannot make medical decisions for yourself. You may be incapacitated, physically or mentally. You may not even realize that there is a decision to be made. You may be fearful and ready to give your unqualified trust to caregivers—I know I did that too, when faced with lung cancer, especially when doctors believed the cancer had already spread to my liver. At that moment, making decisions for myself became a crushing burden.

When we place our trust in someone else's care, though, that trust imposes great responsibilities on the caregiver. If we see that our trust is violated, then we need to take back decision making for ourselves and our loved ones. Remember that the system would have sent Helen Keller to an asylum, where her true genius would have forever gone ignored and unappreciated, had not Miss Sullivan worked her miracles of caring.

Ultimately, *"What makes you feel well?"* is a question for *you* and only *you*; it is not ultimately answered by anyone but *you*. Even when you place yourself in the care of others, *you* must still be in charge of your own wellness. That is a hugely important lesson of these stories of infant teething medicines too. The systems and institutions of health care and the laws that empower them must permit *you* to decide.

Sometimes the system and its laws may be protecting you from hurting others or protecting you from hurting yourself. Be grateful for that protection, for the sake of others and for the sake of your *true self*—the side of your self that feels love and wants wellness. In the end, you cannot truly feel well by hurting others or by hurting yourself, but only by helping and healing.

Other times, however, if the system does not let you decide for yourself, then the system may be substituting its judgment for yours, pretending to know what makes *you* feel well. That is not right and should not be accepted; in those cases, the system and its laws need to be changed. Sure enough, you can get it wrong, but as the stories of Tylenol® and Mrs. Winslow's Soothing Syrup teach us—as do so many other stories from stomach ulcers to beriberi, lime juice to marijuana—the system can get it woefully wrong too.

———

My own stomach began aching when I was just a small child. The pain varied in intensity, but it was sometimes so severe that I would sit doubled-over, clutching at my gut, rocking back and forth, praying the pain would soon end. What was wrong with my stomach was a mystery to me. *I just knew that I did not feel well.*

At first when I would tell my mother and father, they regarded it as a common childhood "tummyache"—a nonspecific ailment afflicting many children. From time to time, most adults know what a tummyache feels like too.

When acute ache turned into chronic complaint, my concerned parents sought medical help. First, they talked with general-practice pediatricians, who in turn recommended more specialized physicians. Each time, the doctors would ask me questions, examine my body, and take tests. In one of the more memorable visits, when I was about six or seven years of age and living in Brooklyn, New York, I remember drinking some disgusting chalky-tasting barium liquid concoction, donning a hospital gown, and then having my tummy X-rayed.

From a child's perspective, the medical process seemed to be a *name game*. What the doctors were most interested in naming was the medical condition that was making me hurt. They wanted a word more serious-sounding than *tummyache*. The name game was challenging and it could be fun, but all I really wanted was to feel well again.

I learned lots of new words during the name game. There were new words for my body parts and new words for the tests they gave me. There were words like *diagnosis*, which seemed to be how doctors declared victory in the name game; words like *symptoms*, which is how I'd describe the way I felt to the doctors; and words like *treatment*, which the doctors told me would follow diagnosis and then make me feel better. I remember the doctors also using new words like *duodenum* and *diverticulitis*, and these words held such allure that they still linger in my mind today, although I've come to learn that they had nothing to do with my gastric distress.

No one ever really won the name game, because the doctors could not find anything wrong with me. Despite all their questions, their physical examinations, their X-ray pictures and tests, my tummyache stumped the medical experts. Some doctors suggested to my parents that the pain was all in my imagination. In secretive voices meant to confound my childish ears, these doctors called it a *psychosomatic* illness, a name that was popular in the fashions of medicine back then.

Ironically, in the way that false secrets can become more alluring than a truth plainly told, their hushed tones triggered childhood curiosity that made me listen a little more closely. I remember being fascinated with the notion that an aching pain could be the product of my mental imagination. I remember thinking too that if these doctors were correct, then perhaps I could learn how to control the pain with my mind too, like a cartoon superhero.

Even as I marveled at the suggestion of the mind's superpowers, there was something about the "psychosomatic" suggestion that bothered my childhood sensibilities. Perhaps it was the smug arrogance of the doctors who made this suggestion to my parents; they wielded their diagnosis as if it was a condemnation of me, instead of their own inability to win the name game. I remember thinking that *"even if"* my tummyache was in my own head, it did not make my pain any less real; I just wanted to feel well again, and I thought that was the sole reason I went to these doctors.

The doctors persevered, continuing their tests and consultations, and after all was said and done, their best collective medical advice was this: *Avoid eating peanuts and corn.* They said that these particular foods, or foods like these, might be getting stuck in little pouches hidden in my digestive tract. They said that peanuts and corn might be causing a painful inflammatory condition they called *diverticulitis.* They couldn't be sure, they explained to my parents and me, and sometimes they used the word *diverticulosis* instead, but this diagnosis was their very best guess for winning the name game.

My parents dutifully heeded their medical advice, and they banned my further consumption of corn and peanuts, or at least they tried for a while. Both of these foods were childhood favorites of mine, so it was not easy for me to accept the medical diagnosis and the doctor's preventive treatment protocols. I especially liked the peanuts roasted and salted in a jar, which my parents now kept hidden in the kitchen cabinet and only took out of hiding when special guests came to our apartment—this jar of peanuts could signal the start of a party! Similarly, another delight of childhood, now banned, were summer trips to a farm market for fresh corn on the cob. My mother would boil the corn New England style and serve it piping hot with salt and pepper, oozing sweet creamery melted butter. Yummy!

No more corn or peanuts, said my parents—it was doctor's orders.

Trying to accept that I could no longer eat these special foods, I consoled myself that I still had lots of other favorites to enjoy— like milk and cookies or chocolate cake and ice cream! *You scream, I scream, we all scream for ice cream!* The thought of these childhood delights still excite my taste buds. Thankfully, I rationalized to myself, the doctors had not taken away these other favorite foods, so very popular with me and most other children I knew in the America of my youth.

So, for a while, I heeded the doctor's orders and my parent's wishes and refrained from eating peanuts and corn, but I still got sick, dou-bled-over in pain, with the same violent stomachaches as always.

One day my parents caught me sneaking some of the salted pea-nuts from the jar. Their first reaction was surprise that I had won the game of hide-and-seek, discovering the jar's secret location. Then, they scolded me, lecturing me about how I needed to follow the doctor's orders and not eat peanuts. I protested that the peanuts didn't make me sick, confessing how I knew that already because I had eaten the peanuts before and didn't get sick, not once. Besides, I explained, I was still getting the tummyaches even without eating peanuts. With rational logic, I announced that I was going to continue to eat those peanuts, and with childhood defiance, that's just what I did.

It was like speaking truth to power, and though a small child, I felt energized and alive in taking a stand. My childhood exercise in Thoreau-like civil disobedience made the peanuts taste even tastier. It was as if I was standing up on behalf of little people everywhere, resisting the arbitrariness of a health-care system that wasn't helping me feel well and taking charge of my own wellness for what seemed like the very first time.

———

"It is easier to maintain good health," Dr. Kenneth Cooper had famously said, *"than it is to regain it once it is lost."*[10] Dr. Cooper advocated prevention, in much the same way that my childhood doctors did when they told me to avoid certain foods. Prevention is good solid advice for wellness and remains a pillar of the wellness movement.

Prevention can mean different things to different people, however, and the same preventive formula does not work for everyone. For example, the recommendation of my childhood doctors that I avoid peanuts and corn to prevent my stomachaches was erroneous. I did not have the conditions they diagnosed, and besides, in the way that medicine can be like fashion, medical thinking today ironically now believes that eating foods like corn and peanuts may in fact *lower* the risk for diverticulitis.

Prevention is also the name of a venerable wellness magazine, first published by wellness pioneer J. I. Rodale in 1950 and still going strong as I write this. Though *Prevention* magazine was founded several years before Dr. Dunn coined the word *wellness*, J. I. Rodale's clarion message to his readers was that focusing on prevention would inevitably lead to their own wellness. Rodale especially believed in the connection between the quality of our foods and the quality of our health. In fact, J. I. Rodale was so inspired after reading Sir Albert Howard's seminal 1940 book *An Agricultural Testament* that he bought a farm in Pennsylvania, adopted sustainable farming practices like composting, rejected the use of then-common pesticides and synthetic chemicals, and began publishing the first of his influential wellness magazines, *Organic Farming and Gardening*, in 1942.

As in the example of J. I. Rodale and Sir Albert Howard, inspiration is contagious. *Inspiration can leap magically from heart to heart, and it changes the direction of lives.* It is one of the most powerful forces known to humankind, buoying our spirits during times of trouble and adversity and propelling ideas and achievement forward. It is a necessary ingredient for invention and creativity, and it can move nations too, in monumental ways that violence and fear cannot. As this book will discuss later in more detail, inspiration makes us feel profoundly well.

The wellness movement owes J. I. Rodale a debt of gratitude for inspiring so many with his visionary publications and magazines. The wellness movement also must give thanks for Rodale's willingness to stand up for his beliefs. To put it mildly, Rodale was controversial in his day. He was routinely ridiculed by the health-care establishment for the organic and vegan-centric diets he advocated, and he was openly mocked by agribusiness institutions for the organic farming practices he used. Even the US government vigorously prosecuted a lawsuit against him, for his claims about diets and their health consequences that did not conform to then-prevailing medical fashions.

Speaking truth to power is never easy. It takes courage and conviction and often requires a heaping dose of quixotic foolishness for good measure. J. I. Rodale was persecuted, but he persevered. Today, sustainable organic farming and local foods are far more popular and widespread than in the last century, and the trend is still growing by leaps and bounds. Good food is now routinely seen as part of good preventive health.

Indeed, what began as a vicious no-holds-barred competition between rival systems of "organic" and "scientific" agriculture has led to the mainstream food industry widely adopting many of J. I. Rodale's farming practices. The food industry had no choice really. Once label-reading consumers wanted to know *how* and *where* their foods were grown and *which* chemicals and *what* poisons were being used in agricultural production, then change needed to come simply to meet market demand. J. I. Rodale understood that avoiding poisons on our farms—like Dr. Harvey Wiley understood that avoiding poisons in our foods—is an important way to preventively maintain good health.

Of course, "prevention" is not just about the quality of our foods and our farms; there are other formulas to preventively maintain good health too. In the 1950s, as Rodale began publishing *Prevention* magazine, Dr. Jonas Salk became the world's most celebrated figure in medicine, introducing a vaccine against polio. Dr. Salk reinforced for most physicians that what we do to protect our health today can preventively determine our wellness tomorrow.

A decade later, in the 1960s, respected physicians like Dr. Cooper began talking about a preventive health-care formula of *"proper exercise, diet and emotional balance."* Today many other experts have added their own contributions to this prescription for preventive health—a good night's sleep, certain vitamins and supplements, handwashing and toothbrushing, and a humane workplace, to name but a few.

Dr. Halbert Dunn, who won the name game for his word *wellness* in the late 1950s, saw prevention in a somewhat different way. *"The preventive path of the future, both for medicine and public health,"* Dunn wrote *"inevitably lies largely in reorienting a substantial amount of interest and energy toward raising the general levels of wellness among all peoples."*[11] In other words, Halbert Dunn inverted the formula, reversing cause and effect. Dunn suggests that by focusing on wellness, prevention inevitably follows. That which makes us feel well ultimately prevents disease and infirmity.

The notion is intriguing, but philosophers might say that whether prevention leads to wellness or wellness leads to prevention is just a tautology. Zen masters might say that cause and effect are indistinguishable, part of the same *yin-meets-yang* unity that we mistake for duality. Either way, whether you begin by seeking wellness or start by trying to prevent disease, your destination is the same.

The real point is to begin—preferably in this moment of time that we call *now*—and then to continue your preventive wellness journey step-by-step. With each careful step, you still need to vigilantly ask yourself the question: *What makes you feel well?*

———

As I told the story in an earlier chapter, I met "Doctor Dan" Bernstein while I was still in college and dating his daughter, and he was the first to suggest I try a pink bismuth compound to relieve my stomachaches. It turned out to be a godsend, providing welcome relief.

Armed with this pink medicine to finally treat my acutely aching stomach, I began to think about prevention, to prevent the pains before they started. I was a young man in my early twenties and wasn't ready to accept a ceaseless cycle of disease and affliction, remedy and recovery, so I began to investigate the hidden connections between the foods in my diet and the pains in my gut. These connections might seem simple and obvious in hindsight, especially in a chapter of a book tracing the links between diet and wellness, yet the pains seemed so frequent and so unrelated to any particular food that no one had suggested there might be a root cause.

My first big clue came when I was in my midtwenties, living as a law student in Manhattan. I had just begun dating my future wife, Jane, who loved good pizza—it is still one of her very favorite foods. She particularly enjoyed eating authentic brick oven pizza at a famous Italian restaurant on Bleecker Street in Greenwich Village—thin, crunchy New York-style crust, loaded with fresh mozzarella cheese, red ripe tomatoes, and aromatic garlic essence—yum! I enjoyed both the food, which was both affordable and delicious, and especially the time getting to know Jane, even as we waited on long lines to get into the landmark pizza restaurant.

To my chagrin, I noticed that my stomach sometimes hurt violently after eating this tasty Greenwich Village pizza. This was not a new revelation—long before I met Jane, I had noticed that my stomach hurt after eating pizza; but then again, I noticed how my stomach hurt after eating lots of other types of food too, so I hadn't singled pizza out as a source of my gastric distress. Now that I had to excuse myself to the restroom at the end of dates with my future wife, I became acutely aware of a correlation between the pizza and my stomachaches.

Maybe it was Jane, and not the cheesy pizza, that really got my attention.

At some level, I may have already known that eating cheese provoked my gastric distress. It wasn't just pizza that hurt my stomach; it was gooey nachos, crackers and cheddar, and lots of other foods I enjoyed that contained cheese. Though I may have known this fact about myself, I refused to admit it to myself. Denial avoided the need for proactive prevention, the need to avoid these foods in my diet.

Sometimes the simplest things for each of us to admit—obvious things we should know about ourselves—can be buried under layers of self, hidden away deep inside. Reconciling different sides of self is a fundamental aspect of our wellness. These conflicts, deep within us, often lead to disease and infirmity. It's difficult to feel healthy, peaceful, and well when aspects of our self are unknowingly at odds with one another. Sometimes the unreconciled conflicts in our personality lead to anger or jealousy, which seem to bubble up from nowhere. Other times, the disconnect manifests as anxiety or depression, with a general sense that you are not satisfied with who you are or are not comfortable within your own skin. It is extremely important to recognize the sides of yourself pulling you in different directions, even when these internal conflicts within you may seem trivial or inconsequential.

I needed to ask myself why I was willing to eat pizza even though on some level I knew I'd likely be sick afterward. Part of me may have enjoyed the communal experience of shared food. Eating pizza let me be one of the kids at a party, accepted as part of a larger group. I thought it was a way to please my future wife, since she liked pizza so much and it showed her that we enjoyed the same tastes and experiences. A part of me wanted to continue eating the food that made me sick, to avoid a sense of loss.

Another part of me feared the feelings of rejection if I refused to eat the food that everyone else was enjoying. Rejection of a group conformity can risk ostracism and cause feelings of social deprivation and loss. The feeling is no different for a boy rejecting pizza at a party than it is for the scientist challenging dogmas of medicine. *"Everyone was against me,"* Dr. Barry Marshall had said of his heretical discovery that stomach ulcers were bacterial in nature, *"but I knew I was right."*[12] It takes courage and conviction to rise above fears like rejection, ridicule, and ruination. It is not easy to choose to be well when other parts of your self pull you in another direction, away from wellness. Some people sickened by beriberi would still choose to eat white rice to conform to the customs and norms of their community, even if they knew on some level that brown rice could make them feel well again.

So, on some level, I rationalized eating pizza, being part of the party, even though I may have understood, on some other level, I'd likely be in the bathroom later that evening clutching my stomach in pain. Our fears can motivate our choices, and in hindsight, I suppose that my stomach pains seemed preferable to feelings of rejection back then.

That was until Jane came along. When she began to see me sick after eating pizza together, she *cared enough about me* to be concerned for my well-being. That helped me value my own health and wellness, for her sake. So when I *cared enough for her*, I began to care more about myself. She allowed me to make the difficult choice to say, *"No cheese, please"*—to order a cheeseless pizza or something on the menu without cheese.

The part of ourselves that feels love is the same part of self that chooses wellness. It prioritizes wellness above any fears, like loss and rejection. It is the most profound and truest part of our self, our highest and best part, and it knows how well it makes us feel to give love unconditionally. It knows that to give is also to receive, so it chooses wellness *for others*, not just *for self*.

The part of your *self* that truly feels love and cares for others is not the self-obsessed part of you. Indeed, it stands in stark contrast to self-obsessed parts of self—like greed, gluttony, lust, sloth, vanity, pride, wrath, and envy, sometimes called mortal sins or given other names that suggest the worst parts of our nature. These parts may seem to lead to happiness for a short while, but these egotistic, narcissistic, and self-obsessed choices leave us feeling empty and sick inside. These choices move us further away from love and wellness.

You may not even be aware of these competing parts of your self, but they are there in all of us, to greater or lesser degrees. If you think that there is no love and wellness within you or if you think that you are without fear or ego, then look again, and look more closely, for within us all are the same human ingredients. *"I have found that there is no ingredient of the human race which I do not possess in either a small way or a large way,"* Mark Twain wrote, recognizing these many human sides of himself. *"When it is small, as compared to the same ingredient in somebody else, there is still enough of it for all the purposes of examination."*[13]

Confronting mortality forces many people—myself included—to examine many sides of self and to embrace the part that loves and cares and wants wellness. This loving part of self reveres all of life as the special blessing that it truly is. That's one reason why confronting life-threatening illnesses and infirmities can paradoxically be so life-affirming, full of wellness.

As Twain suggests, it is not necessary to face your mortality in order to see all these parts of yourself. These parts of you are already there, already within you, for purposes of self-knowledge and self-discovery if you are devoted—like Twain—to undertaking the examination. It may sound simple, but it is never easy. Twain himself claimed in his Autobiography that during the last quarter century of his life, he was *"pretty constantly and faithfully devoted to the study of the human race—that is to say, the study of myself, for in my individual person I am the entire human race compacted together."*[14]

The very first step in balancing sides of yourself to move you toward feeling well is to become *aware* of these varying sides of yourself. Only when you understand these sides of yourself can you consciously choose a healing side over a destructive side or choose prevention instead of feeling rejection.

There are choices in how you live and how you love, whatever your circumstances, even when it comes to pizza. Though she loved pizza, Jane helped me make a conscious choice to stop eating it. She encouraged me to make these healthy choices for myself because she loved me. Because she cared about my health, she wanted me to be well.

Because I loved her, I wanted her to be well too. If another food made her sick—her skin breaks out in hives from strawberries—I didn't want her to eat that food either. We wanted each other to be happy and enjoying favorite aspects of life. I didn't want her to stop eating pizza any more than she wanted me to stop eating strawberries. We both wanted each other to feel well. To do that, we needed to make ourselves feel well too.

"No cheese, please." Even if I forgot, Jane would remind me, in the way you do when you care about someone else.

Chapter 9

TAKING GOOD CARE

For *you* to feel well, you need to genuinely care about the wellness of *others*.

If you are like many people, this simple notion may sound strange to you or even counterintuitive, difficult to understand. You may mistakenly believe that your health is confined to your physical body and may view your outermost layer of skin as a boundary separating you from the environment beyond you. You may have no care or concern for the wellness of the people and planet beyond those illusory lines of demarcation.

Being proactive about your own health is an important first dimension for your wellness, but it is not enough. As a second dimension, you must also be proactive about the health of your environment. This means embracing not only good *self-care*, but good *selfless* care.

———

This second of the three keys (dimensions) to understanding the meaning of wellness may seem difficult to grasp, but it is a simple lesson. In one ancient variation of this lesson, found across diverse cultures and traditions, we are taught to *"do onto others as you would have them do onto you."* This *Golden Rule* applies to our personal relationships as well as to our interactions with Earth and its many inhabitants.

Truly, it is a simple lesson, but it has not been an easy one for humankind to learn. Maybe the reason we find the lesson so difficult is in its *application* to the business and routines of daily life. Not seeing the practicalities of the lesson, we pretend that selfless caring for others is just a beautiful notion or perhaps a naive and romantic dream. We war against one another, and we war against the environment. As devastation spreads, we are reminded of the urgency of taking good care of others and reminded how the lesson applies to our own health and wellness. Soon after peace and prosperity seem restored, sadly, we may forget the lesson and are forced to learn it all over again.

"Oh, when will they ever learn?"[1] Pete Seeger wondered aloud in his classic folk song about the impact of war and environmental destruction, entitled "Where Have All the Flowers Gone?" Pete is a favorite son of the Hudson Valley where I live, and he passed at the age of ninety-four while I was still writing this book. Born a few months after the end of the First World War, Seeger served in the US Army in the Pacific during World War II. *"Oh, when will they ever learn?"* is a sad lament, yet offers hope that we might yet learn.

As the wellness movement accelerates, more and more people have made great leaps forward in their understanding of this simple lesson. Realizing that the health and wellness of their environment is deeply connected to their own health and wellness, they take care of both. They are reminded that to give is to receive, that both giving and receiving are indivisibly connected in another Zen-like unity at the heart of an illusory duality. They discover that selflessly caring for others, with no expectation of reward or return, benefits their own wellness—often in unexpected and miraculous ways.

On some deep and intuitive level, you probably understand this lesson too. You know how good it feels to have someone care about you and how good it also feels for you to care about someone else. You may appreciate how selfless caring feels qualitatively different—to both giver and receiver—than when strings and conditions are attached.

As more and more people learn this lesson, a remarkable thing is happening—humanity itself is slowly evolving in wonderful and historic new ways. This evolution is a bit like our species finally realizing that Earth revolves around the sun, revealing new paradigms that transform our awareness of ourselves. As we learn to apply this simple lesson, doors to health, happiness, and wellness can open for us all. These doors were never locked; we just didn't realize that the doors were there, waiting to be opened.

———

One of my favorite expressions of this simple lesson, about caring for others as ourselves, comes from John Donne, a poet who penned his words in 1624. Donne was also a priest and a lawyer, in the great Renaissance tradition that encouraged humans to exercise their full potential across diverse fields, like a DaVinci or Michelangelo.

In the Middle Ages in parts of England, there was a custom to ring a church bell when someone died. Hearing the clanging sound of the death-knell bell, townspeople would be naturally curious to know who had passed on. In the gossipy way that we pretend other people's bad news has no bearing on our own lives, they would ask one another for whom the bell tolled. *"Perchance he for whom this bell tolls may be so ill as that he knows not it tolls for him,"* Donne answered. [2]

"Any man's death diminishes me," John Donne mused, deeply understanding how our own wellness depends on the wellness of others, *"because I am involved in mankind, and therefore never send to know for whom the bell tolls; it tolls for thee."* Donne observed that we each suffer along with the sufferings of others because we are part of one another, profoundly connected to one another. *"No man is an island, entire of itself,"* he explained, for *"every man is a piece of the continent, a part of the main."* [3]

John Donne's insightful realization was prompted by the death of a beloved daughter and his own near-fatal illness. Suffering can instigate true learning, and this learning helps us evolve toward wisdom and wellness. Truly, if we do not learn from our own suffering, then we cannot expect to feel well even during periods of good health.

While confronting your own mortality might propel such insight, as was true in my own life when I grappled with diagnosis and treatment for lung cancer, there are countless others ways to learn John Donne's lesson. Some reach this understanding through reverence for the natural world or by participating in a selfless charitable enterprise and seeing how good that makes them feel inside. Others learn by finding true love, by having a child or a pet, or by mindfully choosing to transcend their ego and fears. The realization can come spontaneously, through an epiphany, revelation, or chance encounter, or it can arrive gradually, through a wide variety of experiences, events, and educational teachings, like reading the poetry of John Donne.

It would be a mistake to confuse John Donne's beautiful poetry as mere words. We can read his poem and recite its verses, yet ignore their meaning and practical application to our own lives. Even as the refrain *"for whom the bell tolls"* rings in our head, we can go about harming others—hurting ourselves in the process, never realizing what we are doing. *Forgive them, for they know not what they do,* was a lesson taught by Jesus of Nazareth even while being crucified.[4]

It can take a dramatic and frightening event, like a crucifixion, to comprehend a simple lesson. In the history of humanity, throughout the world, there was no greater dramatic or frightening experience to learn from than the Second World War.

Not only can the origins of the wellness movement be traced to this horrific war, but this historic event forced the nations of the world—at some level of awareness—to finally acknowledge the simple lesson about the importance of caring for others as ourselves. The Second World War produced evolutionary advances in our collective understanding of how the environment in which we all live affects the health and well-being of us all.

Even if you lived far away from the battlefields, you could not feel well as war raged on. All across the globe, soldiers were *"marching in admirable order over hill and dale to the wars,"* to borrow words of Henry David Thoreau from his famous Essay on Civil Disobedience.[5] It didn't matter what side of the war you were on, for all of these soldiers—whether celebrated as heroes or reviled as enemies—laid waste to villages and farms and turned factories and cities to rubble. Their actions and intentions produced what Thoreau described as *"a palpitation of the heart"* for all of humanity.[6]

How could our hearts—and our health—not be affected by this caustic environment? World War II terrified us with the threat of total annihilation from atomic bombs and shocked consciences with the brutality of innocents slaughtered in concentration camps. Humanity witnessed incomprehensible violence, atrocities, degradations, diseases, famines, and displacements. The sound of bells tolling all across planet Earth was deafening, and it made us all sick.

———

The war's end was another chance to take good care of one another and the environment we share. It was another chance at good health for people and the planet, so health-care representatives from around the globe gathered together in an earnest attempt to apply the lessons learned from the war.

On April 7, 1948, a day still celebrated as World Health Day, delegates of nations from north, south, east, west, and in the middle, international friends and foes of differing religious, philosophical, ideological, and economic beliefs, all joined together to ratify and adopt the constitution of the World Health Organization. It was a day worth celebrating, and 194 nations in total have each declared these same words of solemn principle about the importance of good health and what that means.

They declared how *"health is a state of complete physical, mental and social well-being and not merely the absence of disease or infirmity"*; how *"the health of all peoples is fundamental to the attainment of peace and security"*; and pleaded for proactive participation by the public, declaring how *"informed opinion"* and *"active cooperation on the part of the public"* are *"of the utmost importance in the improvement of the health of the people."* These constitutional declarations reminded the world how *"the ability to live harmoniously in a changing total environment is essential."*[7]

These declarations were not empty platitudes to World Health Organization delegates, like a poem without meaning, for the words were forged in the deadly crucible of a world at war. The simple principle *how our wellness depends on our environment* became obvious after World War II, so it was easily embraced by founders of the World Health Organization.

Many others since have understood the truth of this elemental principle. It was understood by hippies hugging trees in the 1960s and 1970s—and it was understood by private equity banking professionals during my white paper presentation. As I explained how caring for our environment was the second of three keys to understanding the wellness movement, these financially astute men and women nodded their heads in obvious agreement, observing the similarities between consumer movements toward *wellness* and toward *environmentalism*. They acknowledged how businesses that embraced these movements used similar marketing and branding, and how words like green, sustainable, natural, cruelty-free, cage-free, holistic, organic, and biodynamic were associated with both the wellness and environmental movements.

When presenting this second dimension of the wellness movement to these business-minded investors, I didn't mention Donne's meditations on how *no man is an island, entire of itself*, although his insights were relevant and applicable to the topic. I knew that Donne's poetry might seem too fuzzy for their analytical financial minds, so I respected a formal line that wasn't really there, knowing you can call the same thing a "key" or a "dimension" and it should not really matter, for a thing is a thing. I was able to discuss the other Dunn, but when all was said and done, both men revealed the same *meaning*.

Both men taught lessons how we are profoundly connected to our environment and how our environment affects our health and well-being. One Donne used poetry and religious meditation, and the other Dunn used statistical charts and scientific graphs. Though expressing meaning in different ways, Donne and Dunn both found the same meaning from sources of personal inspiration, each turning a tragedy into hope for the future. In turn, both men inspired future generations with words of profound meaning.

John Donne's poetic meditation about a bell tolling was inspired by the tragedy of a daughter's death and his own near-fatal disease, yet his inspiration inspired countless generations of poets, priests, philosophers, statesmen, and novelists, among them Ernest Hemingway. Hemingway's novel *For Whom the Bell Tolls* honors Donne's inspirational insight in the book's epigraph as well as its title; the setting was the bloody Spanish Civil War, where Hemingway had been a journalist, and it was written in 1940 as World War II began, and the same lesson was about to be painfully learned again.

In turn, Halbert Dunn's health-care prescription was inspired by the tragedy of this second global war and the words of declaration and constitutional principle of a new World Health Organization. In the way inspiration leaps from heart to heart, Dr. Dunn's inspiration gave the world a new word—*wellness*—which then inspired a movement. Movements begin with groups of inspired people, who inspire still more people.

Inspiration is powerful, and it can change the course of history or the course of your own life, but inspiration is unpredictable. It cannot be measured or managed. It cannot be logically explained or legally controlled. Though inspiration is where *true meaning* can be found, there is no assurance that this meaning will be revealed to the uninspired. You can *know merely things* without being splendidly familiar with *the meanings of them*, like reading Donne's poem without being moved emotionally by it.

If you have already been inspired for wellness in your life, the simple notion that *"our wellness depends on our environment"* may seem obvious to you, but it was not a common understanding in medicine and health care back in 1950s America. Dr. Halbert Dunn needed a better way to explain the unfamiliar concept to his scientifically minded peers, so he drew a scientific-looking chart, with two lines for a *"health"* axis and an *"environmental"* axis, which he named *"The Health Grid."* [8]

Dr. Dunn divided his health grid into four separate quadrants, showing how your body's health can be poor or good and how the environment in which you live could be favorable or unfavorable. With its four boxes of comparison, it graphically illustrated how living in an unfavorable environment, like a war zone, negatively affected health and well-being. The grid showed how a good environment could help even sick people get to a better state of *"protected poor health"* and how individuals could have *"emergent high-level wellness"* even in a very unfavorable environment.

Of course, the most desirable of the four quadrants on Dr. Dunn's health grid was when good personal health was combined with a favorable environment. Halbert Dunn called this optimal fourth quadrant *"high-level wellness"* and he believed it should be the goal of the entire health-care system. Because the system and institutions of health care were focused on disease and infirmity, Dr. Dunn knew that it was not the goal of health care, so he urged that we gradually refocus on the new goal. *"As the goal, at first seen far above us, becomes clearer and stirs response from deep within us,"* Dunn envisioned *"we will reach out toward it and fight for high-level wellness even as we have fought so valiantly and so long against sickness and death."* [9]

The goal of high-level wellness requires the health-care system to examine the relationship between a patient's health and environment. That examination goes well beyond diagnosing diseases and requires health caregivers to learn about and improve the patient's environment.

Ask whether that goal is being achieved in your community or in an era of managed health care. In America today, with insurance reimbursement mandates that manage the time allotted for patients to speak with their own doctors, most health caregivers do not have sufficient time to get to know a patient's environment—much less do anything about it, like recommending ways a patient can help improve their environment. Ironically, even as our physicians and hospitals learn more about the connection between a patient's environment and his or her personal health, Dunn's goal of high-level wellness may seem further out of reach for a "managed health-care" system than ever before.

If the system does not embrace the goal of high-level wellness for you or if the system cannot achieve that goal because of its inflexible managed-care rules, regulations, and laws, then ultimately *you* must embrace that goal for yourself. *It is your health, and you are in charge of your own health!* Proactively taking charge of your own health requires you to proactively take good care of your environment too.

Do what you can do! Your environment benefits from your selfless care, and caring for your environment benefits you as well—sometimes in surprising and even magical ways, like the way that to give is to receive.

———

There may be more to your environment than you realize, and your environment may be affecting your health and wellness in ways that you might not expect.

If you start to consider the many aspects of your environment that affect your wellness, you might include people you know and people you don't. You might consider the air you breathe, the water you drink, rivers, oceans, mountains, and valleys. You might think of the plants and animals that share Earth with you and the cultures and values that share it too. You might think of foods, farms, and natural resources, as well as cities, towns, and historic places. Your environment also includes your schools, hospitals, governments, charities, finances, and businesses too.

Dr. Dunn wrote in his seminal essay on High-Level Wellness that a healthy environment includes not merely *"the physical and biological factors of the environment but also socioeconomic components affecting the health of the individual."* [10]

Recognition of these many components of our environment has come slowly and often comes grudgingly. For too long, we would not admit that we needed to take better care of our environment and would scarcely admit that our environment affected our health either. Perhaps this resistance resulted from a romanticized and heroic myth that individuals should be able to conquer their environment, instead of being affected by it.

One obvious way that our environment affects our health is through the *stress* it places upon us. Today, the notion that stress causes disease may seem like simple common sense—but as we have seen time and again, what becomes simple common sense is not always obvious nor understood.

It was once a radical concept—roundly rejected by the medical establishment—that the stresses of our environment can cause illness and disease. The connection between stress and disease was first described by Hungarian János "Hans" Selye in 1926, during his second year of medical school at the University of Prague. Selye believed this connection was "ridiculously childish and self-evident," yet he wondered "why nobody had ever given this syndrome any special attention." Hans Selye recollected too, how his medical school professors and classmates openly mocked his theories, calling his ideas as stupid and meaningless. [11]

Despite this ridicule, Hans Selye was determined to prove the connection between stress and disease, which he wrote *"struck me as the most fundamental problem in medicine."*[12] Determined to overcome the derogatory environment of his judgmental professors and peers, he emigrated to Canada soon after finishing medical school and began to specialize in endocrinology, which allowed him to scientifically test the effect of stress on the body's hormonal response.

Ten years later, in 1936, Dr. Selye had gathered enough evidence to again present the basics of his theory to the medical and scientific community. In a widely read letter published in the prestigious scientific journal *Nature*, he identified *"noxious agents"* and other stresses and strains on the body's immune system as a cause of disease.[13] For his simple commonsense genius, some compared Hans Selye to Albert Einstein. Indeed, according to biographer Denis Brian, Einstein himself personally congratulated Dr. Selye for his contributions to finding a "unified theory" of medicine, in this stress research, which Dr. Einstein believed was not unlike his own search for a "unified field theory" of physics.[14]

However, not all scientists of the era were as visionary as Albert Einstein. For a very long time, Dr. Selye continued to be ridiculed by his health-care colleagues. In a 1974 interview in *People Magazine*, Selye recounted how "when I first expounded the stress theory, it was more viciously attacked than anything since Freud...Now it is in every medical textbook in the world." [15] We are fortunate indeed that Selye persevered and continued in his research and study, eventually writing over fifteen hundred scholarly articles.

"Stress in health and disease is medically, sociologically, and philosophically the most meaningful subject for humanity that I can think of" said Selye[16] and he soon realized how we experience both *negative* and *positive* stresses in our life. Some stresses create disease and infirmity, yet other stresses promote satisfaction and well-being. This realization opened new paradigms of insight for Selye, not only about the cause of disease but about the relationship of our *external* environment to our *internal* mental processing.

For instance, Selye wondered aloud whether lab rats were being affected by the substances injected into them—or by the stressful trauma of the injection itself. Think, for yourself, about how *you* respond to such stressful traumas. We all have different internal attitudes and reactions when it comes to experiencing external stress. This new way of looking at the connection between our external environment and our internal mental state has wide application beyond medical science—perhaps one reason that health care has been slow to embrace the connection between stress and disease.

Before his death in 1982, Dr. Selye published *Stress Without Distress* in 1974, promoting a meaningful "philosophy of life" as a means to improve our health and well-being. [17] You may wonder how a philosophy of life is relevant to medical studies, but Dr. Selye understood how those lines of separation were illusory. He wrote the book while still a dedicated scientific researcher and medical professor at the Université de Montréal.

———

Finding your own way to reduce harmful stress—modifying your internal reactions to stress, or reducing external causes of stress in your life, or both—is essential for your health and wellness.

This may be more important than ever before, given Dr. Dunn's observation how the fast-paced *"tempo of modern life"* and its steadily increasing *"demands on the human being and his society"* are negatively affecting our health and wellness, creating new varieties of disease and dysfunction. Dr. Selye would say that you need to *adapt* to your stresses, so that the stress doesn't cause you any *dis*tress. It is good medical advice that can prevent illness and infirmity from occurring in the first place.

When it comes to reducing harmful *dis*tress, once again *one size does not fit all!* Meditation, prayer, yoga, massage, exercise, sports, biofeedback, painting, pottery, hobbies, therapies, support groups, music, volunteerism, entertainment, knitting, gardening, bathing, resting, relaxing, pausing, playing, petting, breathing, smelling the roses, savoring small successes, absorption in a task, showing gratitude, tuning in, sharing, and caring—these are just a few of the many stress-reduction techniques that can work wonders for your wellness.

It bears repeating that there are many varied ways to ease stress internally—some seek social camaraderie, others seek quiet solitude; some dive deeper into work, others need to walk away from their jobs. Become mindful of the stresses in your life and the way that you react to them, so that you can seek to reduce the *dis*tress they cause you. The old adage that *"laughter is good medicine"* is true too, easily understandable because of laughter's remarkable ability to reduce stress *internally*. [18]

While some control stress internally, others try to control their *external* environment. Of course, some external stresses are unavoidable, but as the wellness movement accelerates, more and more people seek to minimize the more egregious and controllable of these external stresses. We can seek peace instead of the negative environment of war. We can encourage workplace environments to be free of harassment. We can promote schooling that is free from bullying. We can pursue economic environments that emphasize fair trade.

Changing these aspects of the environment improves our collective health and well-being. Ask yourself what can *you* change about your environment for the benefit of *all?*

———

Changes to our external environment can be subtle and small, yet can still profoundly affect our health and well-being. Hospitals learned this simple wellness lesson, for example, by redecorating their cold, drab, barren, institutional walls with warm, soothing, healing paint colors and inspirational artwork.

I remember how a large regional hospital proudly told me they were adopting these wellness-promoting paint colors for their walls, as they considered my nomination to their hospital's board of directors. I hadn't sought the nomination—I'm often reluctant to serve on boards and as a lawyer have ethical issues to consider when I do—but I was touched and flattered by the gesture, since the nomination came from some nice friends of mine, who were already on the regional hospital's board of directors.

"It's an exciting time for the hospital," one of these nice friends told me. She said that the hospital board was overseeing the construction of the first brand-new hospital to be built in New York State in a quarter century, and she had arranged a VIP tour for me of the new facilities. She then explained how the hospital board was expanding, along with the new construction.

She told me that my friends on the hospital board, including its chairman, all thought I would be a great fit for the expanded board because of my wellness background. I had previously served with some of these friends on a community venture capital fund board, so they knew of my background in wellness, as well as my business and legal qualifications. "The hospital board," my friend told me, "understands the importance of wellness for the new hospital; they know it's a very important subject with patients and consumers." She encouraged me to consider the nomination. "What a great contribution you could make to the hospital's environment, promoting the interest of wellness on the board!" she gushed.

"Even the colors of the new walls will be changing—no more dull beige and gray rooms!" she exclaimed, gleeful at the possibilities for increasing wellness at the hospital. "Think about it, Steve," she urged.

I agreed to consider it and complimented her on the plans to change the environment through something as simple and obvious as wall decor. Conversationally, I remarked how there were a lot of fascinating new color and light therapies available in the wellness market before this friend—an analytical chemist by educational training—began excitedly telling me of her own experiences with various wellness therapies. Meditation, aromatherapy, yoga, and reiki were among her many passionate wellness interests.

I wasn't surprised by her admission of seeking wellness in her own life, not at all. I already knew some of her fuzzy side from our participation on the community venture capital fund's board together. On that venture fund board, chaired by our mutual friend Dennis Barnett, we were encouraged to be ourselves, to be fuzzy as well as formal. Dennis himself combined the formality of a major in the US Marines and a corporate chemist with the fuzziness of a devout Christian soul who personally helped comfort and assist both me and my son Nicholas during our troubled time of teenage intervention.

Looking back, I realize that the sharing of our fuzzy sides was what made this otherwise formal venture fund's board so spirited and collaborative—and so very pleasant to serve on. The sharing of our whole selves led to many deep and lasting friendships, among them with fellow director Antonio Varano, who of course became my business partner at Lotus Energetics Management—and with whom I presented the white paper to the private equity investors.

Though these board members could be fuzzy at times, they were all highly accomplished people who knew how to use formality to govern boards—formalities like corporate laws, rules, resolutions, constitutions, and evolving best practices—and they knew that formalities like these could help resolve board disputes. Board disputes can get quite ugly and messy and can be personally unpleasant—unwell and unhealthy, you might say. But even for noxious board disputes, the *dis*tress and *dys*function must eventually be resolved for the ultimate health and benefit of the corporation that the board serves.

As a practicing lawyer with more than thirty years' experience, familiar with both the boardroom and the courtroom, I prefer to help *avoid disputes* before they start, knowing that, as the saying goes, an ounce of prevention is worth a pound of cure. Sometimes, however, disputes cannot be avoided, but even then, once disputes begin, you need to *fight ferociously to end the dispute* fairly and finally. If the environment in which you live is not healthy, then you must find a way to improve your external environment even as you adjust your internal mental state. It doesn't matter how dire the situation or how messed up the environment—wellness must be found *for all* to *benefit all*.

Strong leaders know that. As World War II raged on, President Franklin Delano Roosevelt said: *"We have faith that future generations will know that here, in the middle of the twentieth century, there came a time when men of good will found a way to unite, and produce, and fight to destroy the forces of ignorance, and intolerance, and slavery, and war."*[19] Even as bells tolled and battles raged, even in an environment filled with death, destruction, fear, and hatred, Roosevelt spoke words of healing and wellness.

"Unless the peace that follows recognizes that the whole world is one neighborhood and does justice to the whole human race," the president declared in the same address given on February 12, 1943, *"the germs of another world war will remain as a constant threat to mankind."*[20] Conflicts and disputes—whether a board dispute, a litigation, or a world war—cannot ultimately be about retribution, reprisal, hatred, or fear. The aim of resolving these disputes fairly and finally must always be about unity and wholeness.

And so I considered my friend's request—she who had encouraged me to *think about it*—and I agreed to go forward with the nomination to the hospital board. I did so because I believed I might be able to help move a large regional hospital toward better health and wellness for its patients and the communities it served and maybe help influ-ence other hospitals in the long run to do so too.

This was my hope and vision for that hospital board nomination, although I learned long ago that we can't always affect our environ-ment in the ways we want. Knowing that, I went through the cor-porate nominating process anyway—which included submitting résu-més, attending interviews, and meetings over lunch, as these formal processes often entail—until the hospital board eventually *rejected my nomination.*

My dear, polite friend who had encouraged me to *think about it* was embarrassed and contrite. She told me that some of the direc-tors on the hospital board who opposed my nomination were medi-cal physicians who believed I took wellness "too far." They were unnerved and disturbed by my résumé's expansive list of wellness business ventures—or *ad*ventures, as I like to say—which included nonconventional health-care treatments like homeopathy and energy medicine.

"Does he understand that the hospital has to comply with health-care rules and regulations?" was the concern of these oppositional directors. "Of course he understands that," my friend said she responded in defending me; "he's a smart lawyer and a businessman, and I know that because we've served on boards together and I've seen him in action."

Rejection stings as surely as the trauma of injection to a lab rat. Like with any stressful situation, I've learned that it's your *internal* reac-tion to the stress that you can try to control for the sake of your own wellness. Mostly, I just wanted to ease the discomfort of my apologetic friend, who tried her best but felt bad about the outcome. Borrowing an old Groucho Marx joke, I told her not to worry, that I wouldn't want to join any club that would have me as a member. She laughed, and I laughed, and it was good medicine for us both.

It was a lost opportunity, of course, for both the hospital and me, but I knew there would be other opportunities and that I needed to *accept the things I could not change*—to borrow a very meaningful line from Reinhold Neibuhr's oft-quoted serenity prayer.[21] When changing the landscape of your external environment, it's important to be pragmatic as well as proactive.

For the regional hospital, changing the color of their drab walls was enough of a start, an important step on their own journey toward wellness. We've all become sadly accustomed to institutional fearfulness when it comes to people's wellness, but for me, the wartime words of President Franklin Delano Roosevelt are like the sound of bells tolling, for *"the only thing we have to fear, is fear itself."*[22]

You can seek to change your environment rapidly, or you can do it slowly, but your wellness demands that it must change. It's up to you to do your part to help.

———

My daughter Melissa, who illustrated the cover to this book and provided the artwork for my previous book on *(((tuning)))* too, decided she wanted to study art therapy at the university she was attending, one of the oldest academic institutions in New England.

The university was well known for its open-mindedness, which was a major reason she chose to go there in the first place, but unfortunately for her, they did not offer any courses in art therapy in their educational environment. This was surprising to Melissa, and to me too, since this university was known as an educational innovator, especially well known for its environmental studies programs.

By volunteering at a local hospital while attending the university, Melissa had already learned firsthand how healing and therapeutic art can be. She spent countless hours drawing pictures and creating artwork with sick children and had coauthored a coloring book to help these children overcome their fears of hospitalization and surgery; it was called *art for the heart*. The illustrated coloring book story, designed for the child's own interaction with crayons, offered a comforting lesson for frightened children awaiting surgical procedures. It was a wonderful way to help *dis*tressed kids find wellness through their health-care ordeal, and now my daughter wanted to learn more about art therapy in formal university studies.

Because the university didn't offer any courses in art therapy, Melissa proactively sought to *adapt* her educational environment. Going through her university's "create your own field of interdisciplinary study" approach, she organized an independent course on the subject under the supervision of the university's psychology department.

Melissa asked me to read the final paper she wrote for the course, which I did, and I was stunned by the beautiful unity she brought to the topic. Her paper combined insights and knowledge from many areas, including psychology, philosophy, medicine, religion, spirituality, art, and anthropology, to help show why artistic expression can be of great therapeutic value for patients. She even *applied* what she learned to a concrete situation involving art therapy for the elderly in nursing homes.

I told my daughter that I would give her an "A+" on the paper (*and yes,* I'm a proud father, *although no*, I'm not an easy "A"), but I also pointedly warned Melissa that not every professor would feel likewise. The paper was so holistic in its breadth and scope that I said professors who insist on imaginary lines separating fields of study—like Hans Selye's own professor in medical school—might give her a mediocre grade or even a failing one. It was clearly not a traditional psychology paper, I reminded her.

She submitted the paper, and when her grade came, she was crestfallen; the psychology professor did not even give her the courtesy of a "gentleman's B" grade. What's more, the written comments explaining the low grade made it clear to me that the professor just didn't get it. In my opinion, it showed how the professor had read the words but didn't grasp the *meanings* of them. Melissa was again proactive; she spoke to the professor to better understand the professor's point of view and learn from it, as well as to see if she could improve her grade, which she did through some extra credit—but the experience taught her even more valuable lessons.

Some environments directly oppose and challenge your wellness, but you are still part of these environments and you still need to do your best to seek wellness within them. Even when the environment becomes unhealthy and unproductive, it is essential to take care of your environment for the sake of your own wellness, and when the time is right, to have the courage to proactively change the environment.

Melissa took some time off from this New England university and I saw how she created a positive environment for herself in the midst of a negative environment. After a year, she decided to transfer to another university, where she could better study the things she wanted to learn about and improve her educational environment. Now she's learning how *artistic creativity* can improve our *physical environment*. I think that's a bit ironic, since it imaginatively pushes the narrow boundaries of what her former New England university described as *environmental studies*.

———

Our environment includes much more than what some limit environmental studies to—yet the wellness movement cannot be separated from the *environmental* movement, or what some call the *"green"* movement.

Like the word *wellness*, the words *environmental* and *green* can mean different things to different people. One size does not fit all when it comes to the

148

meaning of these words. They can mean clean air, fresh water, and uncontaminated soils. The protection of species and biodiversity. The reduction of industrial pollutants, agricultural pesticides, and consumer waste. More efficient use of natural resources. Recycling and adaptive reuse of manufacturing goods, materials, and by-products. The advance of sustainable technologies and renewable industries. The development of nontoxic products, services, solutions, and energy. The improvement of damaged and threatened ecosystems. The restoration and conservation of habitats. More generally, these words can signify a basic recognition of individual and societal responsibilities toward Earth and its many inhabitants.

Recognition of the many ways to be *green* has come slowly and grudgingly, as was the case with Dr. Selye's recognition that the stresses of our environment affect our health. In the years following World War II, publicity around news stories revealed one type of environmental catastrophe after another—real-life stories that affected the air, water, land, and species that inhabit Earth, including our own species.

With each big news story, large numbers of ordinary people became worried that their own health and well-being were compromised along with the environment. Each story focused public attention, heightened our awareness, spurred political action, and forced pioneering legislation, all of which helped better protect and promote public health and wellness. The history of the environmental movement would require a book of its own, but here are a few of its many notable stories:

- In 1952, a few years after the end of World War II, thickly polluted air, heavy with sulfur-laden fumes from coal furnaces, hovered for five days over the British capital, causing respiratory illness and death for thousands. The public concern from the environmental catastrophe of the "Great Smog" of London prompted the United Kingdom's first major Clean Air Act and affected clean air legislation around the world.
- In 1962, the same year that another poisonous smog hovered over London, biologist Rachel Carson published a best-selling

book, *Silent Spring*, that showed how the pesticide DDT was killing entire populations of birds, including America's national symbol, the bald eagle. The concern prompted new pesticide regulations and new concern about endangered species, and her book is often cited as a primary catalyst for the birth of the American environmental movement.

- In 1964, with the election of President Lyndon Johnson, came the inauguration of Lady Bird Johnson as America's First Lady. She campaigned tirelessly to end littering in America, to plant wildflowers and trees, and to find other ways of beautifying the nation. The publicity she received made the public begin to realize that throwing their trash alongside the highway was hurting us all.

- In 1969, the waters of Ohio's Cuyahoga River, thickly polluted with oily toxic waste, caught on fire. The American public was shocked by the sight of a burning river, as reported in the cover story of *Time Magazine*. Earlier that same year, the sloop *Clearwater* set sail on her maiden voyage to promote the cleanup of New York's Hudson River, and the ship became an instant international symbol of clean water. The Clearwater organization had been founded a few years earlier by Toshi Seeger and folksinger husband Pete Seeger ("Where Have All the Flowers Gone?"). Public attention on the cleanup of these two rivers and then others spurred the US Congress to adopt the Clean Water Act in 1972.

- By 1978, beginning with local stories by investigative reporter Michael H. Brown for the *Niagara Gazette* that spread to the national media, it was discovered that a neighborhood of homes known as Love Canal, near Niagara Falls, New York, was built over a toxic chemical dumpsite. As news spread of the health repercussions of Love Canal, including severe birth defects, mental illness, and urinary tract diseases— along with the stark realization that there were hundreds of contaminated places like Love Canal all across America— Congress adopted the Comprehensive Environmental

Response, Compensation, and Liability Act, sometimes known as "Superfund" cleanup legislation.

In each of these examples and countless others, at first we pretended that our physical environment did not affect us at all, until the environment became so grim that our pretenses were shattered. At that moment, when publicity scared us into action, we viewed the environment as an *oppositional* force, something that needed to be combated and controlled. Just as we battled and imperiled our environment, now we would battle and vanquish the pollution. Instead of taking good care in the first place, now we would go to war to correct the problems we created for ourselves.

The simple connection between the environment and our health should be obvious by now, yet we continue to pretend that our environment does not affect us, and we wait until our environment becomes menacing before becoming proactive. Taking good care from the start would be so much healthier and easier for us all than fixing a problem once it advances to the stage of crisis management. *"It is easier to maintain good health,"* as Dr. Cooper famously reminded us, *"than it is to regain it once it is lost."*

Perhaps in Albert Einstein's oft-repeated definition of insanity, we are doomed to repeat the same mistakes and learn their same lessons over and over again, like being stuck in a strange recurring loop. Indeed, it was not until 2013 that a cancer research agency within the World Health Organization *"definitively"* concluded that outdoor air pollution is carcinogenic and poses a much greater cancer risk than even secondhand tobacco smoke. Did anyone stop to grasp the obvious—that spewing poisons into the atmosphere is harmful to our collective health?

We don't need to treat the environment as if it were an oppositional force, to be warred against and systematically controlled. We can treat the environment as what it is—something outside our bodies, yet indelibly connected to ourselves, that connects us to one another and to the planet. We can begin to recognize how we are not separate and apart from our environment.

———

The realization that you are part of your environment changes the way you interact with your environment.

Food is a good example of our interconnectedness with our environment. We are undeniably dependent upon our environment for our food—what we eat, drink, or absorb into our bodies comes from our environment. As we consume these foods, they become physically part of us. Food can sustain us, make us well, or make us ill.

Whether you've thought about it or not, we are all immersed in our environment's culture and its cuisine. Sometimes that immersion becomes clearer when you are a tourist in a strange environment, with a different culture and different cuisine. The local food can be the best part of an unfamiliar environment; it can be the worst part too if you don't enjoy new culinary experiences or if you're intolerant or allergic to the local foods.

You don't need to be a tourist for this principle to apply. Even if you are a local resident, enjoying your native cuisine, your health and wellness are still affected by the foods of your environment. This is true of the place you live today and the foods common to that place, just as it was true in Asia in the 1800s, where white rice replaced brown rice in everyday Asian culture and cuisine, unintentionally creating deadly beriberi epidemics.

When I learned how to politely say, *"No cheese, please,"* for the sake of my own digestive health, I learned something fundamental about my environment—how it is a part of me and I am a part of it.

The culinary culture of the United States, where I live, enjoys cheesy pizza as a staple of common diets. It's not just pizza—cheese is an ingredient added to a wide and growing variety of everyday foods, like burgers, sandwiches, pastas, eggs, salads, and tacos. I enjoy living in America and enjoy American culture, and I enjoy spending time with friends and family who enjoy pizza and other cheesy American foods—but I don't enjoy the feeling when any of that food makes me physically ill.

When I finally realized that eating pizza and other cheesy foods was not worth my personal stomach distress, I realized that I needed to change the way I interacted with my environment and its foods. That change may sound simple, but it was not easy.

It became more difficult than I could have ever imagined when I realized that I was allergically intolerant of *all* dairy foods—milk, cream, and butter, along with cheese. Dairy was everywhere in my American environment! It was found in foods that you might not expect and added to other foods reflexively and compulsively for flavoring. Until I adjusted to my environment and until my environment adjusted to me, being dairy-free in a land of milk and cheese was not easy at all.

Allergic or not, I was part of my environment. As a child, these foods nourished and comforted me. It's funny, but when my childhood doctors told me to stop eating corn, it was good medical advice—despite their misdiagnosis of diverticulosis—because I enjoyed eating corn with lots of *creamy butter!* By consuming less corn, I consumed less dairy to upset my stomach. Unfortunately for my stomach, though, my dairy consumption didn't stop with corn—I dolloped sour cream on baked potatoes, slurped creamy New England clam chowder, and guzzled cold dairy milk with milk-chocolate chip cookies.

Today, knowing of my severe dairy allergy, I no longer eat these foods, but they remain delicious childhood memories. My mind's taste buds can fondly remember them, and the thought of these foods still excites comforting memories for other senses—like the happy sound of an ice cream truck driving down our street, ringing its jingly bells, as the neighborhood children all screamed for the truck to stop. I was one of those screaming kids, gathering around the truck to taste its creamy frozen dairy treats, though I now realize how the ice cream made me sick. For whom does a bell toll?

Not a single doctor during my childhood—not one—ever suggested dairy foods could be the cause of my stomach *dis*tress. Like my parents, these doctors were themselves immersed in the cultural messages of the health-care system and the dairy industry, absorbed into the prevailing wisdom of their environment, which said that milk and dairy products were essential for every child's good health and development, building strong teeth and bones. Maybe all that milk *did* help me grow tall and strong, but it also gave me violent stomachaches. Since giving up dairy entirely, I've also realized how it made my nose stuffy and my chest congested, all chronic ailments of my childhood too.

No man is an island, and it turns out I'm not alone. I've seen statistics that estimate that as much as 60 percent of the total world population may be allergic to milk and dairy products, although the figure varies by severity and by ethnicity. If you look at population percentages as actual numbers of people, that means many millions of dairy-intolerant people, like me, live in cheesy environments. Many of these millions of people haven't even realized they are allergically intolerant, and until they learn how to politely say *"no cheese, please,"* they too will be sickened unknowingly by their environment.

Taking care of our environment for good health is not a lesson about just food—but when it comes to foods, the same concept applies to much more than just dairy.

For example, gluten is a hot food topic and a wellness concern for millions of Americans today. Gluten is found in wheat and other common grains. Like dairy, it is a staple of American cuisine, an everyday ingredient in everyday foods you'd never expect it to be in. Gluten allergies and intolerances vary from mild to severe; for those afflicted, eating gluten can cause a range of symptoms, including stomach distress, rashes, moodiness, disorientation, even infertility. A significant percentage of the American public, perhaps 10 or 20 percent or more, are gluten-intolerant; estimates vary, along with varying definitions of gluten sensitivity.

Any way you count the percentage, even if it's just a single percent, it means there are millions of gluten-intolerant people. Some of these people still unknowingly eat foods that make them ill; others have learned to give up the hot buttered wheat bread and biscuits that are a staple of American cuisine. As these people seek a healthier gluten-free environment for themselves, their environment has begun to respond, with more restaurants and groceries suddenly offering gluten-free food choices. The trend is accelerating, along with the wellness movement.

There are many more everyday examples from common foods revealing our inseparable connection to the environment and how we must take good care of our environment to take good care of our own health and wellness. When I was growing up, peanut butter and jelly sandwiches seemed to be everyone's lunchtime favorite. Children with peanut allergies, though, must learn to interact with their environment to avoid these foods. This avoidance is essential, because severe intolerances to peanuts or tree nuts can cause swelling of their eyes and throats, even death from anaphylaxis.

As our awareness grows, the examples seem to multiply. Many people in American culture are now giving up diets loaded with sugars and fats. These ingredients are also common to the American food environment, found in greasy burgers, supersize fries, sweet soda pops, rich gooey dessert treats, and many foods you'd never expect. Those who are intolerant of these everyday American foods may experience symptoms like diabetes, heart disease, obesity, and sluggishness, among others.

The solutions—giving these foods up, moderating intake, or find-ing medicines to treat the allergy—may seem simple, but they are not easy. Despite all of these allergic intolerances, these foods still nourish and comfort many people, who want to make their own food choices. Look closely enough, and lines blur again—for different people, the same substance can be a nutritional food or a deadly poison. What heals can also harm, in the way that milk may have strengthened my bones even as it upset my stomach.

Indeed, people often continue to eat the foods of their environ-ment even as they realize that a food is making them ill. We all pick our own poisons from time to time; or perhaps there are no other good options available in the environment. Sometimes foods that harm are the only real chance for belly-filling comfort. I'd still drink a glass of dairy milk too, if that truly was the only way to satisfy my hunger or my only choice for nutrition. Mostly, though, I do have other choices, and I have made a decision not to drink dairy milk. I try to adapt to my environment and ask my environment to adapt to me too.

—

Dr. Selye would say that adaptation to an environment's stresses is necessary to avoid personal *dis*tress, just like evolutionary adaptation is necessary for species survival.

He would remind us that there are both *internal* and *external* ways of adjusting to the environment and that both methods can be proactive. Both methods of adaptation involve taking good care of yourself and your environment, and both can dramatically improve your wellness.

For me, the first step in adjusting *internally* to my food environment was accepting and forgiving my own dairy intolerance. If I wouldn't accept that aspect of myself, how could I expect the environment to accept me? Serenity is found in the acceptance of things that cannot be changed, including one's own allergic intolerance to certain foods. As you strive for self-improvement, there are aspects of self that define who you are—you are who you are, with all your glorious imperfections! For me, despite all denials, whether I liked it or not, I remained dairy-intolerant.

There were denials, to be sure. On some personal level, I could not believe that childhood favorite foods—trusted parts of my environment—were making me sick. As the evidence mounted and I could not honestly deny the connections and correlations I saw between my consumption of dairy and my stomach distress, I just wouldn't admit it to myself. Maybe it was habit, conformity, or nostalgia; maybe it was hunger, gluttony, or addiction. Maybe there were other reasons why I would not accept what I could not change, and find my own serenity in the essential first step of forgiving myself. Whatever the reasons, until I *internally* accepted my own dairy intolerance and forgave myself for it, I denied myself the chance to cure what ailed me and find good health.

I needed to make external adjustments too. Adjusting *externally* required me to respectfully ask my food environment to accept and forgive my dairy allergy. At first, it seemed my environment denied my dairy intolerance just like I had done internally for myself. Even though I would ask politely and explain informatively that I could not eat dairy, the environment could turn oppositional. Waiters would sometimes sneer at me disapprovingly and ignore my requests for dairy-free food. Recalcitrant chefs would sometimes spitefully put butter and cheese into my food despite my earnest request.

I'm sure they had their reasons. Maybe these food service workers did not believe in dairy intolerance or believed the dish tasted better with cheese. Maybe my requests created problems in their kitchen, or the server didn't know the ingredients and couldn't be bothered to find out. Maybe the environment's intransigence was based on petty and narrow beliefs that everyone enjoys the same foods and has the same wellness needs, the mistaken notion that *one size should fit all.*

Whatever the reasons, I needed my environment to accept and forgive my dairy intolerance as I learned to do for myself. So I asked and kept on asking, with the courage to change the things I needed to change about my environment. Sometimes, with good humor and spirit, I would laugh about my need to avoid dairy, knowing the biblical proverb that a cheerful heart is good medicine and a crushed spirit saps your strength. *"Give my friend my cheese—he can have my extra,"* I'd good-naturedly say to the waiter, so that my cheese would be given to some other patron, who'd enjoy it more. Or, like the old Catskill vaudevillian Henny Youngman, I'd joke, *"Take my cheese—please!"*

Henry David Thoreau himself may have enjoyed my *shtick* of nonviolent civil resistance to dairy in my foods. Thoreau was right—civility to oppositional forces in your environment takes good care of both you and your opponents.

As the wellness movement grows, there's been quite a lot of civil resistance influencing our culture and its cuisine. Resistance has come from people who are dairy-intolerant, gluten-sensitive, nut-allergic, or sugar-overloaded, among many others, all proactively seeking good health and wellness for themselves. These people all want a more forgiving environment, one that gives them the foods they need to feel well. All seek to find internal and external ways of adapting, both for themselves and their environment.

With all this bottom-up resistance by ordinary people seeking to be well, an *extra*ordinary thing began to happen. As people demanded wellness from their environment, their choices for wellness multiplied. That's part of the process of *adapting* too—as you adapt to your environment, your environment begins to adapt to you. There is an ebb and flow to the pattern of adaptation because you are part of your environment.

An environment that begins with opposition and denial can grow increasingly understanding and tolerant. I have found that to be true for my own dairy allergies. Over time, I noticed how it became far more common for a waitress to conscientiously explain to the chef that a customer has a dietary need and for the chef to thoughtfully alter a recipe and cook with appropriate nonallergenic substitutes when the dish is made to order, or explain politely that the dish is already made with dairy, so I can choose another dish that won't make me sick.

When we speak up, persistently and politely, about what makes us well, the environment adapts toward our wellness. The pattern changes in degrees to create new patterns of wellness over time.

———

An environment that takes good care of wellness needs is not just about tolerance for differing foods and diets. An environment that takes good care of wellness needs is not just about being green and cleaning up the pollution in someone else's neighborhood, as it is not just about openness to medicines and therapies that may seem odd or alternative.

As we grow in understanding for the wellness of others, we sweep away prejudices and biases against people who are just trying to find a way to feel well themselves. Other people may believe opposition and war is the way to wellness, but even when war becomes necessary, tolerance and forgiveness remains essential to our common wellness. Tolerance does not excuse wrongs, but it directs appropriate response, allowing even ferocious enemies in war to thereafter build enduring friendships and strong alliances, as was the world's actual experience after World War II.

Zero tolerance is an *oppositional* policy; its very name demonstrates intolerance, and intolerance always perpetuates an intolerant society. Even where the intolerance is directed at things that you may find wrong or misguided, adding more darkness can never bring the light of understanding. To be sure, wellness requires forgiveness, but the power of history is that forgiveness does not mean we must forget.

Indeed, we cannot forget—we must *never* forget. For wellness to grow after the Second World War, and for wellness to accelerate today, we must remember some things long forgotten, like how to live together and take good care of each other.

If you demand tolerance and understanding for your self to help you feel well, then you must learn how to be tolerant and understanding to help others feel well. If you exercise empathy, you will see empathy grow around you, for as you learn how to take good care of others, it becomes possible for others to learn how to take good care of you.

In other words, if you want your environment to take care of your health, then take good care of the health of your environment. Try as you might to separate your health from your environment, the two cannot be separated.

They were never separate from the start. They are connected, as are we all.

Part B

WHOLENESS

Chapter 10

BE CONNECTED

As the second part of this book begins, it is more important than ever to recognize that lines designed to separate need to be blurred—if not erased altogether—to discover the heart of wellness for yourself.

It may seem strange that something as important as your own wellness can depend on blurring or erasing a line, but wellness requires thinking, understanding, and just plain being *based on connection*, not the mistaken separations that lines can bring. Said another way, lines cannot separate what remains connected together, and misguided attempts to impose separation upon your wholeness can leave you feeling disconnected, depressed, empty, or sick. Wellness requires nothing more—and nothing less—than a restoration of wholeness.

As you wonder what all this really means, you may already intuitively understand how separation is *not* wholeness and how wellness *needs* wholeness. Since antiquity, humankind has sensed that too, and wondered why it is so. You might explain wholeness with similar or suggestive words—like holistic, holism, unity, omnipresence, ubiquity, unified field, communion, completeness, or connectedness—and these words are also at the heart of many of humanity's oldest religious, spiritual, and mystical traditions.

Perhaps because of those ancient associations, you may believe that omnipresence or completeness is confined only to the sacred or sublime, or you may think this holistic unity is nonsensical, illogical, or nonscientific. Sadly, you may even insist connectedness somehow does not apply to *YOU*. These erroneous thoughts and misguided beliefs about your wholeness—*our* wholeness really—are more pervasive and more poisonous than you may realize, and must now be gently corrected and then released, like a flawed line that needs to be blurred and then erased.

That simple goal is at the heart of this second part of the book.

———

The historical significance of the worldwide wellness movement is that it gradually restores wholeness to a wide range of mistaken separations. As the wellness movement grew from the lessons of the Second World War and then accelerated into the third millennium, it began to blur and erase varieties of lines that had obscured our wholeness.

Many of these lines had long been drawn dogmatically, and in many cases accepted for centuries unthinkingly. For instance, hard lines drawn among people that segregated and discriminated based on wrongful and illusory labels and categories (like skin color or sexual orientation), slowly blurred and erased during this historic period of the wellness movement. In hindsight, the absurd fiction of these lines should have been obvious, and over time, fewer people clung to the hurtful lines they once drew with their own minds. As separations between people gradually dissolved, newfound connections transformed human relationships, marking a revolutionary advance of human conscience and consciousness.

As communities of people move towards wholeness, society itself is transformed, often in easily perceptible but logically inexplicable ways. For example, pundits are now puzzled by the widespread drop in violent crime rates across America; recognizing the profound significance of the statistic, social scientists have tried in vain to find the cause. Though this drop in violent crime "stands as one of the more fascinating and remarkable social phenomena of our time" according to Inimai M. Chettiar of the *Atlantic* magazine, it remains "a big, if happy, mystery"[1] to social scientists accustomed to explaining things with their tools of linear measurement. And yet the cause of this revolutionary social transformation should be obvious—as lines blur between people, it leads to a rise in empathy, kindness, and just plain niceness. You don't need statistical analysis to see how violence declines as we learn to see each other as whole people to be respected, not as objects who can be viciously attacked.

Indeed, whenever and wherever lines are blurred, the gradual restoration of wholeness augurs revolutionary changes that transform institutions as well as people. You may recall stories from the first part of this book that remind you how blurring a simple line of thought and belief helped transform institutions like medicine *(e.g., bacteria are all harmful or cannot live in the highly-acidic stomach)*, agriculture *(e.g., using poisons in farming has no impact on the quality of our food)*, education *(e.g., Helen Keller was an unruly wild child that needed to be restrained in an asylum)*, or law *(e.g., homosexuality is a deviant behavior that should be legally punished)*. In each of these stories, holistic connection evolved understanding, which then radically changed the institutional wisdom.

This same pattern of wholeness transforming institutions also applied to business and commerce, which as you may recall was the subject of the white paper I wrote. As I presented the economic data to logical private equity financial professionals, it seemed self-evidently obvious to them how *wholeness was the third of the three keys* to understanding the wellness movement. Foods marketed to wellness consumers spoke of being "whole" and healthcare services targeted to wellness patients described a "holistic" approach. Words of unity and connection appeared in the names of wellness companies, the mission statements of wellness enterprises, and the packaging of wellness products. The data also showed how lines had blurred between foods, medicines, drugs, and cosmetics, and between once-separate channels of commercial distribution and legal regulation, transforming the business landscape and providing remarkable opportunities for wellness entrepreneurs.

Of course, I was not the only person to see this transformation in commerce. Prominent economist Paul Zane Pilzer described the seismic business change as *"The Wellness Revolution"* in his best-selling book of the same name, heralding the incredible possibilities for monetary growth and profit in the book's subtitle *"How to Make a Fortune in the Next Trillion Dollar Industry."*[2] In ways that neither Professor Pilzer's book nor my own white paper mentioned, though, restoring wholeness also offered incredible opportunities for *personal growth and prosperity*. It may be uncommon for an economist like Pilzer or a lawyer like me to say how money cannot measure some things, as the tools of both our professions emphasize linear analysis and evidence-based metrics. However, you may already intuitively understand that some of the things that we treasure most in life—like love, inspiration, fulfillment, and wellness—can never be measured with lines like that.

It may also be helpful to remember that lines are not inherently bad—so long as you don't lose the connection amidst their separation. Lines can aid in economic evaluation, legal enforcement, or scientific measurement. Lines can provide amusement and entertainment, like the punch lines of a joke or the field lines of a sport. They can be useful in defining, classifying, and comparing, so they can be constructive and productive—so long as the lines do not obscure a deeper understanding of our essential wholeness.

Unfortunately, though, oftentimes the lines we draw—or allow others to draw for us—limit our perception of the whole. Unable or unwilling to see beyond the lines, we overlook or ignore the majesty of our holistic unity; this can be true too even for people who believe in wholeness and intuitively sense its connected unity. Perceiving wholeness can be like seeing the tip of a truly gigantic iceberg, where our vision of the iceberg becomes limited by the surface water lines of the ocean. You may sense the enormity of the iceberg, but the lines of surface appearance can limit what you actually view and understand of its whole.

If you find the analogy of the tip of an enormous iceberg rising above the ocean's water line helpful to perceiving the majesty of our wholeness, then you should extend the analogy further. As the historic wellness movement accelerates, it is as if the ocean waters recede to expose much more of the enormous iceberg to view, even for people who are unable or unwilling to see what lies hidden beyond the lines of surface appearance. To extend the analogy still further, it is useful to remember that the surface water lines of an ocean do not really exist—the line is actually a fictional construct that we take for granted. In truth, the ocean tides ebb and flow, its waves crest and crash, and its waters froth and foam, so the ocean's surface is not really a line and cannot truly be measured that way. Our gradual recognition of this mathematical truth is an important story in the history of the wellness movement too, told later in part B of this book.

For now, the point is this: If you allow your perception of wholeness to be blinded by lines, then the lines themselves become the type of pernicious, prevalent thoughts and beliefs that must be gently corrected and released, as is the goal of the second part of this book. Each of us may have different illusory lines at this very moment keeping us from wholeness, but the goal of blurring and erasing them is the same for us all. That goal is like a guiding star for a navigator steering a small boat in a vast sea in the darkness of the night sky; it provides perception where eyes alone cannot see.

Blurring lines and then erasing them altogether always leads toward healing wholeness, and should be vigilantly pursued for the sake of your own wellness as well as the wellness of others.

———

It may sound simple, but it is not always easy. You may take the lines for granted, or cling to them reflexively. Sometimes the lines are self-imposed, and other times, the lines are culturally or legally reinforced. You can imagine these lines exist because everyone else seems to believe they do too. You may habitually and falsely assume that the whole can be separated into the sum of its parts.

What's worse is that the systems, processes, habits, customs, rules and routines of your everyday life can all be built upon illusory lines—organizing and institutionalizing mistaken separations that forget our connectedness and dishonor our wholeness. When this happens, the lines can be so deeply embedded in our thoughts and beliefs that it becomes extremely difficult to remember that the lines are there, or how and why they got there in the first place. It can become more difficult still to remember that these now-forgotten lines are mere hidden illusions that keep us from the *truth*.

It is as if we constructed false premises and then built faulty towers upon these pillars of mistaken separation. Toppling a pillar of separation, which may have held strong for centuries, can be like a simple game of dominoes, in which other pillars fall one after another, bringing a new age of greater awareness. When these false pillars begin to topple, everything else we believe can rapidly change. That is why restoring wholeness can be so very revolutionary and transformational. What becomes obvious in hindsight can be but a simple perception overlooked and ignored for centuries—until no longer overlooked or ignored anymore, changing entire paradigms of thought and belief.

If that sounds fuzzy or difficult to comprehend, remember that for centuries we unthinkingly believed that the sun revolved around Earth, a view dogmatically enforced by the systems and institutions of the time. Through a telescope, Galileo Galilei understood how Earth move around the sun, defying the entrenched belief system of the times. Like dominoes, Galileo's simple astronomical observation toppled pillars of knowledge, one by one, as adherence to

Church doctrine and law gave way to rational and logical methods of seeking truth.

The event is still celebrated today as the start of the scientific revolution and the beginning of the Age of Enlightenment, which historians generally consider to be a two hundred year period from 1600 to 1800. Of course, Galileo Galilei was not the first person in history to make the astronomical observation that Earth revolved around sun. The great Nicolaus Copernicus had seen the same thing generations before him; Copernicus, however, did not have to suffer the wrathful consequences that a visionary's clear perception can sometimes provoke. Copernicus escaped the Church Inquisition because he was wise enough to publish his astronomical masterpiece *De Revolutionibus Orbium Coelestium* on his deathbed.

Galileo, however, was very much alive when he perceived how Earth was not the center of the celestial universe, so he had to face the vengeful consequences of his clear vision. According to the actual minutes of the Inquisition and the Special Injunction issued thereafter, in February 1616, Galileo was instructed to "abstain completely from teaching or defending this doctrine and opinion or from discussing it," recanting his opinion that "the sun stands still at the center of the world and the earth moves," and "if he should not acquiesce, he is to be imprisoned."[3] This edict of February 1616 was a couple of months before the great playwright William Shakespeare died; as Shakespeare wrote in Hamlet, Act II, Scene II: "Doubt thou the stars are fire; Doubt that the sun doth move; Doubt truth to be a liar; But never doubt I love."[4]

Perhaps the passionate love of truth that burned inside Galileo compelled him to persist in his astronomical beliefs—to secretly doubt that the sun doth move as his Inquisitors insisted it did, and slyly sidestep the Church so he would not be a liar doubting truth. After 1616, his sneaky strategy worked for a while but it caught up with him in 1633, when Galileo was forced to stand trial for heresy. Threatened with execution in a court proceeding, and hoping to save his own life, Galileo relented to his Inquisitors, formally declaring Earth fixed and stationary in the cosmos, renouncing legally and denying publicly what he plainly saw with open eyes and knew with an open heart. As the trial came to a close, his very life spared despite the ordeal of Inquisition, Galileo is said to have uttered under his breath, *"Eppur si muove*—And yet it moves." [5]

Whether or not Galileo actually said those words, his now-famous wisecrack seems to embody the spirit of the Age of Enlightenment—a historic period when false pillars of knowledge toppled one by one, forever changing human understanding of ourselves and our place in the universe. *And yet it moves.* Galileo's supposed punch line was just a simple sarcasm by a man condemned for speaking truth to power, yet some truths can transform us by making us laugh even as they make us think.

Comedy buffs might describe the type of humor that points out an obvious truth *"the elephant in the room."* It's the truth that we ignore or deny, pretend not to see, are blind to, or refuse to discuss, but it's still there. Our connected wholeness is a lot like that too. Ignore it, pretend not to notice, turn a blind eye, refuse to address its true meaning—but it's still there. Its simple truth leads to a revolutionary transformation of understanding too, heralding a historic new Age of Awareness.

———

Even if it's still the elephant in the room, our connected wholeness now has an important place in science. The scientific study of holistic systems and processes is sometimes called the study of *ecology.*

Ecology has been applied to earth sciences, biological sciences, environmental sciences, human sciences, genetics and population sciences, climate and meteorological sciences, agriculture sciences, natural resource management, and a growing number of other academic fields. In each of these scientific disciplines, ecology reveals hidden cycles and relationships within systems that somehow are linked together in a greater whole.

In one early and infamous example, ecology demonstrated how a single substance moved through the environment, connecting supposedly separate parts of nature in hidden and unexpected ways. Rachel Carson revealed in the book *Silent Spring* how the DDT poison we sprayed to kill an insect pest unintentionally decimated America's national symbol, the bald eagle, nearly to extinction. We ignore the connected nature of the whole at our own peril, and ecology teaches that *even when the connections are hidden from our view, they are still there.*

This example of unwittingly poisoning a national symbol to the brink of extinction is by no means unique. One of my personal favorite stories of hidden ecological connection involves the systematic eradication of prairie dogs by cattle ranchers and governments in the vast grasslands of North America.[6] Some estimate that there were once *tens of billions* of prairie dogs living in their elaborate communal prairie dog "towns" of burrows and tunnels throughout the wild grasslands that stretched from Manitoba, Canada, through the West-Central United States, down to Chihuahua, Mexico.

Prairie dogs are small mammals, inviting anthropomorphic comparison. They stand on two legs, have openly affectionate relationships with one another, and expressively communicate complex messages to one another too—including colors and characteristics of objects—in a prairie dog language of yips and chirps and barks that we're only beginning to decode.[7] They seem like nice kindly creatures, with busy social lives.

To the governments and the ranchers, however, these prairie dogs were a threat to cattle. Their theory was that prairie dogs competed with cattle for the grasses that fed them both and that prairie dogs dug holes that posed a dangerous grazing hazard for cattle. The theory seemed logical enough in the way we draw fictitious lines of separation to make sense of things, and prairie dogs were given a new name—*varmints*, furry pests to be exterminated like vermin—as a ferocious *oppositional war* commenced against them.

Them varmints were killed primarily by mass poisoning from a nerve toxin that led to the animal's painful convulsive death. Eliminated from 99 percent of their previous habitat, the prairie dog population was reduced to less than one-thousandth of 1 percent of their previous numbers. Perhaps not surprisingly, most of the survivors are distressed and diseased. It is among the most systematic and intentional species eradications in all of recorded human history, all to make the lands safe and productive for grazing cattle.

What makes the cruel story one of my favorites to illustrate how the environment is holistically connected in unpredictable and surprising ways is the story's great irony. With the prairie dogs gone and the brutal war against them successful in its goal of eradication, the once-fertile grasslands began to turn into dry mesquite desert, making the land in many places unfit for cattle—and unfit for eagles, chickens, coyotes, ferrets, and other once-common grassland species, which vanished along with the prairie dogs in the changing desert landscape.

It turns out that prairie dogs actively cultivated the land, like farmers of the grasslands. They gnawed at the roots and stems of water-depleting mesquite plants, controlling their growth and spread, and their burrowing aerated and turned the soil, enabling nutrient-rich grasses to thrive. With their demise, the land itself changed.

If you're looking for another comic punch line, perhaps the cruelest irony of this story is that domestic cattle, like their wild bison cousins, actually seem to *prefer* to graze on the healthy vegetation around a prairie dog town. Had anyone bothered to look, the cattle could be seen happily and harmoniously *coexisting* with them varmints!

The bottom line, if you are still thinking in lines, is that tens of millions of acres of grassland habitat were needlessly and wastefully destroyed, all because we foolishly believed the whole could be reduced into the sum of its separate parts. Back then it seemed like *simple subtraction*: "grassland habitat" *minus* "prairie dogs and pesky burrowed holes" *equals* "surer footing and more grass for grazing cattle"—and yet the mathematical equation was wrong, flawed in its basic premise. You cannot separate a natural habitat, oblivious to its connected whole.

———

Whether told in a story of prairie dogs and grasslands, pesticides and the near-extinction of a national symbol, or countless other true stories, it should be easy to understand why *ecology* is such an important and practical science when it comes to taking care of Earth and our natural environment.

The very first Earth Day in my home state of New York took place on April 22, 1970, and a young ecology professor teaching at Long Island University helped to organize the event. Back then, Gerald J. (*"Jerry"*) Franz was one of a handful of ecologists with a bona fide academic background in this still-emerging environmental science. He spearheaded a march of six thousand students, converging on Brooklyn's Prospect Park. As the assembled marchers waved Earth Day banners and demanded protection for the environment, Governor Nelson Rockefeller rode in on a bicycle, greeting Professor Franz and the cheering crowd, to formally declare New York State's first official Earth Day.

From teaching ecology and planning Earth Day, Professor Franz eventually became the first chief of Environmental Permitting at New York City's Planning Department. After that, his next phase of life was as a private businessman, cofounding a consulting firm that obtained environmental permits for projects like Manhattan's Trump City, South

Street Seaport, and Metrotech Center in Brooklyn. When I met Jerry Franz, he had moved on to yet another phase of life, helping green tech and wellness businesses grow and prosper through their own connected cycles. We connected too, and Jerry is now a good friend and has been a partner on many business adventures.

I once asked Jerry the source of his inspiration to become an environmental scientist. I often ask people about their inspirations because I like to understand what motivates people to do what they do. I know how an inspiration can change the course of a life, and in the magical way that inspiration leaps from heart to heart, how one person's inspiration can change the course of other lives too—even the course of history, as might be said for that very first Earth Day.

"Years before the first Earth Day," Jerry answered, "I was in college as a premed student listening to a professor give a synopsis of the biology areas of study when he came to one I had never heard of—*ecology*." Jerry is the type of person who becomes intrigued by the meaning of words he doesn't know. He is a teacher who has taught at every level of the American educational system from kindergarten to postgraduate university, but who never lost the desire to learn as a student. "I was moved by the word *ecology*," he explained to me, "how everything is connected to everything else."

Everything is connected to everything else! It is a staggering concept if you've never heard it before or if you've never spent a moment to appreciate the enormity of its meaning. Although its wisdom is ancient, it was new to the syllabus of a biology class at Brooklyn University, where premed Jerry Franz attended. Not everyone understood the holistic concept back then, and not everyone understands it today, but it inspired Jerry to become an ecologist.

Jerry also recalled his Jewish mother's reaction when he told her the news. "Her son, the doctor" was now going to be "an ecologist." To Jerry's mother, ecology was not part of medicine, and it was not what doctors do. It was barely a word in her vocabulary. *"Doesn't that have something to do with garbage?"* she asked her son, bursting into tears.

Jerry's mother was correct. Ecology does have something to do with garbage, because garbage is part of the whole equation. It doesn't matter whether the garbage is the dead carcasses of billions of poisoned prairie dogs in the once-expansive North American grasslands, or the plastic waste we discard that is now swirling around the vast dying corridors of the Pacific Ocean. Whether the garbage is what we discard on Earth or whether it is the mess we make in our own lives and our relationships with others, garbage has its consequences.

You can try to hide your garbage or pretend it does not exist, you can refuse to address the mess you've made or deny it affects you, but it's still there, like an elephant in the room.

There are other elephants in the room too—*even the elephants themselves.*

As I write this, elephants inhabiting the African forests are being brutally murdered by poachers, who use military assault weapons to attack the remaining herds of these enormous animals. These beloved and iconic creatures are now facing extinction, and in the way that *everything is connected to everything else*, these attacks have visibly changed the African forest and all who inhabit that landscape.

Turns out that the elephant, like the prairie dog, is what ecologists call a "keystone" species, on which the health and vitality of an entire ecosystem depend. The loss of these gentle giants affects seed dispersal, vegetation control, and plant diversity, among other hidden but essential systems and cycles of the African forest. The loss of the forest landscape, in turn, threatens survival of many other animal species in this connected ecosystem, including humans engaged in commercial ranching and subsistence farming. To borrow another Pete Seeger lyric, "Turn! Turn! Turn!" but hope *it's not too late.*

How can we continue to ignore these connections of the greater whole? Whether oblivious blindness or delusional denial, the problem stems from our fictitious separation of the elephants themselves. It is a problem of *dis*connection and, to borrow a word from medical psychiatry, *dis*sociation. It begins when we don't see the wholeness of the *real elephant* in the room. If you open your eyes and are willing to look, it is obvious that elephants are highly intelligent, devoted, compassionate, and self-aware. They have phenomenal memories—some say an elephant never forgets—and they mourn their dead.

Look at the real elephants themselves, see their wholeness as living beings, and then the murderous acts of the poachers become crimes of unspeakable atrocity and unconscionable brutality. Whether disconnected or dissociated, the poachers won't or don't see the real elephants they attack. To the poachers, the elephants are *merely objects*, valued only for their separate body parts, especially their ivory teeth and tusks.

Ironically, it is the wholeness of the elephants as living beings, including their emotions beyond their physical body parts, which now changes the African ecosystem. Many of these elephants are terrified and traumatized—not surprising for creatures that vividly remember attacks upon them and still grieve for lost loved ones. An elephant's feelings may seem fuzzy, scientifically immeasurable and unquantifiable, but these palpable fears disrupt their historic migration and mobility patterns, necessary for the elephants to fulfill their keystone ecological function. When elephants are prevented by fear from roaming the African forest, *in turn*, the landscape changes and the forest begins to disappear.

If that seems odd or unscientific, recall how Dr. Hans Selye observed laboratory rats react differently to the traumas of their injections. The rats couldn't control the external stress, but in some rats there was greater internal *dis*tress, which manifested into *dis*ease and *dys*function. That's true for the laboratory rats, suffering from the stress of a needle and syringe, as it is true for the forest elephants, suffering from the stress of brutal attacks upon their herds—as it is true for us humans too, suffering from the stresses of our own lives. The way we process our internal feelings and emotions is part of our wholeness. It is part of the essence of who we are.

If you still don't understand the connection, ask yourself how the sudden and brutal murder of your own family members or loved ones, like the elephants experienced, might affect *you*? You might retreat to a place you feel safe and secure, or you might insistently try to go about your daily routines. You might become physically ill, unable to cope with everyday life. You might dissociate from your feelings and emotions, or you might seek counseling and camaraderie for those feelings. You might not have any idea how you'd be affected by such a horrible event, and I hope that you do not have to find out. If you do suffer the nightmare of that ordeal, I pray you find peace and wellness for the *whole of you.*

———

Are you the sum of your own separate body parts—like the ivory tusks and teeth of an elephant—or is there more to the *whole of you?*

To see the great truth of your essential wholeness, spend a moment thinking about yourself. You have many body parts—some visible like your skin, others hidden like your beating heart—but there are other parts of you too, like parts of your personality and sides of your self. Perhaps only a few people know about some of these parts of you; maybe there are other aspects of self that only *you* know about *you*, or so you think.

These different parts may all seem separate, yet they are all a part of *you*, connected together in the indivisibly whole person that is *you*. To see that's true, notice how if even a small part of yourself—like

177

your toe or your pride—suffers distress, discontent, dysfunction, or disease, it can make the *whole of you* ache and hurt.

It's like an age-old story, told in different variations, about different parts of the body bickering about who should be in charge. Each separate body part made the case for its importance. The brain argued how it did all the thinking, the eyes how they guided the body through sight, the stomach how it converted food into energy for the body, the legs how they allowed the body's mobility, and so forth, until the asshole spoke up. All the other body parts laughed at the little asshole, at the outrageous suggestion that it should be in charge of the whole body. So the asshole shut itself tight, and after a while, the brain couldn't concentrate, the eyes were crying, the stomach was cramping, the legs were shaky, and so forth, until all these body parts finally relented from the painful siege, allowing the asshole to be in charge of the whole body. What seems separate can be connected in unexpectedly painful ways.

That may seem funny, reminiscent of Doctor Dan's suggestion about how opinions are like assholes, but it reminds us to look for connections that may not be immediately apparent. Look again at the whole of you from different angles, the way you might observe Earth differently from sea level or a mountaintop or from outer space. If you do not take care of your *whole* self, notice how parts of you will become sick or unbalanced and eventually affect the whole of you. Notice too how you can take away certain body parts, like lose a limb or a lobe of a lung, or take away some parts of your personality, like your anger or your fear, yet you can remain a *whole* person.

As you get to know your self better, you may also notice that in order for you to feel *whole*, you must attend to certain essential parts of yourself. These essential parts are at the heart of who you are, like the parts of you that feel love and wellness. They are part of your wholeness, unlike the anger and fear that take you away from wholeness.

If you are not accustomed to thinking about your wholeness, this may all seem strange and uncommon. Even with the wellness movement gaining momentum and acceptance, you may still think of wholeness as something that only applies to foods or ecosystems. That may be true, but *your wholeness begins with you.*

If you habitually create or enforce fictitious lines of separation within yourself—as we all do sometimes—you may not realize this wholeness within yourself. The more you look, the more you'll realize how you are not just a sum of your body parts.

———

Don't expect your connected wholeness—truly, *our* connected wholeness—to be the focus of the systems and institutions of science, medicine, and health care. These authorities aren't accustomed to thinking this way, so top-down recognition that we are more than the sum of separate body parts has come slowly and reluctantly, when at all.

Historically, that's quite understandable. Ever since the Age of Enlightenment, scientists have sought to understand the whole of things by reducing them into separate parts. During this remarkable period of history of the 1600s and 1700s, great luminaries of science and reason revealed secrets of human and celestial bodies alike through the process of rigorous *separation, observation,* and *analysis* of parts of the whole.

The iconic Sir Isaac Newton, for instance, made sense of the whole of the physical universe by breaking it down into separate forces like gravity and motion in his classic treatise *Philosophiae Naturalis Principia Mathematica*, published in Latin in 1687. A few years after Isaac Newton's death, the whole of Earth's natural environment— all of nature herself—was separated painstakingly by Carl Linnaeus of Sweden. In 1735 Linnaeus published his comprehensive *Systema Naturae* in Latin, revealing a *"system of nature through the three kingdoms of nature."* The book organized everything into hierarchical categories, starting with the three "kingdoms" of animals, plants, and minerals, and continuing, per the book's title, *"according to classes, orders, genera and species, with characters, differences, synonyms, places."*[8]

Carl Linnaeus and his assistants catalogued thousands of species, and gave each their own unique two-word Latin name. Linnaeus classified human beings, for example, as *Homo sapiens*. It was a prodigious accomplishment identifying a "system" for all of nature, meticulously drawing lines to separate each of nature's varieties of living things, and for this celebrated achievement, Linnaeus was elevated to the aristocracy—knighted like Sir Isaac—taking the noble name of Carl von Linné.

The process of separating the whole into its parts, even for *nature* itself, can be enlightening indeed. At first, diligent observation brings greater awareness and understanding. Even the mere *naming* of a newly discovered species, for example, leads to better appreciation of the species, because new words convey new meanings not easily conveyed without a word.

Over time, though, the process of separation blinds us to the truth. We draw false lines of separation that never really existed in the first place— like Linné's fictitious lines of *"classes, orders, genera and species, with characters, differences, synonyms, places"*—that woefully distort our view of reality. These erroneous assumptions and harmful misconceptions are then perpetuated, passed down unthinkingly through many future generations. This pattern holds for scientists, scholars, ordinary folks, and powerful institutions alike, who become mistakenly attached to the lines they learned from others, and who then aggressively defend these fictitious separations, often in the name of "science" or "precedent" or "conformity."

This problematic pattern persists, even when the *real truth* of our connected wholeness should be as obvious as an elephant in a room. New discoveries make it difficult to defend these imaginary lines, but we still do.

Even Carl von Linné (née Linnaeus) discovered new things that challenged the very separations he imagined in *nature*. To his credit, Linnaeus diligently continued to observe nature throughout his life, and the more he *looked*, the more he *learned*. The new data compelled Linné to repeatedly rethink and revise his own *Systema Naturae*, constantly drawing and redrawing his lines of *nature* anew, so that by the time of his death in 1788, he had published thirteen major new editions of his original 1735 book.

The process of looking and learning is admirable in anyone and possible for everyone. Looking and learning—not the fiction of lines—is what truly advances scientific understanding. Of course, like the tip of an iceberg, there was much hidden from Linnaeus, as there is much hidden now. Today there are *millions* of species identified—a number exponentially greater than the *thousands* Linné observed and imagined. Some discoveries defied classification in his *Systema Naturae*, like newly discovered life-forms with characteristics of both animals and plants, which blur the lines between the supposed Linnaean kingdoms.

What is a "kingdom" anyway before the majesty of nature? Nature herself does not pay heed to these imagined hierarchies and fictitious lines, which belie the beautiful connections and imperfections in all of life. Discover a new life-form that doesn't neatly fit into a tidy checkbox, like a creature that seems both plant and animal, and we often label the new discovery an *"anomaly."* We push the disruptive data to the side, pretending the discovery somehow does not apply, returning to the same comfortably fictitious lines of separation, like plant or animal.

In other words, although these new discoveries should give us pause, reminding us the separations don't make sense, we still cling to the same old lines and boxes. Indeed, many hundreds of years after Linnaeus first created his *Systema Naturae*, even as it became apparent that *nature* herself had no regard for his illusory naming system, intelligent scientists still devotedly adhere to the Latin binomial nomenclature convention of categorization. In grade school, I remember being compelled to memorize the fictional Linnaean lines of *kingdom, phylum, class, order, family, genus,* and *species* with the mnemonic device of <u>K</u>ing <u>P</u>hilip <u>C</u>ame <u>O</u>ver <u>F</u>rom <u>G</u>eneva, <u>S</u>witzerland!

That childhood memory now strikes me as funny, tickling my fancy all these years later, as I ask myself the real question that most teachers discouraged me from ever asking: *Does it really matter?*

———

To some people this discussion may seem impertinent. Those who believe that knowledge increases as data accumulates, filling up the boxes that science has already built for our understanding, may even be angered by the discussion. But that is more of the same old conformance to the comfortable lines of fiction we fabricate.

That observation is not new, and was observed by Professor Thomas Kuhn in his groundbreaking 1962 book *The Structure of Scientific Revolutions.* In that best-selling book, Kuhn introduced the phrase *"paradigm shift"* to the popular culture, helping us understand the true nature of scientific advancement. It turns out that science does not advance our understanding in the way most thought it did.

Kuhn examined the patterns of *"normal science,"* which he defined as "research firmly based upon one or more past scientific achievements, achievements that some particular scientific community acknowledges for a time as supplying the foundation for its further practice."[9] As an example of further practice, think of the many scientific generations inspired by the noble Linné and then building on his foundational achievement of fitting newly discovered life forms within rigid lines and tidy boxes of a *Systema Naturae,* classifying and categorizing by kingdoms and species and such.

"Mopping up operations," said Professor Kuhn, *"are what engage most scientists throughout their careers. They constitute what I am here calling normal*

science." Mopping up is about conforming to the boxes. *"That enterprise seems an attempt to force nature into the preformed and relatively inflexible box that the paradigm supplies."*[10]

This is why normal scientists cannot see the elephant in the room: they cannot see beyond the preformed and inflexible boxes that the scientific paradigm supplies. *"No part of the aim of normal science is to call forth new sorts of phenomena; indeed those that will not fit the box are often not seen at all,"* continued Kuhn, explaining how otherwise brilliant scientists can be blind to an obvious truth. *"Nor do scientists normally aim to invent new theories, and they are often intolerant of those invented by others."*[11]

———

This pattern of intolerance holds true even when it comes to the truth of an elephant.

As the story was told in the international science journal *Nature* in 2013, the revolutionary new discovery of DNA sequencing was applied to examine a fetal specimen of an elephant preserved in a jar from the 1700s. It wasn't just any ordinary elephant fetus examined—it was the one used by Carl Linnaeus himself to classify the archetypical *Asian* elephant species, *Elephas maximus.*

DNA sequencing sleuths, testing an amino acid marker from the fetus, revealed that the specimen in the jar was not an Asian elephant, but was actually the *African* elephant, once known as *Elephas africanus.* Quite literally, Linnaeus failed to see the real elephant in the room…or in this case, the elephant sample in the jar.

Did this new data convince the Linnaean taxonomists, those scientists who classify and name such species? As DNA detective Dr. Tom Gilbert of the University of Copenhagen, a leader of the team that discovered the fetal specimen's misclassification, described, "I was imagining the chaos we were about to unleash on the [Linnaean] systematists when they find out their type specimen is the wrong thing." Dr. Gilbert wondered aloud, "Would *Elephas maximus* become the new Latin name for the African elephant, forcing taxonomists to come up with a new name for the Asian variety?"[12]

As Professor Kuhn predicted—*"those that will not fit the box are often not seen at all,"* Kuhn said—there was no rethinking of the illusory lines already drawn. *"Unfortunately, they're wily creatures, taxonomists,"* DNA detective Dr. Gilbert soon learned, *"and they've always got loopholes."*[13] These "normal scientists" simply pushed Tom Gilbert's data to the side, refusing to see the elephant for what it truly was.

It wasn't the first time for the elephant either. Once upon a time, Carl Linnaeus and his assistants missed the fact that there were *two* types of African elephants, both easily observable, unless of course you don't see the obvious. One inhabited the African savannah, and the other roamed the African forest (until of course their ecologically essential roaming stopped from fear of brutal attacks by poachers with military assault weapons). Armed with the new and incontrovertible data that there were really *two* African elephants, the scientific arbiters of Linnaean lines needed to split the existing *Elephas africanus* into two new species of African elephant.

The problem was that, based on the constructs of Linnaean lines and boxes, a species once established cannot be further split into *two* new species. Conformity controlled conduct, so scientists changed the genus (Geneva!) of the elephant instead of its species (Switzerland!), a nice example of what Kuhn called *"mopping up operations."* The original species of *Elephas africanus* became *Loxodonta africana*, for the savannah elephant, and *Loxodonta cyclotis*, for the forest elephant. In other words, the elephants got fictitious new lines and fictitious new names in a taxonomic makeover of a fictitious construct from a fictitious 1735 *Systema* that missed the connected whole of *naturae* and that missed the whole of the elephants besides.

Lines and boxes, constructs and conventions, all serve useful and important purposes if they help us learn and grow—tall tales and mythologies can help us learn true meaning too—but the danger is when we become rigidly attached to the fictions we create. *Ever believe a lie and then try to build on its shaky foundation?*

As a circus ringmaster might say, drawing the crowd's attention to the real elephants parading in the center ring of the big-top tent for delighted children of all ages to look and learn from: *"Folks, you can't make this stuff up!"*

———

What is true for the elephant is also true for us humans. We created lines of separation for ourselves that are not real, and then we stubbornly clung to these fictions, even though these lines inhibited true understanding of our holistic connection.

In his *Systema Naturae*, Carl Linnaeus separated his newly named human species of *Homo sapiens* into four *subspecies*. The noble Linné carefully proceeded to describe each subspecies, using scientifically formal-sounding Latin names to correspond to the four separate geographic continents these supposed human "subspecies" inhabited. To these continents, he then attached colors—*white, yellow, red, black*—and followed these color lines with other *"characters, differences, synonyms, places"* he observed or imagined.

It shocks today's conscience, but Linné said that some human *"subspecies"* were *"very smart"* while others were *"foolish."* Then he attributed mental, emotional, and personality differences to each fictitious subspecies of white Europeans, yellow Asians, red native Americans, and black Africans, using descriptive words like *"ill-tempered," "contented," "melancholy," "serious," "lazy," "impassive," "greedy,"* and *"crafty."*[14]

Belonging to a subspecies apparently came with a fashion sense too, and Linné wrote how some subspecies were *"covered by tight clothing"* and others *"covered by loose clothing"* and how some used *"paint"* and others *"grease"* in cosmetic makeovers. According to Linné, each subspecies governed themselves differently too. The subspecies of white Europeans, to which the noble Carl von Linné belonged, was supposedly *"ruled by laws,"* while the other subspecies were *"ruled by custom"* or *"ruled by caprice"* or *"ruled by opinion."*[15] I don't know about you, but I'm a lawyer and visibly appear to be of white European descent, yet I still find myself ruled by custom, caprice, or opinion, as well as by law, from time to time.

I've observed in myself, as Mark Twain observed in himself, *"that there is no ingredient of the human race which I do not possess in either a small way or a large way,"* and even when small in myself, *"there is still enough of it for all the purposes of examination."*[16] Within me, as within us all, are all the attributes Linné ascribed to each supposed subspecies. At times, I can be *"very smart"*; yet at other times, no matter how I strive for wisdom, I can be *"foolish."* Truly, you just have to look a bit closer within your self and within others.

Not everyone is willing to look and learn, and that *unwillingness* is the real dilemma for humanity. Look how long we humans mistakenly clung to these erroneous subspecies boxes, with their wrongful color lines of white, yellow, red, and black! Believing the imaginary lines of separation between us, we objectified and stereotyped one another, repressing and enslaving and murdering one another. It took oppositional wars, fought with the weapons of violence or the resistance of disobedience, to finally blur these color lines, even if they are not yet erased altogether.

It is important to remember that these lines weren't really there in the first place. They were fictions all along, falsely separating us against ourselves. Like a house divided against itself, these lines could not stand.

The reasons why we cling to these false lines—whether security, conformity, habit, mistaken logic, rationalization, greed, insecurity, *whatever*—these reasons truly do not matter. What matters is that we blur the lines and then erase them altogether.

Let that be your bottom line, if you still need lines.

———

Don't blame Linné for the lines and for the mistaken separation that followed.

Wellness requires forgiveness, not blame nor anger—and besides, it wasn't just Linnaeus who imagined these fictitious lines. It was the *underlying approach* of most of the "foundational" scientists and thinkers of the Age of Enlightenment during the 1600s and 1700s. After the Age of Enlightenment, it became the *underlying approach* of most of the "normal" scientists and scholars who built on their foundational achievements. Over the next several hundred years, they constructed systems and institutions of science, medicine, health care, business, law, and government, all based on similarly mistaken lines of separation.

When the error of one specific line was discovered by scientists or finally acknowledged—like a line misclassifying elephants or mischaracterizing human beings—then according to the underlying approach of the Age of Enlightenment, new lines would be drawn instead. "Mopping up operations" is how Professor Thomas Kuhn described the process in *The Structure of Scientific Revolutions*.

Wellness, however, requires a new paradigm that embraces our wholeness. The connection of unity can never be found with lines. Think about that powerful concept again for a moment, because it changes the way you see healthcare, science, government, and so many other systems and institutions built upon linear foundations.

Indeed, if you are seeking better health through wellness, you may soon realize that the very notion of *connected wholeness* can be at odds with those physicians and health-care professionals who forget the whole of *you*, preferring to divide you into separate body parts for diagnosis and treatment. In the bottom-up ways of the wellness movement, you must proactively prod your doctors to use new tools and to embrace new holistic paradigms, based on the wholeness essential to wellness. Your physicians can continue the very best scientific observational and measurement practices of the Age of Enlightenment, but they must reject medicine's foundational fictions of separation in a new Age of Awareness.

You are a whole connected human being, not just the sum of your body parts.

———

How did this underlying approach of separating your body parts for diagnosis and treatment become the foundational approach of "modern" medicine?

In some ways it can be traced to a single remarkable man at the beginning of the Age of Enlightenment. William Harvey was an English physician, formally educated at the prestigious University of Padua in Italy, considered the most advanced medical research institution of its day. In 1628, Dr. Harvey published a landmark scientific book in Latin, entitled *Exercitatio Anatomica de Motu Cordis et Sanguinis in Animalibus*, translated as *An Anatomical Exercise on the Motion of the Heart and Blood in Living Beings*.

The book set the standard for all Western medical doctors and is still followed by physicians today. For his amazing accomplishments and his insights on the motion of the heart, Dr. William Harvey was named one of the *"Ten Most Influential People of the Second Millennium"* by Dr. Arthur Schlesinger Jr. [17]

Schlesinger himself was an iconic historian[18] and an influential advisor to presidents like John F. Kennedy—he was called the "court historian" of Kennedy's Camelot—as well as a confidant to many other world political elites, celebrities, and thought leaders. Dr. Schlesinger was influential in my own life too, and I was privileged to have met him, although I'm not sure he ever really knew my name.

For a brief but shining moment in time, I worked alongside him, seeing Arthur Schlesinger nearly every day as we both researched and wrote our separate histories at the small Franklin Delano Roosevelt archival library in Hyde Park, New York. As we sat near each another at the small research library's tables, I could see his approach to his work; I could feel it and sense it too. He always seemed methodical and mindful, and I observed how he would diligently gather facts and then ruminate on their implications, deeply engrossed in his own thoughts. I could almost see the wheels turning in his distinguished graying head as he traced the evolution of ideas in history.

When Arthur Schlesinger was about to receive the first of his Pulitzer Prizes in history (for "The Age of Jackson"), he was interviewed by Robert van Gelder for the *New York Times* book section, in an article published on March 10, 1946. Asked about his underlying approach to history, Dr. Schlesinger explained *"What primarily interests me... is the relationship between thought and action—the course that ideas take as they travel from the mind"* of one person *"into the mind"* of another. He believed it was these ideas traveling from mind to mind that determined the course of history; these ideas, said Schlesinger, were the true *"powers"* that affected our *"social conditions,"* that gave us our *"laws"* and directed our *"accepted axioms for conduct and judgment."*[19]

If physician William Harvey was one of the *"Ten Most Influential People of the Second Millennium"*—as Schlesinger said he was—it was because Dr. Harvey's powerful ideas about medicine traveled from mind to mind across the globe and far into the future. Harvey emphasized linear separation, like other scientific greats of the Age of

Enlightenment; physicians that emulated William Harvey's example divided the whole body into separate anatomical systems and parts for further identification and observation. In other words, Dr. Harvey supplied what Thomas Kuhn called *"the foundation"* for *"further practice"* in the areas of medicine and health care.

Maybe another reason William Harvey was so influential was his focus on the heart. The *heart*, perhaps more than any other body part, has folklore of its own. Some say the heart represents the love at the center of our whole being. Others say it holds the essence and spirit of humans, as of all things. The heart beats and pulses and is commonly seen as the source of life and vitality. Its energy is often understood as radiating outward, encompassing the whole, which is why getting to the heart of the matter explains so much; I myself embraced that understanding when seeking the heart of wellness and the history of the wellness movement.

To discover the truths of the *heart*, Dr. Harvey used the tools of the Enlightenment and wrote that his purpose in writing *the Motion of the Heart* (in Latin as then customary, translated here into English) was to focus *"the light we have made to shine"*[20] on the darkness of ignorance, in *"order that what is true may be confirmed, and what is false set right."* To do that, he wrote in his landmark medical book that it was *"imperative"* to recognize *"what has been thought of these things by others in their writings, and what has been held by the vulgar and by tradition."*[21] In other words, Dr. Harvey was not interested in vulgar folklore, but in medical science.

William Harvey said his approach to discovering truths of the heart was based on *"dissection, multiplied experience, and accurate observation."*[22] Dissection creates physical separation with its surgically precise and razor-sharp lines, and Dr. Harvey encouraged physicians to slice the whole into thinner sections for even better understanding; he wrote how *"it would be proper to look more narrowly into the matter, to contemplate the motion of the heart and arteries."* By observing what was narrowly separated, he said, is how you *"investigate and discern the truth."* Dr. Harvey's approach to truth demanded *"greater and daily diligence and investigation," "frequent inspection of many and various animals," "collating numerous observations,"* and *"frequent appeals to vivisection, and much ocular inspection."*[23]

How influential are Dr. Harvey's ideas? Look how far and wide they have traveled—from mind to mind over the course of many generations—since 1628 when William Harvey published his medical text on *the Motion of the Heart.* Look today at hospitals, clinics, physicians, and health-care professionals narrowly separating and observing the body's functions and purposes, dividing the body into circulatory, respiratory, pulmonary, digestive, endocrine, urinary, reproductive, neurological, skeletal, and many other systems, and further dividing by skin, bones, blood, glands, heart, spleen, brain, eyes, ears, and many other parts, all observed by experts and medical specialists with narrow focus, in isolation of the whole. Dr. Harvey earned his spot on the top "Ten Most Influential People of the Second Millennium" for good reason—his Enlightenment tools and techniques of *"separation"* and *"observation"* have surely advanced medicine and health care, as they have surely advanced other fields like science and law.

This book unabashedly celebrates the contributions of William Harvey's ideas towards today's understanding of medicine, just as it expresses sincere gratitude for the accomplishments of Carl Linnaeus towards today's appreciation of nature's amazing diversity. We continue to build on the approach of these pioneering Enlightenment scientists, just as we continue to use their customs and practices, like using Latin in their scientific words and phrases. That custom and practice continues in professions like law too, where—*ipso facto*—a word or two of Latin conveys the *meaning* at the heart of something meaningful.

But this book also acknowledges their approach misses something meaningful at the heart of it all. Even with Harvey's tools of *dissection, vivisection,* and *ocular inspection,* a surgeon can narrowly dissect and observe my grandfather's ulcerated stomach—yet still not see the *H. pylori* bacteria that caused his disease. If surgeons draw lines that bacteria can't grow in acidic stomach environments, then they won't find them there. Even after erasing that set of lines, finally seeing the bacteria in the stomach, if they believe that all bacteria in the stomach are harmful germs, then they'll hurt the ones needed for healthy digestion.

You have to be willing to look farther than you can see with eyes alone, to look past lines of belief you draw for yourself or others draw for you. Otherwise, the information gathered through separation and observation can be meaningless, overlooking and ignoring the whole in its entirety. Professor Thomas Kuhn said that information *"that will not fit the box are often not seen at all,"* and when new data doesn't fit into our tidy boxes, with its lines of separation, we can miss seeing a microbe, or we can miss seeing an elephant.

We can miss much more than that.

———

Here's a riddle: What part of you cannot be dissected with a sharp scalpel nor separated with a bright line? *Here's a clue:* It's among the strongest and most powerful parts of you, yet is best observed and understood only through your wholeness.

If you need to think about this riddle, then you are probably using your *mind*. Your mind differs from your physical brain, although the two may intersect and connect. Your mind includes the thoughts and ideas that historian Arthur Schlesinger said travel to other minds and can change the course of history.

How can you separate and observe the nonphysical mind?

You could use the foundational approach of the influential Dr. William Harvey, with *"dissection"* and *"frequent appeals to vivisection, and much ocular inspection"* but such tools of the Enlightenment do not seem especially helpful to observe and understand the mind. My own mind, like yours, cannot be observed with visual investigation, and frequent *"vivisection"*—which is how scientists unemotionally describe live animal dissection—won't allow you to see an animal's mind as it is cut by a knife either.

Perhaps if you look closely at the animal, observing the *dis*tress you cause it by cutting it while alive, you may begin to understand that the whole of the animal is more than the sum of its parts—that it is more than a two-word Latin species name or a check-box in an imagined hierarchy of an Linnaean animal kingdom. You might begin to understand, in the way that Dr. Hans Selye observed caged laboratory rats reacting to the *dis*tress of an injection, that the subject in the experiment is more than just the sum of its separate animal physical parts. You might even empathize with distressed laboratory rat's thoughts and emotions as a living whole being, not just an object in an experiment.

In the 1700s, hundreds of years before Dr. Selye's observation, Carl Linnaeus wrote that he considered humans superior to the rest of the animal kingdom because of what he called our *"morality"* and our *"magnificent mind"*[24]—and if that is how you draw the lines, and arrange your tidy boxes, then you will not see how the laboratory rat shows *morality* with its *magnificent mind* too.

A groundbreaking study entitled "Empathy and Pro-Social Behavior in Rats," published in 2011 in the journal *Science* revealed how a laboratory rat will free its caged fellow rats and then share its food. As Peggy Mason, Jean Decety, and Inbal Bartal, the article's authors at the University of Chicago, wrote, "They freed cagemates even when social contact was prevented. When liberating a cagemate was pitted against chocolate [that the noncaged could have kept to itself]" the rat freed its fellow rat and then "typically shared the chocolate."[25] These experiments have been repeated in other studies and in other contexts, such as a rat preventing a fellow rat from drowning even before feeding itself (that particular study by Nobuya Sato and researchers at Kwansei Gakuin University in Japan was published in 2015).[26]

These studies have also been repeated for other species—including of course elephants—shattering the narrow-minded bias that *only humans* possess "morality" and a "magnificent mind." Indeed, although we humans are capable of great magnificence and morality too, we have also historically enslaved and imprisoned one another, hoarding food and prized possessions as crumbs for ourselves.

Despite such data, an animal's magnificent mind—like our own—does not appear anywhere in the *Systema Naturae* of Carl von Linné or the anatomy charts of Dr. William Harvey. It does not appear in the scientific achievements of other great Enlightenment thinkers, like the chemistry tables of Antoine-Laurent de Lavoisier or the physics equations of the great Sir Isaac Newton. Indeed, the absence of these nonphysical aspects of the mind in science led some Enlightenment scientists to consider animals and humans as *machines*, made of separate mechanistic parts, separating mind from body as if the mind didn't exist at all.

The scientific geniuses of the Enlightenment should have known that *"mind"* exists, because they used their own magnificent ones to influence the minds of their peers, and their minds still influence ours today. Their minds, in cooperation with their hands and eyes and other parts of their whole being, wrote books communicating their powerful ideas, which traveled far and wide.

The enlightened Sir Isaac Newton, for instance, appears as the number-two most influential person of the second millennium on Arthur Schlesinger's "top ten" list. Newton, with his laws and equations for the physical universe, is still highly regarded among scientists, but in this third millennium, he's not quite as influential as he once was. There have been revolutionary shifts in our understanding of physics, thanks to Albert Einstein, as well as quantum physicists, string theorists, and many other scientific revolutionaries of their day—much like the scientific acceptance of our connected wholeness will inevitably shift our understanding of physics yet again.

However, even if Sir Isaac's star is waning among "normal" physicists, he remains part of the popular culture, celebrated for an iconic image of an apple falling from a tree and hitting him on his head, to suddenly reveal to him the hidden laws of gravity. The story may be true—maybe so, maybe not—but the image itself continues to influence. It is a metaphor of an *Aha!* moment of discovery and inspiration that rational logic could not provide all by itself. Neither that *Aha!* image nor the many contributions of Sir Isaac Newton to physics, though, was good enough for Newton to earn first place on Schlesinger's list.

Number one on Schlesinger's list, as the most influential person of the second millennium, was none other than William Shakespeare, also known as the Bard of Avon. The *bard* is not a royal designation, like the knighting of Sir Isaac or von Linné, but rather a populist name of honor given to a people's poet, who hailed from a town in England on the River *Avon*. Though the criteria for Schlesinger's list may be complex, it is easy to see why Shakespeare is so influential. His plays and stories, with their universal themes and powerful metaphors, make us *feel,* they make us *think*, and they continue to be adapted and readapted for new audiences each generation into this third millennium.

Maybe playwright William Shakespeare bested scientist Sir Isaac Newton for top spot on Schlesinger's "most influential" list, because the Bard of Avon seemed to understand something about the *whole* of humanity—including our *minds*—that the brilliant scientists of the Enlightenment somehow did not. I'd even say that Shakespeare understood *the complexion of our beating hearts* in ways that Dr. William Harvey did not, and that science and medicine still do not.

———

195

If you're still scoring, comparing and contrasting with linearly precise measure, William Harvey was number ten on Schlesinger's list, and it is likely that he and number one, William Shakespeare, actually knew each other personally or at least knew about each other in the small elite circles of London, England, of the early 1600s.

In 1604, shortly after graduating from the prestigious University of Padua in Italy (where Galileo, number five on Schlesinger's list, was then a professor teaching astronomy and geometry), young Dr. William Harvey began settling into his long, prominent medical career in London, marrying the daughter of King James I's personal physician, Dr. Lancelot Browne. By 1605, when Shakespeare's *The Merchant of Venice* was being performed for King James I in 1605, Dr. Browne may well have been in attendance at Shakespeare's play, along with his daughter Elizabeth and new son-in-law, Dr. Harvey. With so many in the king's court knowing of these prominent newlyweds, it surely must have delighted the crowd to hear the play's pivotal news of *"A messenger with letters from the doctor, new come from Padua!"*[27]

The Bard of Avon always knew how to amuse an audience, to make them laugh and applaud for themselves, even as he challenged their understanding of what it means to be human. Unlike Harvey, Shakespeare never traveled to Italy, much less Padua or neighboring Venice, the setting of the play, but that did not prevent the playwright from knowing his way around town. It is also unlikely that Shakespeare ever met a Jewish moneylender like the play's famous character Shylock, but that did not prevent the bard from knowing human nature, for Jews as for the whole of us.

Back in 1605, when the *Merchant of Venice* was being performed for King James and his court, Jews were still demonized in London, having been formally expelled from England since King Edward's Edict of Expulsion in 1290. Shakespeare appealed to his audience's prejudices in creating a villain like Shylock, someone to draw *boos* and *jeers* from the crowd, a vile person who wanted to exact a *"pound of flesh"* for a loan gone unpaid by Antonio, the Christian merchant of Venice, who was the play's title character.

Look a little closer, though, and the Jewish villain Shylock appeals for recognition of our common humanity. He asks for empathy and understanding, for recognition that we are all living beings with many sides of self, not objects separate from one another:

> *"Hath not a Jew eyes? hath not a Jew hands, organs, dimensions, senses, affections, passions? fed with the same food, hurt with the same weapons, subject to the same diseases, healed by the same means, warmed and cooled by the same winter and summer, as a Christian is? If you prick us, do we not bleed? If you tickle us, do we not laugh? If you poison us, do we not die?"* [28]

Shylock defends the *"pound of flesh"* he desires from Antonio with the same zero-tolerance vengeance that Antonio displayed toward him and his fellow Jews. As his character proceeds to explain, the price of treating another person as an object is to be treated as an object yourself:

> *"If you wrong us, shall we not revenge? If we are like you in the rest, we will resemble you in that. If a Jew wrong a Christian, what is his humility? Revenge. If a Christian wrong a Jew, what should his sufferance be by Christian example. Why, revenge. The villainy you teach me, I will execute, and it shall go hard but I will better the instruction."* [29]

This speech in Shakespeare's *Merchant of Venice* is all the more remarkable, not only because the bard defied the stereotyped caricature of a Jew in an age of rampant anti-Semitism, but because he saw the connections of our wholeness in an age of separation. Through the character of Shylock, Shakespeare reveals the vicious and connected cycles of victimization and villainy, another example of the Zen-like unity of seeming opposite dualities holistically containing the seeds of the other.

Even today, *The Merchant of Venice* speaks the language of wellness and is one of the many reasons for Shakespeare's enduring influence well into this third millennium. Our connected holism applies to Jews and Christians living together in medieval Venice, as it applies to the anatomical organs and parts living together in our own bodies today.

Remember the old story of body parts arguing over their importance, while forgetting the wholeness that connects them together? Shakespeare told a different version of the same old story[30], recalling "a time when all the body's members rebelled against the belly" for lazily eating and drinking, "idle and unactive," and "never bearing like labour with the rest."

The belly "thus accused" first admitted to eating all the food "because I am the store-house and the shop of the whole body." The belly then reminded the other body parts what it does with that food; that "if you remember, I send it through the rivers of your blood, even to the court, the heart, to the seat o' the brain; and, through the cranks and offices of man, the strongest nerves and small inferior veins from me receive that natural competency whereby they live: and *though that all at once, you, my good friends,*" the belly concluded.

Shakespeare told this story of the belly's connection to the whole body in the play *Coriolanus*, which he wrote around 1608. It was just a few years after the performance of *The Merchant of Venice* for King James I, and the setting of *Coriolanus* was also in Italy, though ancient Rome instead of Venice. You may believe you are separate and apart, the stomach is saying, but we are all connected together and we are whole. "*No man is an island, entire of itself,*" as John Donne mused years later in 1624.

————

In the ways of Shakespeare, this story of the belly's connection to the whole body was a moral lesson about the importance of caring for others, and Shakespeare's *Coriolanus* began with a scene of public riots over an imperial Roman general's withholding of food from the poor.

Feeding the poor was not merely a moral lesson for imperial armies of ancient Rome; it was a pressing issue for England in Shakespeare's own day, as it remains today. It is likely that Shakespeare was inspired to write Coriolanus by riots over the enclosure of public lands used by peasants to feed themselves, and resulting shortages of grain, most notably the Midlands corn riots of 1607, which engulfed the bard's home county of Warwickshire. In this period of the early 1600s, the government began taking measures to address the growing problem of poverty in England.

How we define a problem is often the most important step to solving it. At first, the poor in England were seen as villains for their presumed idleness and indolence. To combat the aristocratic discomfort of seeing beggars on the streets without food to eat, English laws swept the poor out of sight, hoping to keep them out of mind. Under the Vagabonds and Beggars Act of 1495, during the reign of Henry VII, as well as similar legislation of the 1400s and 1500s in England, the poor were compelled into forced labor, banished, tortured, or even hanged.

The *Poor Relief Act of 1601*, also known as the *Elizabethan Poor Law* or the *Old Poor Law*, was an ambitious accomplishment of redefinition in a country where privileged members of society did not think about the poor at all and, when they did, tried to mask poverty through punishment and expulsion. It was adopted in the reign of Queen Elizabeth I, who came to believe that many of the poor were victims who should not be blamed for their circumstances, and were deserving of Christian compassion instead of moral indignation.

Queen Elizabeth was deftly able to effect these changes in attitude about the responsibility of the whole of England toward its poor because she was at the height of her power and influence in 1601.

She had consolidated her formal control over England's network of church parishes with the Elizabethan Religious Settlement of 1559; this religious proclamation declared the independence of the Church of England from the pope in Rome and made Elizabeth the *supreme governor of the Church of England.* As *Her Majesty the Queen,* Elizabeth also exercised formal authority over the country's network of justices of the peace, wisely building on foundations established centuries earlier by King Richard the Lionheart.

Besides controlling these formal levers of church and state, Elizabeth ruled with the fuzzy power of the English people's love and gratitude. "I do not so much rejoice that God hath made me to be a Queen, as to be a Queen over so thankful a people," the Queen herself proclaimed in what is known historically as the "Golden Speech" she delivered to Parliament in 1601, just a few months after passing the Elizabethan Poor Law. There is nothing more valuable than love, the Queen declared, "for I do esteem it more than any treasure or riches; for that we know how to prize, but love and thanks I count invaluable. And, though God hath raised me high, yet this I count the glory of my Crown, that I have reigned with your loves." [31] To this day, many royal-watchers consider Elizabeth I to be England's most beloved monarch over its long history; she was nicknamed *Good Queen Bess* or the *Virgin Queen*—who never married because she married England herself.

Able to effect changes through both formal control and fuzzy power, Queen Elizabeth I redefined the problem of poverty by using the under-lying approach of the new Age of Enlightenment. First, the poor were narrowly separated and divided into classes and categories, and were then sent to systems and institutions based on these supposed separations. The queen entrusted these jobs of separation and administration to the parish churches and the justices of the peace under her control.

The separations under the Elizabethan Poor Law were stark and decisive, like other line-drawing characteristics of Enlightenment think-ing. There were the "deserving poor," seen as victims of circumstances beyond their control, such as famine or other economic catastrophes; and the "impotent poor," who could not care for themselves, such as the sick, infirm, or elderly. At the other extreme, still seen as villains, there were the "idle poor," or worse, "vagrants or sturdy beggars," who continued to be legally harassed and persecuted. The poor, now classified into these rigid boxes, were then sent to narrowly focused institutions—"hospitals," "almshouses," and "orphanages" for the impotent and deserving poor, and "workhouses" and "correctional prisons" for vagrants and the idle poor. [32]

Just two years later, in 1603, after forty-four long years on the throne, Queen Elizabeth died. However, the separation of the poor based on these categories and classifications did not die with the queen. Her chosen successor, King James I, continued the policies of the *Poor Relief Act*, as well as continuing Elizabeth's policies of extending royal control over the systems and institutions of both British church and state.

The new king strengthened the State, becoming the first monarch to simultaneously wear the crowns of England, Ireland, and Scotland in what would eventually become the United Kingdom, and he commissioned an official English-language Bible, still known and widely read as the *King James Bible*, further Anglifying and controlling the Church of England, further distancing the church from Rome. In the realm of good King James, both "top ten" influential Williams—William Shakespeare and William Harvey, each born during the reign of his predecessor Queen Elizabeth—also flourished. The new king became the chief patron of Shakespeare's royal repertory company, renamed *The King's Men* in 1603, and became chief patient for Dr. Harvey, who was named King James's *physician extraordinary* in 1618.

King James himself died in 1625, prompting proclamations of *"The king is dead! Long live the king!"* in the way that the influence of a life goes on, even in death.

———

This history of the early 1600s—the historical beginning of the Age of Enlightenment—might seem strangely misplaced in a book on *wellness*. Most people would consider this period to be little more than dusty, musty old history and may not understand why this old history is included in a chapter devoted to our connected wholeness.

We often take for granted how thoughts and ideas from the distant past inform our understanding in the present day. When we speak of the "top ten" influential persons of the second millennium, for example, what we really mean is that these people's thoughts and ideas survived their death and continue to affect the way we think, even into this third millennium. Like pebbles tossed into still water, their ideas and thoughts reverberated far into the future, in ripples that spread outward, sometimes gaining or losing momentum as they met with other waves of influence.

Uncovering the foundation of our thoughts and ideas is invaluable, especially if we're stuck in a rut, trapped in an unproductive loop of making the same mistakes over and over again. Finding the false premises of our ideas allows us to reboot our thinking, to finally break free and move forward. It's like realizing there is no color line separating us; only by revealing this false premise are we are able to join together and heal the mistaken divisions of humanity. To gradually restore holistic unity in all facets of our lives and institutions, we need to acknowledge these other lines of separations, many of which have their foundations in the early Enlightenment. It is too easy to take these separations for granted, never realizing how or why the lines were ever drawn.

Though the *Old Poor Law* of 1601 may seem a relic of the distant past, nearly forgotten by history, it is the early foundation of the modern welfare state. Understanding *welfare* is important for understanding *wellness*; quite literally, welfare began as an old English expression of concern for well-being. *"Fare thee well, great Heart!"* wrote Shakespeare[33], a few years before 1601, and helping people fare well during life's rough passages is still a primary purpose of welfare today.

In other words, when citizens are faced with difficult times, with conditions like poverty and hunger, how does a government help their well-being? Queen Elizabeth's approach to welfare in 1601 was the same approach used by enlightened scientists like Dr. William Harvey, and it began with *separation*. Separate the poor and hungry by some defined characteristic trait—*impotent, idle, deserving, or vagrant?*— so that the systems and institutions can narrowly administer to them based on these separations—*hospital, workhouse, almshouse, or prison?*

Welfare has surely evolved since the *Old Poor Law* of 1601; there have been newer poor laws adopted, and even descriptions and phrases like *poor law* and *poor relief* fell out of fashion. There have been newer categories and classifications for the welfare system since the early Age of Enlightenment, and the lines and boxes drawn by Queen Elizabeth in her Old Poor Law have been redrawn and mopped up many times, but at its heart, *welfare* still relies on separation.

The premise of separation, however, was flawed from the start. You may believe that only those poor people seen as *impotent* or *deserving* are worthy of *empathy, compassion, charity*, and *generosity*, to be administered by hospitals, almshouses and orphanages—but all people are deserving of such kind treatment. Even the *idle* poor or criminalized *vagrants* respond better to rehabilitation and recovery if treated with generous empathy and charitable compassion. Similarly, you may be believe that only poor people characterized as *idle* or *vagrants* require *industry, duty, purpose*, and *responsibility*, to be administered by workhouses and prisons—but again, all people need to feel a sense of dutiful purpose and responsible industry, even the elderly and infirm.

The fundamental flaw in the foundation of the Enlightenment's welfare system is that people cannot be separated into *"deserving"* and *"undeserving"* categories without treating people like *objects*. Treating people like objects severs the healing wholeness of human connection. It may seem fuzzy, but without holistic connection, there is anger and angst, sickness and sadness. When you treat another person as an object, it does not just diminish the other person; it diminishes *you*.

Look inside yourself. Observe how you have parts that feel deserving, with other parts undeserving. See how some parts of you seek industry, and how other parts seek compassion, purpose, and empathy, all to greater or lesser degrees. As Mark Twain suggested, there is still enough of each trait in you for purposes of examination.

To be sure, you might define words like *industry, compassion, purpose,* or *empathy* differently than I do, but these words—and words like them—are all words of *action*, so what is truly important is that *you exercise each of these aspects in yourself.* One size does not fit all! Ask yourself, honestly, whether you have exercised those parts of yourself today and whether you exercise them each and every day. If you are seeking wellness, then you should feel industrious, be compassionate, find purpose, and show empathy, all in ways that make sense for you in your daily life.

If you engage in honest self-examination, you will observe how exercising *all* of these traits— as Shakespeare said, *all at once, you, my good friends*—allows you to feel connected and whole. Notice how traits like empathy, purpose, compassion, and industry are all joined together within you and notice too how these traits join you to others. Separate from *any* of those essential parts of yourself, and you will notice how you feel fragmented and empty inside.

Surely self-examination will teach you this, but if you are the type of person that needs an expert to tell you how to feel well, then listen to Dr. Halbert Dunn, the physician and biostatistician who coined the very word *wellness* in the 1950s; he bluntly explained in his seminal essay on High-Level Wellness, how *"wellness can never be achieved in fragments, ignoring the unity of the whole."*[84]

———

If you still doubt how ideas from the early 1600s continue to influence your ways of thinking, erecting unseen barriers to your own wellness, then you may need to focus on how those ideas traveled through time and space to your present day and place.

As Aristotle taught, *"If you would understand anything, observe its beginning and its development."* Even if you never thought to ask those questions before, you might be surprised to learn where some of your own customs and conventions come from and how they evolved over time. You might similarly be surprised to learn how lines of separation became part of the foundation and fabric of today's systems, institutions, laws, and values. Understanding these lessons of history, you may ask if you really need to make the same mistakes over and over again, realizing how a change toward wholeness and wellness is possible for both you and the systems and institutions around you.

The *Old Poor Law* of 1601 required medical institutions of England to care for the *"impotent poor"*—like the elderly, sick, and infirm, considered deserving since they could not care for themselves—so English hospitals and physicians of the early 1600s were now legally required to charitably accept those deserving of medical attention. Even the famous Dr. William Harvey, then chief physician at London's St. Bartholomew's Hospital ("Barts" as the hospital is still called today) was required to take an oath of charitable devotion to these deserving poor, swearing, "in God's most holy name" not to do *anything for the poor but such good and wholesome things as you shall think with your best advice will do the poor good.*[35]

This charitable oath required Dr. Harvey and Barts to steer clear of monetary conflicts and corruptions, to use their "best advice" to "do the poor good, without any affection or respect to be had to the apothecary."[36] In other words, even way back in the 1600s, the apothecaries—the medieval equivalent of druggists and pharmacists—were considered medical merchants who sold more of their merchandise with a doctor's recommendation. Enlightenment thinkers understood how the apothecary might use the powers of "affection or respect" to sway a doctor's "best advice."

Unlike hospitals and physicians, the apothecary drug merchants had no duty to do only "good and wholesome things." They were sworn to the separate goal of economic profits and were given a corporate monopoly in 1617 to single-mindedly pursue these narrow financial objectives. King James I himself took credit for creating a corporation for the druggists: "I myself did devise that corporation and do allow it. The grocers, who complain of it, are but merchants; the mystery of these apothecaries were belonging to apothecaries, wherein the grocers are unskillful; and therefore I think it is fitting they should be a corporation of themselves."[37]

The King spoke these words defending his controversial decision to grant a monopoly over medicines before a populist House of Commons in 1624. This was four years before Dr. Harvey anatomically separated the motion of the heart, but by 1624, the separation of business-only purposes into corporations— narrow legal entities sworn to seek only monetary profits—was old news.

One of the first and most successful early corporate entities was the English East India Company, which received a royal charter from Queen Elizabeth in 1600. Its business charter clearly declared its pecuniary purposes: "for the increase of our navigation, and advancement of trade of merchandize" and to "bring into this our realm of England, from the said East Indies, or from some other parts, beyond the seas, out of our dominions great or greater value in bullion of gold or silver, or of foreign coin." Their guiding creed—to profit monetarily from trade—was to be had "for every voyage, the first voyage only excepted."[38]

Think for a moment about the effect of this narrow separation into benevolent or mercantile purposes. While charities like Barts hospital were sworn to *do good*, freeing themselves of economic corruptions and considerations, business corporations like the East India Company were sworn to *do well*, their wellness measured solely by the accumulation of gold, silver, and monetary riches. One institution was sworn, in these early years of the 1600s, to focus on traits like *compassion* and *generosity*, while the other was legally mandated to focus on traits like *industry* and *economy*.

Surely, as is true for ourselves, each of these qualities is important and meaningful, and all are worthy of vigorous pursuit—but from the beginning, with the swoop of a Virgin Queen's quill pen on a corporate charter and an Old Poor Law in the early 1600s, these qualities were *divided* and *disjoined* and *dissociated*, entrusted to separate institutions. It was an enlightened experiment, narrowly separating entities and systems along qualitative lines.

———

At first, by pursuing one aspect of humanity to the exclusion of all others, singular goals were advanced. Each institution's narrow focus set new standards for excellence in the pursuit of the trait selected. New skills were developed, to accomplish their separate purposes, and new metrics were mandated, to track performance of these separate goals.

Separation seemed so rational and logical, so full of good common sense, but then *something unexpected happened.*

It happened in the midst of all the fantastic accomplishments of these institutional entities with their special purposes. It happened as surely as the slaughter of elephants brought the financial rewards of ivory, though it sacrificed the whole of the elephant's life and, perhaps surprisingly, the forest in which the elephant dwelled. It happened because even Good Queen Bess with her formal authority and fuzzy love could not separate what is already indivisibly connected together.

Hospitals focused solely on *charity* and *compassion* and *goodness*, without regard to *industry* and *economy* and *trade*, found themselves cash-strapped and unable to administer medical care to their communities. Often the hospital's dilemma was emphasized when expensive medical equipment was needed or when health-care personnel became insufficient for a growing population, and the hospital did not have the economic means to buy the equipment or service the whole of the community.

Corporations focused solely on *industry* and *economy* and *trade*, without regard to *charity* and *compassion* and *goodness*, found themselves destroying the very things that made them wealthy. Often the corporation's dilemma was emphasized when its managers and leaders became corrupted and disgraced by the lure of riches, degrading the whole of the business from the inside out.

Some of these lessons were learned early on, way back in the Age of Enlightenment, but we chose to ignore their deeper meanings. Instead of embracing our connected wholeness, we just redrew the lines and mopped up the boxes. We mistakenly believed that the very separations that created the crisis could now solve it. That recurring mistake—*trying to solve the problems of separation with even more narrow separation*—is being gradually corrected by the holism of the wellness movement.

The remarkable history of the East India Company is illustrative. Single-mindedly pursuing the corporate charter granted by Queen Elizabeth in 1600 (to advance *"trade of merchandize"* and deliver *"great or greater value in bullion of gold or silver"*) the East India Company grew and grew, eventually controlling an estimated 50 percent—*fully half!*—of all the world's trade. Separated from any charitable purpose, narrowly concerned only with its profits, and backed by the king's military might, it exploited vast colonies of consumers for economic gain.

In one such colony, the Bengal region of Asia, the East India Company plundered and looted the countryside until an estimated *ten million people* died of famine in the 1770s. It may have just been callous indifference, but with so many dead in Bengal and so many lives destroyed, the East India Company was widely rebuked in its native Britain.

Among the East India Company's harshest critics was the Scotsman Adam Smith, who first published his famous *The Wealth of Nations* in 1776, the same year America declared its independence. He was a major influence on America's Founding Fathers, especially James Madison, Thomas Jefferson and the nation's first Treasury Secretary, Alexander Hamilton[39], and he is still regarded as the father of modern economics today. Adam Smith was much more than a narrow economist, though. He understood how economics was holistically connected with philosophy, politics, ethics, and psychology, and argued that the East India Company hurt the people of England—as well as those of Bengal—because the East India Company excluded others from competing in the trade; it inflated prices to make "extraordinary profits" and committed "extraordinary waste" because of its "fraud and abuse, inseparable from the management of the affairs of so great a company."[40]

Bengal was a horrible tragedy, with a staggering death toll, but it was just one of many uncaring excesses of a company that measured success solely in monetary riches. For example, the corporation's steep profits would cause American colonists to protest in 1773, throwing the tea the East India Company imported from China into the Boston Harbor in a revolutionary tea party that still influences Americans today. Similarly, in the next century, the East India Company fought wars to continue to export opium to China, which it processed in factories in Bengal from cultivated poppies. Like the morphine opiate in Mrs. Winslow's Soothing Syrup, opium can be medicinal, recreational, poisonous, pleasing, highly addictive, and extraordinarily profitable, *all at once*; you cannot separate its benefits from its costs. To do so would be just as dissociative as seeing an elephant only as a set of ivory tusks, or see corporations as only a vehicle to make money.

Seeing the destruction wrought by the East India Company in places like Bengal, Boston, and China, some economists narrowly separate the East India Company from other companies.[41] Some have even a created entirely new mopped-up category box for the East India Company that they call a *"sovereign-backed monopoly."* This newer and narrower categorization may help explain the magnitude of the East India Company's commerce and carnage, but its lines of separation are still illusory.

To greater or lesser degrees, *all corporations* are sovereign-backed and competitively advantaged. Not all corporations are granted the king's armies for their conquests, like the East India Company, but most are granted the tax collector's favoritism or protected in some other way by the government's laws. Sovereign-backed monopolies are more common than you think too; the government grants exclusive monopolies for patents, trademarks, and even copyrighted materials like this book. At the most basic level, for commonplace corporations and everyday entities—bearing legally fashionable letters like LLC, LLP, L.P., P.C., Corp., Co., Inc., or Ltd.—the sovereign's laws protect its owners from personal legal liability. Ordinary people don't have the same limited legal liability as do corporate legal fictions empowered by the sovereign government. Protected legal status is an awfully nice gift from a sovereign ruler, don't you think?

The problem arises, though, when these generous gifts from the sovereign hurt others, harming the whole, just so the corporation itself can seek riches. In a later edition of *The Wealth of Nations*, written in 1784, Adam Smith reached this same conclusion: "To hurt in any degree the interest of any one order of citizens, for no other purpose but to promote that of some other, is evidently contrary to that justice and equality of treatment which the sovereign owes to all the different order of his subjects."[42] Looking all around him and seeing the way most corporations used their special status to harm others, Adam Smith saw "the absurdity and hurtfulness of almost all our chartered companies." [43]

Look around you, in your own community, and you may see the same thing Adam Smith observed hundreds of years ago. You may see business corporations polluting the environment with the by-products of their manufacture, or companies selling shoddy, wasteful, overpriced, or harmful products or services to unsuspecting consumers. You may see corporations exploiting and endangering their labor force or blighting supportive communities by closing productive factories. You may observe corporations lobbying and influencing lawmakers and regulators for further selfish advantages.

These companies may each be demonstrating admirable traits of *industry* and *economy* and may be doing well financially, but they remain separated from commensurate qualities of *compassion* and *caring*. Like people, corporations need to be connected to the greater whole to be well.

———

As the wellness movement accelerates, increasing numbers of corporations understand the importance of honoring our connected wholeness. Corporate pioneers of wellness include Stride Rite Shoes, which provided day care for the children of its employees in 1971, and Ben & Jerry's Ice Cream, which in the 1980s opposed bovine growth hormone in its dairy cows and implemented a business model for *"caring capitalism."*[44]

In connected ways, I personally remember the Stride Rite chairman, Arnold Hiatt, who championed corporate day care as a good business practice, even though some financial analysts of the time ridiculed day care's costs as diluting shareholder profits. Hiatt was my college girlfriend's uncle and Dr. Dan Bernstein's brother-in-law. Uncle Arnie once explained to me how he had real-life obligations to the employees who worked at his company, as well as to the other communities that relied on him as he relied on them—his company's vendors, customers, and neighbors—in addition to his stockholders. Sometimes business could not be measured in mere profits, he told me.

Hiatt didn't quite understand the opposition to his way of thinking—but you know what doctor Dan said about opinions—but a little opposition could not stop Uncle Arnie. He grew Stride Rite Shoes through acquisitions of Keds and Sperry's and other brands until it too was gobbled up in waves of connected mergers that spread Hiatt's message of corporate holism far and wide. Ben & Jerry's too was acquired by a brand giant, Unilever, that specifically agreed as part of the purchase of the iconic ice cream maker to maintain the socially minded missions of founders Ben Cohen and Jerry Greenfield, who, in connected ways, both grew up in my wife Jane's hometown of Merrick, New York.

The holistic approach to business continues to spread rapidly in many ways besides mergers and acquisitions. It has spread from the top down as a growing generation of corporate leaders adopted the holistic mantra of doing good, not just doing well. Like much of the wellness movement, corporate change has also come from the bottom up as growing pressures of the consuming public demand that companies be built around holistic values, not just monetary profits.

Legally speaking, though, that holism can be a problem, since corporations were built on pillars of separation that date back to the 1600s and are written into charters, laws, and customs. *"Having chosen a for-profit corporate form,"* explained Chancellor William B. Chandler, III, chief judge of the Delaware Chancery Court, a company is then bound by *"duties and standards that accompany that form,"* which *"include acting to promote the value of the corporation for the benefit of its stockholders."*[45]

The Delaware Chancery Court is perhaps the most important legal forum in America for corporations, so the chancellor's words—which stated the obvious about the origins of the corporate form and its pillars of separation—echoed loudly. Chancellor Chandler seemed contrite, apologizing how "I personally appreciate and admire" the "desire to be of service to communities." Nonetheless, it was his job to enforce the centuries-old legal separation between charities and businesses, so he declared "the corporate form…however, is not an appropriate vehicle for purely philanthropic ends."[46]

The chancellor's opinion was written in 2010 in a legal case informally known as *eBay v. Craigslist* that pitted the Internet company Craigslist's desire to be of community service against its legal duties as a corporation, including the duty Chancellor Chandler called "stockholder wealth maximization"[46] in his legal decision. Some legal scholars may say the case was *narrowly decided*, acknowledging how lines in the law are redrawn in small increments; other legal pundits may say the case has *broad implications*, forcing us to recognize that corporations should do more than only benefit the purses of their shareholders. Either way, the legal case struck a chord.

A few years later, in 2013, Delaware adopted a new corporate law, becoming the nineteenth state in America to allow B-corporations. *B is for "Benefit"* and B-corporations are legally required to show their benefit to the whole society, demonstrating what Chancellor Chandler called their "service to communities." In other words, if the "corporate form" is "not an appropriate vehicle" for charitable purposes, then B-corps are an explicit change to that fictional separation. Of course, the vast majority of corporations in America have other letters, like C-corps and S-corps, which may still require fidelity to false pillars of separation.

That does not matter, though, for no matter what letter in the alphabet a corporation uses—C, S, or B—all corporate lines are blurring. If the "corporate form" requires corporations "to promote the value of the corporation for the benefit of its stockholders"—as the chancellor said—the stockholders themselves, as owners of corporations, increasingly demand that qualitative as well as quantitative aspects of "value" be considered. How do you measure value, anyway?

Corporate boards and corporate managers increasingly realize that some monetary profits are not worth their costs. Profits can be earned at the expense of the public's trust, the king's wrath, or the harm they do to others. Think about extreme examples like loan-sharking or profiteering, although the slope of "value" can be slippery indeed. When a corporation changes its *metrics of value*[48], the narrow lines of the "corporate form" begins to blur—some caring capitalists pursue socially-conscious business agendas while other companies charitably donate part of their profits for what Chancellor Chandler called "for purely philanthropic ends." As social entrepreneurship pioneer and my dear friend Robert Tolmach says, you *can* do well by doing good.

———

Legal lines separating business from charity blur in other ways too.

For instance, the wellness movement has seen the rise of social entrepreneurs like Robert Tolmach, a former architect and investment banker who uses his proven business skills to promote important charitable pursuits, and the wellness movement has seen the birth of Wall Street funds focused on investing in socially conscious and green businesses. The latter is sometimes described as *"impact capital"*—acknowledging the positive difference that business can make when investing in our communities in pursuit of worthwhile goals.

The flow of capital can work in reverse too, by moving funds away from socially divisive businesses. Nelson Mandela, the courageous and inspirational leader who helped end the racial color lines of a brutal apartheid South African government, credited the "divestment" activist campaign on American college campuses in the late 1970s and 1980s, which demanded universities and pension funds stop investing in businesses that supported apartheid, as "a key factor in the eventual victory."[49]

The wellness movement has also seen corporate billionaires like Warren Buffet and Bill Gates make *"Giving Pledges"* that commit most of their accumulated fortunes to pursue philanthropic goals. At the time of publication of this book, 128 billionaires have already taken the pledge.[50] As wellness and wholeness become explicit goals of businessmen and women, hybrid new vehicles and ventures have been created, defying centuries-old notions of what "charities" and "businesses" are supposed to narrowly be. For example, Newman's Own Inc., founded by the actor Paul Newman and the writer A. E. Hotchner in the early 1980s, profitably trades in high-quality food products, with wide distribution in groceries and supermarkets, yet it donates all of those profits to worthy charities.

My daughter Melissa worked many summers in the Adirondack Mountains of upstate New York at one of these Newman's Own charities as an art director and counselor at a summer camp for children with life-threatening illnesses. The camp is medically ready for these children, but this wonderful institution is not a hospital, at least not as you might define the word *hospital*. It is a place for *Serious Fun*[SM]— to use their own service mark—where seeming opposites like "fun" and "serious" are connected in a greater whole. In the words of their mission statement, it is a place to "reach beyond serious illness and discover joy, confidence, and a new world of possibilities."

This holistic approach benefits campers as well as counselors, each of whom become givers and receivers of loving care. The campers taught the counselors how gratitude can be found in the immeasurably wonderful gift of a new day, learning through the eyes of a child with appreciation for each moment of bliss. I saw how my daughter Melissa was enriched by the experience, along with her campers and fellow counselors, adding value in ways that can't be measured in silver and gold.

Charities have also benefited from the blurring of fictional lines, though in ways that you might not expect. Previously prohibited from commercial arrangements, charities are now pursuing industry and trade and demonstrating admirable business qualities of corporations. The change has been particularly significant at charitable hospitals, with their own needs to be businesslike in a high-cost, high-demand economic environment.

Legal lines and boxes once prohibited charitable *non-profits* from using *for-profit* business techniques to share knowledge and other resources. The law evolved, especially with the financial needs of charitable hospitals, but the landmark American legal case permitting *charities* to partner with *businesses*, using joint venture structures in pursuit of charitable aims was not a hospital—it was a theater. Shakespeare would surely be proud, seeing theaters thriving in business as in art.

In 1977, the Plumstead Theatre Society of Los Angeles, California, needed to raise money for a big show at the prestigious John F. Kennedy Center for the Performing Arts in Washington, DC. The IRS tax commissioner said the theater's for-profit business arrangements violated their narrow nonprofit charitable purpose, so the IRS voided Plumstead's tax-exempt status. A Federal Appeals Court disagreed.[51] Like Shakespeare, the federal court understood that putting on a great performance takes business savvy, moxie, and a little bit of win-win deal-making and monetizing in support of great art.

Relaxation of strict legal prohibitions against charities pursuing commercial arrangements has led to innovations. In health care, for example, groups of physicians now buy new diagnostic equipment and charge hospitals for their use. Unfortunately, it has also led to types of economic conflicts that compromise health and wellness, like drugs being needlessly prescribed to please a pharmaceutical benefactor or medical tests being needlessly ordered to pay for the new machines. William Harvey would not be proud to see charitable medical oaths breached in the name of commerce, though he would understand the value of having this medical equipment for the hospital.

———

Crossing lines of separation can lead to such abuses unless we see through *eyes of wholeness* and feel through *hearts of wellness*.

Learning how to see and feel in this manner may be difficult to comprehend at first, but it is simple. If human beings are capable of balancing traits like *industry* and *economy* alongside *charity* and *empathy* in the pursuit of their own wholeness and wellness, then hospitals and businesses must find such balance as well. Anything less, and we dishonor the unity of the whole.

Too often when the lines fail us, we replace old lines with new lines. *The solution for separation is connection—not more separation!* For example, in the commercialization of hospitals, it would harm the whole to replace an oath of charity with a new oath for profits.

Truly, all of our systems and institutions—not just businesses and hospitals—need to honor our connected wholeness. A good example are military and police forces, which have long recognized that they need to be a force for peace, to protect and serve the whole of a community of which they are a connected part. When separated and unbalanced, they become capable of tyrannical oppression, using their police and military might to wage war on their own people.

When institutions no longer serve the interests of the whole, they lose their very purpose for being. Becoming disconnected from the communities they serve, these institutions can fail us. Consider prisons, where queens and kings once sent some of the "undeserving" poor under the Old Poor Law of 1601. Poor persons categorized as vagrants, beggars, or deadbeat debtors, were sent to prison to supposedly learn about desirable traits of industry, economy, duty, and responsibility. The guiding purpose of these prison institutions was to *rehabilitate*, and in the 1600s, they were called *"Houses of Correction."* Although the "correctional" label may linger on, over time, many prison institutions lost their guiding purpose.

Today it seems that the real purpose of prisons in many places is the physical separation of criminals from communities—*"incarceration"* instead of *"rehabilitation"*—confining prisoners to keep them out of sight, like dirt swept under the rug, as was the purpose of English laws that predated Queen Elizabeth. Today as I write this, the United States of America has the largest total and per capita prison population in the world.

It is a very alarming and deeply disturbing statistic, but whatever it means to us all, someone must tend to those large prison populations. Some states have sought to more efficiently administrate these massive confinements of people by *privatizing* their prisons—selling jails to corporate prison management enterprises. But what does this really mean? Even through eyes of wholeness, *who* is operating the prisons is far less important than *how* they are being operated. We must ask what *purpose* a prison serves.

If, for example, the new corporate owner views its prison investment like owning a hotel or a rental apartment building, then *"no vacancy"* signs are optimal metrics for revenues and profits. Some state governments have guaranteed the corporate jailers high "occupancy" rates for their jails—meaning people will need to be incarcerated simply to keep the prison filled to some agreed-upon contractual capacity.

This guaranteed incarceration may serve the purpose of *"stockholder wealth maximization"* for corporate jailers—but that is more separation for the sake of separation, without serving the whole of a community.

If we see with eyes of wholeness and feel with hearts of wellness, then we need to understand the holistic benefits of prisons for us all. Prisons can protect you, your family, and your community against criminal harm. They can provide meaningful work for both jailers and prisoners. They can teach important lessons, inside as well as outside a prison's barbed-wire fences, about taking good care of others as well as ourselves. Instead of a separated place to discard the unwanted, prisons can be seen as what they truly are—a part of our communities, connected to the whole of us.

Even corporate prison enterprises might be better served by holistic contracts with the state that compensate them based on measured rehabilitation, instead of assured incarceration. Beyond stockholder wealth maximization, all stakeholders—the governments, businesses, communities, jailers, and prisoners—can strive for *personal potential maximization*. That goal helps everyone feel better. It is the way Miss Sullivan helped awaken the potential in a seemingly unreachable Helen Keller, for you can be banished to an institutional asylum to be out of sight, yet not be out of mind.

———

Separation sickens the places we live and the schools where we send our children.

I've spent time working on real estate development projects with architects, builders, land use planners, and municipal officials, each of whom grumble that suburban sprawl has displaced once-vibrant communities. Whether they realize it or not, the root of their complaints is the very land use system they established. Zoning is based upon sharp lines and rigid boxes that physically separate land uses into classifications and categories, like a fictitious Linnaean *Systema Naturae* for neighborhood communities.

There are zones for "residential," "retail," "office," "agriculture," "industrial," and other aspects of human activity; narrowly divided, this zoning destroys the hidden connections of each to the other, stripping the soul from the neighborhood. As the wellness movement accelerates, these separate zones give way to more holistic planning methods, like "traditional neighborhood" designs, yet I've personally observed municipalities and planners still cling reflexively and unthinkingly to their systems of zoned separation, sadly even in my own hometown.

I've also listened to teachers, educational administrators, and parents, who lament that today's children are not interested in education anymore. *How absurd—all children begin their young lives craving learning!* If you don't think that's true, just watch a toddler seek language and information, and then apply his or her newfound knowledge, often through play and art. It is entrenched educational institutions and systems that have themselves separated learning into narrow fields of compartmentalized study—subjects and objects with no apparent connection to one another or to the whole of learning—until education itself becomes meaningless. *Who wants to learn something that is meaningless?*

Instead of holistic connection, some educators and administrators mistakenly believe the solution is more separation, because that's the way we've approached problems since the 1600s. With new boxes reminiscent of an *Old Poor Law*, they separate and objectify children with the linear metrics of new standardized tests, and then they narrow the fields of study to address the supposed learning deficiencies. For example, they concentrate on subjects like *mathematics* and *science* to the exclusion of classes they deem nonessential, like *music* and *athletics* and *humanities*, but they never understand how all of these courses and studies are indivisibly connected, facilitating one another in the unity of the whole.

These well-intentioned but woefully-misguided educators and administrators miss the most important measurement of all—the child's *internal spark* of discovery and creation. Their lines and boxes and statistical metrics cannot possibly measure this spark, for how can you measure the light of learning, love, and life that knows no limits? Recall how Helen Keller described the process of learning, despite her difficulties and disabilities; she said it *"awakened my soul, gave it light, hope, joy, set it free! There were barriers still, it is true, but barriers that could in time be swept away."* Her words are not just empty metaphor or figurative poetry; they describe the boundless way in which we learn.

Teachers who seek to move beyond the lines and boxes to creatively fan the flames of the child's internal spark—like Miss Sullivan did for Helen Keller—are often shamefully rebuked by educational institutions and administrators mistakenly attached to their rigid separations. As the sparks in both teacher and student are slowly extinguished by the system, the motivation to teach and to learn both precipitously decline.

Not surprisingly, without institutions to support this spark, the students who excel are increasingly the self-educated and the home-schooled. It is *despite* the institutional mandates that some students learn in school, often those who are lucky enough to have teachers or parents who inspire through their own love of learning—teachers and parents who often rebelliously defy the lines and boxes imposed on them by the schools and the system.

———

These are but a few examples. Some separations are so deeply embedded in our institutions and systems, so deeply woven into the fabric of thoughts and beliefs, that we become blind to them. We ignore these separations, as if an elephant in the room.

By now, as you read this, many of these separations should be obvious to see. It has been centuries since the start of the Age of

Enlightenment, and generations since the end of the Second World War, so as the wellness movement accelerates in this third millennium, the elephant in the room is becoming clearly visible—no matter how many people and institutions still ignore it or pretend not to notice. Observe what is separated and notice how these lines and boxes harm our wholeness and disturb our wellness.

You may say, *"That's not the way the system works!"* and I know this all too well myself, as a lawyer working within the framework of systems and institutions that are sometimes rigidly separated, dividing people with lines and forcing people into boxes that make absolutely no sense whatsoever. Yes, indeed, you are correct—*that's not the way the system works!*—because the system itself is built on separation.

So fix these institutions! Help lift their broken edifices from their cracked foundations and gradually move them toward wholeness and wellness, transforming them for the benefit of all. Help the people in these institutions and systems finally see with eyes of wholeness, and help them feel with hearts of wellness. Help them see that separation is as separation does. Be connected, for your wholeness will help heal them, as it heals you.

Fixing what's broken in our systems starts with *you*. You may not move these institutions quickly, but gradually you can proactively move *yourself* toward wholeness and the wellness that it brings. Be connected in your own life. You can do that; surely you can.

———

Begin by moving beyond separation and seeking unity and communion in everyday life. Each and every day, treat others—everyone and everything in your environment—with that same unity and communion, even if they do not seem to reciprocate. Life will seem richer, fuller, more meaningful. It will move you toward wellness.

Open your eyes, open your heart, and open your mind, and you will begin to see, feel, and understand things you did not before. Others will begin to see, feel, and understand things they did not before too, moving beyond lines that you helped blur.

If you still believe you cannot see, feel, and understand these things about your connected wholeness, then you are correct—and you may never see, feel, and understand these things. As Henry Ford, the founder of the Ford Motor Company and one of America's great industrialists, once said, *"Whether you think you can or you think you can't— you're right."* How you think and believe is a proactive choice that only you can make.

Believe you can be whole again, and soon you will be. Whether or not you realize it yet, your connected wholeness is already at the heart of who you really are. It may be buried deep within you, obscured by fictional separations that you interpose, like an elephant in the room, but your wholeness is there, at the heart of your wellness. The unity at the center of you may be like the sun hiding behind dark clouds, perhaps offering only a fleeting glimpse of its brilliant and healing light now and again, but the sun is there nonetheless.

Your connected wholeness never left you. It is you who abandoned it, but this unity at your center welcomes you back with open arms, like an errant child returning to a loving parent. Honestly examine the separations in your own life—in your relationships, family, career, worship, business, charities, hobbies, and communities, in your body, mind, heart, and soul—and begin to heal the divisions and dissociations of each of these important aspects of self. Connect each to the other, together, into the unity of who you truly are.

As the wellness movement accelerates, people are increasingly seeing themselves in these connected and holistic ways. Some of this trend is reflected in what I call the *"hyphen"* movement, because of the type of punctuation mark used to string separated sides of self back in wholeness together. In this way, I might be a *lawyer-musician-father-son-husband-uncle-friend-fighter-healer-hiker-cook-teacher-student-entrepreneur-strategist-writer* and so forth. If you are the type of person who defines others or themselves with singularly and similarly narrow lines, then hyphens connecting *what you do* may help move you past one-dimensional job descriptions toward the multidimensional living being of *who you are.*

Whether or how you hyphenate yourself is your choice. Sometimes, I can focus narrowly on a job of being a lawyer or musician or father for instance—but focusing on an important job does not mean *who I am* is limited by *what I do.* As Shakespeare observed in the *Merchant of Venice*, each of us has *"dimensions, senses, affections, passions"*[52] that come together uniquely within each of us. Qualities of self can be applied to jobs you do, so performing a job can become a genuine expression of your wholeness, a source of wonderful fulfillment.

Job descriptions like "lawyer" or "musician" or "father" may seem to have sharp lines and rigid boxes, and others may expect these jobs to be performed in narrow ways. It may seem that each job is separate and apart from the other, but—to borrow more wisdom from Shakespeare—*"though that all at once, my good friends."* Jobs can be disguised opportunities to cultivate all your *"dimensions, senses, affections, passions"* together and apply what you learn in one job to another.

The connection of one job to another cannot be measured by a checkbox of job descriptions. For instance, a checkbox for *lawyer-musician-father* could comically separates the jobs, since I do not play guitar in court nor cite case law in a rock-and-roll band. But that checkbox would not measure how I might use rhythmic and lyrical words to better tell a client's story and impart meaning to a judge, nor how I might bring skills of legal structure, organization, and collaboration to play and practice songs in a garage with band mates. Changing diapers on a baby and raising children to adulthood may seem to have nothing to do with either music or law, but the patience and commitment cultivated as a parent should be applicable to both.

Of course, some people will continue to treat me in shallow and objectifying ways, perceiving me only as a *lawyer* or *musician* or *father,* defining my personality and essence with the stereotyped sameness of those job descriptions. Those lines prevent them from seeing me, and although I hope I can help them blur or erase some of the lines they project onto me, I refuse to limit myself based on their inability to see me. I strive to bring everything *I am* into everything *I do,* communing in an indivisible unity that connects me to *myself* and to *my universe.*

For a moment, think about the many sides of *you* connected within *you* that connect you to your *universe.* The very word *universe* was coined in the early Renaissance, back in the 1300s, from *uni* ("one") and *verse* ("to turn"). As you *turn to the unity of one,* exercising and balancing all of these diverse sides of yourself in all you do, you will begin to feel a great personal renaissance occur within you. You may not have the unique gifts of the quintessential Renaissance man, Leonardo da Vinci of Italy (and then France) as *artist-engineer-mathematician-musician-anatomist-geologist-botanist-inventor-writer-teacher-and so much more,* but you have your own multifaceted dimensions, senses, affections, and passions in combinations and extents unique to *you.*

Connect sides within yourself, and connect them altogether to your own universe. Even if you don't think you can become a Renaissance person like da Vinci, balancing and pursuing your many dimensions of self has wonderful benefits—like experiencing *wonder!* As lessons learned in one pursuit are applied to other activities, you will experience the childlike joy that comes from opening windows of insight and doors of perception across your universe.

———

You may believe that narrowly focused one-dimensional specialization leads to greater mastery and understanding than broad, interdisciplinary, multidimensional focus, but I'd bet Leonardo da Vinci would disagree. I know I do.

What's truly remarkable about da Vinci is how he applied what he learned in one field of study into others. A popular Internet poll voted Leonardo the people's number-one genius of all time, perhaps because of the breadth of his talents. He integrated mathematical engineering into human anatomy and turned the natural flight of birds into the invention of a flying machine. He studied facial muscles used in emotional expression to capture the mystery of a smile on his artist's canvas and mixed his paints with uncanny knowledge of chemistry to produce his distinctive *"sfumato"* painting style.

Leonardo described his sfumato style, seen in his iconic painting of the *Mona Lisa*, as being *"without lines or borders, in the manner of smoke."*[53] Like da Vinci's genius, his painting style was limitless, unbounded, and infinite. The same might be said of the way Leonardo opened his eyes, his heart, and his mind to see the essential unity of all things. Even an ordinary day spent observing the movement of wildflowers led Leonardo to sketches with stunning detail that both artists and scientists could admire. In da Vinci, art and science came together as one, indivisible and inseparable.

He lived from 1452 to 1519, many generations before the Enlightenment of the 1600s and 1700s, with its narrow separations, lines, and boxes. In the Renaissance of the 1300s to 1500s, Leonardo da Vinci's approach of connecting what he learned into a greater whole—instead of narrowly separating and dividing—was not unusual. Other great thinkers of the Renaissance shared similar belief in the unity of all knowledge.

Among the greatest of these broad, interdisciplinary Renaissance minds was Nicolaus Copernicus, who historian Arthur Schlesinger ranked as number four on his list of the most influential people of the second millennium. You may think of Copernicus as an astronomer who pioneered the then-radical notion that Earth revolved around the sun, but he was a true Renaissance man, with broad focus across many fields of study. Born in Polish Prussia in 1473 and dying there in 1543, Copernicus obtained a doctorate in religious law and had a successful career as a diplomat and administrative official. He was an accomplished painter, known to future generations by his own self-portrait, and was also a physician, mathematician, and economist who pioneered the understanding that the supply of a currency affects consumer prices; his "quantity theory of money" is still used by monetarist economists today. Despite his seemingly diffuse and peripatetic focus, Nicolaus Copernicus distinguished himself in almost all he attempted.

Or consider Johannes Gutenberg, who lived from 1398 to 1468, and was number nine on Schlesinger's list. By applying technologies from different fields—metalworking, the chemistry of oil-based inks, publishing, and agricultural screw-press machinery—Gutenberg created a printing press with movable typeset, forever changing the way information can be shared. Quite simply, if Johannes Gutenberg saw knowledge as divided into narrow fields for specialized focus only, then he never would have invented the printing press, as he did, by connecting diverse fields of knowledge together into one.

The Renaissance examples of da Vinci, Copernicus, and Gutenberg may seem extraordinary, but they are neither unusual nor exceptions to a rule. It would be a mistake to assume that scientific (or artistic!) advancement comes only from specialization, which is to say along specific lines of separation. To be sure, narrow focus and circumscribed study can lead to great competencies—that was true even for these Renaissance geniuses committing their time to study and mastery—but without connection, competency can be little more than *"mopping up operations"* (to borrow Thomas Kuhn's terminology).

Competency is an important goal in and of itself, but it is important to remember that notions of "competency" change over time. Competent physicians treated my grandfather William for his stomach ulcer back in the early 1960s, yet today, a surgical approach to a simple stomach ulcer would not be deemed competent. Many of today's standards for competency certainly will be seen as outdated and incompetent tomorrow, whether we like that or not. No, it is not the competency of specialization that allows Renaissance greats like da Vinci, Copernicus, and Gutenberg to withstand the test of time, continuing to influence and inspire us today.

Creative breakthroughs like theirs require us to gaze towards the infinite, and perceive its unlimited unity. At least that's my observation, in a career of representing and promoting entrepreneurs and artists over more than a quarter century. The most amazing inventions and innovations occur as the insights of one field of study are applied and connected to another. That seems as true today as it was during the Renaissance.

As the end of this chapter draws near, take a moment to ask yourself whether you see through a lens of narrow separation, or do you see with eyes of wholeness?

Be honest, and accept that the question of *how you see* is neither rhetorical nor metaphysical. The question is literal, as it is practical. Changing the perception of *how you see* truly changes *what you see*, and it changes *what you feel* too. If you wish to see with eyes of wholeness, then begin by opening your eyes and your heart.

See as if you were a child, with all of an inquisitive child's joy and wonder of discovery, searching for the hidden connections of knowledge. You can be old or ill or infirm, but you can still see and feel this indivisible unity that is at the heart of your own wellness.

That is really the heart of the matter, and as a final story for this chapter, look again at the motion of the heart. It may seem like a metaphor to say—as I said earlier in this chapter—that playwright William Shakespeare understood more about the complexion of our beating heart than physician William Harvey, but in actuality, can we learn more about the medical anatomy of our hearts by visualizing our connected wholeness than by seeing the heart through the narrow lens of separation alone?

You may recall how Dr. William Harvey—that most enlightened physician of the Enlightenment—steadfastly believed *"it would be proper to look more narrowly into the matter, to contemplate the motion of the heart and arteries."* His Enlightenment approach was to focus *"the light we have made to shine"* in *"order that what is true may be confirmed, and what is false set right"* by dissecting, inspecting, detecting, and selecting anatomical lines and borders.

You may not know this, but Leonardo da Vinci—Renaissance genius of connected thinking, painter of the *Mona Lisa*—contemplated the anatomical motion of the heart and arteries too, but he used an entirely different underlying approach than William Harvey. In visualizing the whole, da Vinci observed *"without lines or borders."* Seeing with Leonardo's eyes of wholeness may seem metaphorical, even beautiful in its *sfumato* style, but what did this connected approach mean for da Vinci's anatomical study of the heart?

Unlike Dr. Harvey, Leonardo was not formally trained in medicine, but he was similarly devoted to discovering the *truth* of the heart, so Leonardo passionately pursued all modes of self-education and all methods of observation—including anatomical dissection. Da Vinci personally dissected a wide range of human cadavers, at first illegally with the bodies of deceased prisoners delivered to him by grave robbers, but eventually with the sanctioned and collaborative assistance of hospitals and physicians throughout his native Italy. Leonardo da Vinci also did comparative dissections and investigations of animals, as did Dr. Harvey, although da Vinci never confined his comparisons to the anatomical.

With vivid artistic detail, Leonardo sketched and described what he learned about the heart and its motions in his journals and notebooks. He did not confine his thoughts and observations to what we might today call "scientific" or "medical" observations. As Leonardo explained in his notebook, in what would later be assembled into da Vinci's Treatise on Painting: *"A good painter has two chief objects to paint, man and the intention of his soul; the former is easy, the latter hard, because he has to represent it by the attitudes and movements of the limbs...The most important consideration in painting is that the movements of each figure expresses its mental state, such as desire, scorn, anger, pity, and the like."*[54] In one famous series of his sketches, he compared anger, as manifested in the snarling expressions of horses, birds, lions, and humans.

Leonardo understood that there are some things—like mental state and the intentions of the soul—that cannot be observed with dissection, vivisection, or narrow separation alone. He knew too that there were other things that could not be observed by surgically slicing the heart open. As one obvious example, the natural flow patterns of blood through the chambers of the heart cannot be revealed with dissection; clearly, the cut of a knife dramatically disturbs the internal motion of blood within the heart. To a medical mind focused solely on surgical separation, discovering how blood moves through the heart may seem like an intractable and insoluble problem.

But da Vinci thought holistically about this problem, and searched for hidden connections between vessel and fluid. Using the tools of a sculptor, he made a plaster mold of a bull's heart to see its contours and shapes, to view it as a vessel for holding the bull's blood. He observed how the blood vessels of the body bore a striking physical resemblance to the veins on the leaf of a tree or the arteries of a living river, and he saw recurring patterns in each of these natural flows, concluding that fluids must flow in comparable ways in each of these vessels, much like the way he saw anger was manifested similarly among different species.

Observing how the water along the river's shore flowed much slower than the water in the center of the watercourse, he realized how it should be that way too with blood flowing through the heart. Returning to the shape of the heart and its chambers, Leonardo visualized its swirling and pulsing flows and built glass models to test his ideas about form and function, and how vessel merges with fluid— *without lines or borders*, as da Vinci said, *sfumato* style.

Leonardo da Vinci also observed how the shapes of blood vessels changed over time. He wrote how changes in health were because of the change of shape of the vessel and how these changes in shape affected the flow of the blood, describing how blood vessels thickened by age and infirmity can cause heart attacks. In the way that all knowledge was unified to Leonardo, with everything connected to everything else, he wrote how *"vessels act in man as in oranges, in which the peel becomes thicker and the pulp diminishes the more they become old."*[55] Such a simple metaphor for what is now known medically as atherosclerosis!

Leonardo da Vinci made all of these observations about the heart and its vessels in a stunningly brief timespan, in the years between 1508 and 1513. Some da Vinci scholars estimate that as much as three-quarters of all Leonardo's journal entries on the functions of the heart were lost or destroyed as his notebooks were separated, disassembled, and rearranged for publication. We can only imagine what other amazing insights da Vinci had regarding the heart and its motions that were lost forever.

———

Whatever Leonardo da Vinci may have written and discovered about the heart and its motion, he did it more than one hundred years before William Harvey published *An Anatomical Exercise on the Motion of the Heart and Blood in Living Beings* in 1628.

This was the seminal treatise that catapulted Dr. Harvey to number ten on Schlesinger's most influential list and displaced Leonardo's beautifully artistic anatomical illustrations of the heart from standard medical school textbooks. For much the same reason, da Vinci is not on Arthur Schlesinger's "top ten" list of the most influential persons of the second millennium. Over time, Leonardo da Vinci's holistic Renaissance methods were seen as good for artistic creation but discredited as unscientific by the "normal scientists" adopting William Harvey's Enlightenment approach of narrow separation and specialization.

These "normal scientists" told us that science could not be art, and that art could not be science, and that only what could be separately measured mattered in the final analysis. Throughout the last half of the second millennium, these normal scientists used Dr. Harvey's narrowly precise diagrams of the heart, not da Vinci's holistically vivid illustrations, in medical schools and on surgical tables.

What has become clear, however, in this third millennium is that Leonardo da Vinci was able to understand things about the motion of the heart—its actual medical anatomy—that Dr. William Harvey did not understand. It turns out these normal scientists of the second millennium, with their narrow separations, were woefully wrong to treat Leonardo's holistic knowledge and wisdom derisively, as little more than the pretty pictures of a Renaissance artist that predated "real" scientific advancement.

As the story was told in an international science journal in 2002[56], by applying the revolutionary new technology of magnetic resonance imaging (MRI) to the motion of the heart, it was finally revealed that blood flowed through the heart *almost exactly* as Leonardo da Vinci said it did. The in vivo MRI images of a beating heart showed the twists and turns of the blood's current, including the formation of vortices in the aorta, that Leonardo had sketched and described in stunning detail. The journal article was entitled "Leonardo's Vision of Flow Visualization," and its authors were a group of distinguished professors with specialties in biology, engineering, mechanics, aeronautics, and art history, associated with world-class universities like California Institute of Technology, Michigan State University, and the University of Oxford. They concluded how "Even our present in-vivo MRI techniques cannot give as much detail as was routinely drawn by Leonardo." The authors described Leonardo's accounts as "remarkable" and noted that *"perhaps the most important finding in his observations is the identification of vortex formation...as a mechanism for the [aortic] valve's closure."*

In other words, Leonardo da Vinci understood how the aortic valve opened and closed *nearly five hundred years before "normal" science could understand the same thing!* In the absence of scientific tools like an MRI, the authors wondered aloud how Leonardo could have known these things about the heart. With cross-disciplinary understanding, these scholars—M. Gharib, D. Kremers, M. M. Koochesfahani, M. Kemp, and M. Zarandi—acknowledged how "Leonardo would not have recognized our contemporary opposition of art and science...in the unity of knowledge sought in the Middle Ages and the Renaissance"; they marveled how Leonardo "knew the power of visualization to be instrumental in depicting knowledge."

What they were really saying is that da Vinci opened his eyes wholly, connecting art and science and all the branches of knowledge to reveal the secrets of the heart.

A few years after this 2002 science journal article appeared, it was reported by the BBC News that a prominent British cardiac surgeon named Francis Wells was using Leonardo da Vinci's visionary drawings and insights to pioneer a new procedure for the repair of another of the heart's four valves, the mitral valve. "It's a complete rethink of the way we do the mitral valve operation," Dr. Wells explained. "What Leonardo was saying about the shape of the valve is important. It means that we can repair this valve in a better way."[57] With proven success in eighty patients, Dr. Wells told the BBC News in 2005 that he was looking at many of Leonardo's other drawings of the body to see if they might similarly help medicine now.

———

There are many ways of describing this holistic way of thinking, learning, and creating, as practiced by Leonardo da Vinci and Dr. Francis Wells. The 1970s catchphrase *"thinking outside the box"* is one description, as is the *"hyphen"* approach connecting job descriptions together to indicate the wholeness of each and every person.

Holism acknowledges that the branches of knowledge, whether art or science, are really part of the same tree. Studying each branch separately can never explain the whole tree nor does it provide a true understanding of a single branch either. To extend the metaphor further, holism requires that we see *the whole of the forest through the trees.* That is an old proverb and this has been a long chapter, but being connected is really as simple as understanding the wisdom of what connects the forest through its trees.

So, what connects the trees into a forest? You can narrowly dissect the forest, grouping and cataloging its parts into stands and glades and canopies, yet still not see the whole of the forest. You can wander through the forest, diligently examining what you believe to be its separate parts, for days or weeks or centuries, and still not see how the trees connect together.

The more you think about it, the connections of the forest may seem a complex and mysterious construct. Having difficulty explaining the connection, it is then tempting to take the connection for granted or relegate its study to some arcane branch of knowledge like linguistics or semiotics or ecology. Eventually you may lose sight of the connections of the forest altogether, ignoring the connections until they become an elephant in the room. On some level, you still know the connection is there, but you pretend not to notice, or turn a blind eye, or refuse to address its meaning.

Observe the forest with eyes of wholeness, and you will see the connection of the forest, and even the connection of the elephant to the forest. You will see the connection of the elephants to one another and of the elephants to humans. You will see the connection of me to you and all of us to one another. You will see connections of even a single butterfly to the forest, and to the weather, and to all of humanity.

Today that is well known as "the butterfly effect"—a term first coined by MIT Professor Edward Lorenz, a *mathematician-meteorologist-outdoorsman-family man-chaos theory pioneer*, based on a short science fiction story by the self-educated *writer-reader-family man-philosopher-futurist-Pulitzer and National Medal recipient* Ray Bradbury. Indeed, the connections predicted by the butterfly effect are not new. Many centuries ago, Leonardo da Vinci said the exact same thing, describing how *"The earth is moved from its position by the weight of a tiny bird resting upon it."*[58] Whether butterfly, bird, or however else Linné may have classified an illusory species line, it is a phenomenal effect, akin to a single flap of an invisible wing transforming everything.

This question of what connects everything to everything else, like a forest through the trees, may still seem complex. It may seem like *"a riddle, wrapped in a mystery, inside an enigma,"* as Sir Winston Churchill once quipped in a BBC broadcast—before he famously added, *"but perhaps there is a key."*[59]

Indeed, if you are willing to look, that key—or dimension, as I prefer to describe it—to what connects everything holistically together is really quite simple, even if taboo to talk about.

Chapter 11

BELIEF

When I was a young child with an aching belly, some medical doctors, unable to pinpoint the source of my discomfort to a dairy allergy, called my illness *psychosomatic*.

They said this strange new word to my parents as I listened quietly and politely to their adult conversation, my hands folded anxiously in my lap. Though I was just seven years old at the time, I can still remember the tone with which they said it. Like a musical tone, a word's inflections and timbre can resonate in memory for a long, long time.

Tone, like other subtle cues and manners—a gesture of the hand, a shrug of the shoulders, an expression on the face, the glance of an eye—can belie the words we use, transforming words of affectionate approval into words of contemptuous scorn. Children try to understand the *true meaning* of these subtle cues, much like Leonardo da Vinci knew how the wry smile of the *Mona Lisa* made us wonder, in Leonardo's own words, about the "intention" of her "soul."[1]

These physicians said this word *psychosomatic* with a tone of derision, and it seemed a stinging insult hurled at a seven-year-old who had unintentionally stumped them from a diagnosis in their medical name game. It felt like these doctors belittled my stomachaches by blaming me. I also remember how they paused for a long while after they used this new word, and that pause lingers in my memory too, the way the ear is drawn to the quiet rest between musical notes of a song.[2] After the pause these doctors explained to my parents, in hushed tones as if children cannot comprehend, that sometimes sickness was *"in the mind"* even though real physical symptoms appeared *"in the body."*

This suggestion, that my mind could produce symptoms of disease in my body, resonated with me even as a seven-year-old, but probably not in the way that the doctors intended.

Resonance is the ability to evoke a sympathetic response. In music, it's why a note played on a piano can make the identical note vibrate on a guitar string from clear across the room. It's why a skilled singer, like jazz great Ella Fitzgerald, can make a wineglass vibrate to a specific note, sometimes until the glass shatters in response. There is a common frequency between musical notes or between the singer's voice and the wineglass, and common frequencies vibrate at the same rate—they *resonate* with one another.[3]

The scientific principle of resonance applies to magnetics, and physicists tell us that all matter—even a wineglass—has signature frequencies vibrating at the molecular level. This basic principle is at work in in vivo magnetic resonance imaging (MRI), which, as explained in the previous chapter, scientists in 2002 used to confirm the vortex motion of blood through the heart as envisioned by Leonardo da Vinci nearly five hundred years earlier.

Resonance works for thoughts and feelings too; some thoughts and feelings trigger resonant thoughts and feelings like empathy or harmony. Simply said, they ring true. By contrast, thoughts or feelings that do not resonate with you trigger no such sympathetic response and may seem empty or false.

Looking back, I wonder what response these childhood medical doctors wanted to cause with their *"psychosomatic"* diagnosis. Medical science tries to isolate cause and effect so it can diagnose and treat. For example, if physicians had isolated the cause of my childhood tummyaches to a dairy allergy, they could have advised me to stop eating dairy foods, effectively stopping the ache. So what effect were these childhood physicians seeking by telling my parents—with me in the room—that my painful bellyaches were all in my mind?

What did their diagnosis really mean at its heart? Were they trying to uplift my spirits with news that there were no physical causes, were they trying to break my spirit with their tone of disdain, or did they ignore my spirit altogether? Did they believe it was a case of hypochondria, a need to complain about irrational fears, and that their diagnosis would eliminate the complaint? Were they prodding my parents to seek treatment for my presumed mental condition? Or were these New York City doctors just New York City sports fans, who believed health was much like baseball as described by Hall of Fame Yankee catcher Yogi Berra: *"Ninety percent of the game is half mental."*

Whatever the reasons for their "psychosomatic" diagnosis, what is clear to me now is how *the words we use* and *the way we use them* are very powerful. Words cause responses we do not intend and often do not cause the responses we intended.

I remember the response I felt to the doctors' psychosomatic suggestion. It resonated *false* from the start, contrary to some innate feeling deep in my heart and down in my gut that there was a physical cause of my stomachaches yet to be discovered. I also remember what resonated *true* to me, then as now. It was the suggestion of the mind's incredible power to make our bodies feel sick or well, to both harm or heal, and that any sharp separation between mind and body was merely an illusion.

———

Physicians sometimes use the word *placebo* to describe a healing cure that is initiated by the mind, without the benefit of *"real"* medicine. In a common example of the placebo effect, a patient is given a sugar pill, but the patient believes he or she is taking a drug of medicinal value. Coaxed by the patient's belief in the doctor's prescription, the patient is healed, and the disease is cured by a *"dummy"* pill—as physicians sometimes call it.

This is not an abnormal or unusual occurrence. The placebo response is routinely said to account for 35 percent—*more than a third!*—of all cures attributed to pharmaceutical medicines. Depending on the type of ailment or the particular clinical trial, that number has been estimated to be much higher, *sometimes more than two-thirds* of all positive results from medicines.

Placebo responses can seem amazing or even miraculous. During World War II, a nurse gave an injection of saltwater to a wounded American soldier, telling the soldier that he was being given morphine to ease his pain, even though no morphine was available to treat the soldier. The placebo of the dummy injection not only relieved the soldier's pain but it somehow prevented the onset of shock from his wounds.

The placebo's battlefield success fascinated the US Army anesthesiologist on duty, Dr. Henry Knowles Beecher; after the war ended, Dr. Beecher researched and wrote a scholarly article on the phenomenon he had witnessed firsthand in wartime. The article was entitled *"The Powerful Placebo,"* and it was published in 1955 in the distinguished *Journal of the American Medical Association.*[4] The article created quite a stir in the medical community, although perhaps not for the reasons you might expect.

The placebo response had been known and well-documented for centuries, but when Dr. Beecher published his article in 1955, American medical authorities routinely trivialized what they could not explain with current science—whether it was the placebo response that relieved a wounded soldier's pain, the *"psychosomatic"* illness that some of my childhood doctors blamed for my stomachaches, or any other mind-body anomaly. Indeed, many of Beecher's colleagues dismissively believed that patients who could be fooled into healing by a placebo were of gullibly low intelligence, mostly female, and not worthy of study. Dr. Beecher debunked that particular myth in his review of the clinical studies, concluding *"[w]e found that there were no differences in sex ratios or intelligence"* between those who reacted to placebos and those who did not.[5]

Henry Knowles Beecher anticipated that his medical colleagues would be skeptical, so he underscored the message that the placebo's *"high degree of therapeutic effectiveness"* was applicable to a *"wide variety"* of ailments. Over and over again in his journal article, Dr. Beecher used words like *"remarkable," "beneficial," "real,"* and *"powerful"* to describe the placebo response. He meticulously detailed the mathematical results of each clinical study, demonstrating that the placebo was true science and not the work of *"quacks."*

"The important point here," Beecher emphasized, *"is that in each of these representative studies, patients and observers alike, working with unknowns (usually 'double blind' technique) have concluded that a real therapeutic effect has occurred."*[6] Despite the scientific data, many in the medical community were not persuaded, so Dr. Beecher spoke directly to these skeptics, using the scientific technique of rational logic. "If, against all the evidence to the contrary, one were to hold the view that placebo is a feeble or useless therapeutic agent," he reasoned, "then the placebo should appear most effective when the test condition is mild...and less effective when pitted against severe conditions."[7] Beecher showed these skeptics that clinically "just the opposite is the case: placebos are most effective when the stress (anxiety or pain, for example) is greatest."[7]

To many readers today, even highly educated physicians, the ability of the mind to heal the body is now simple and obvious. If attitudes have changed about this mind-body connection since Dr. Beecher first wrote about the placebo effect, changing the very tone of the discussion, that is just proof of the great distance we have already traveled during decades of the accelerating wellness movement.

However, when Dr. Beecher wrote his groundbreaking article on the placebo response in 1955, this mind-body connection and the notion of our essential wholeness were routinely mocked. It was four years before Dr. Dunn coined the word *wellness* and nearly four decades before the investigative journalist Bill Moyers broadcast his influential television series in 1993 entitled *"Healing and the Mind"*—a Public Broadcasting Service (PBS) series that many observers credit as forever blurring the line between mind and body, slowly opening the eyes of even serious scientists in America.

Many eyes are still closed today, though, refusing to see what should have been obvious all along. Indeed, lines drawn over centuries are not easily blurred, much less erased altogether.

———

The line between our bodies and our minds can be traced to another mistaken separation from the Age of Enlightenment.

René Descartes of France drew this imaginary line many centuries ago. Descartes was an intellectual giant who wrote his *Discourse on the Method of Rightly Conducting the Reason, and Seeking Truth in Sciences* in 1637. As his book's title suggests, Descartes believed that *"sciences"* held the key to *"truth,"* and his goal was to develop better tools of *"reason"* and a better *"method"* of scientific proof.

For truth-seekers of the early Enlightenment, Galileo already had convincingly demonstrated how *"truth"* could be revealed through *"sciences"*—but only if you used the right tools and the right method. Using the tool of a telescope and the method of mathematics, Galileo proved the *truth* that Earth revolved around the sun. Of course, the *truth* was not any less true before Galileo's discovery—Earth always revolved around the sun whether we understood it or not—but the right tools and the right method made proof of the *truth* possible.

Just a few years before Descartes wrote his *Discourse*, Galileo was accused of heresy and subjected to the trials and tribulations of the Inquisition for not adhering to religious orthodoxy as the sole source of *truth*. Galileo's ordeal of 1633 frightened Descartes enough to delay publication of his *Discourse* until he was persuaded that he was safe from the Inquisition by living in the more tolerant Netherlands. Once published, though, Descartes's *Discourse* became a seminal work of the Enlightenment, revered by scientists and scholars as the foundational philosophy of the scientific method.

According to the celebrated method of Descartes, everything not "proven" through scientific investigation must be skeptically doubted and disbelieved. Where dogmatic religious orthodoxy once reigned supreme in seeking *truth*, now hyperbolic doubt ruled! Descartes established *"doubt"* as the linchpin of the scientific *Method of Rightly Conducting the Reason*. It was an amazing and game-changing accomplishment, providing a philosophical method for scientific advancement.[8]

In addition to his new *Method*, René Descartes also gave science new mathematical tools. He invented Cartesian coordinate geometry—"Cartesian" being a Latinized form of his name "Descartes"—which allowed scientists to mathematically analyze and compare their observed data as points and lines on a page. Descartes stated his reason for developing this geometry in Part Two of his Discourse on the Method: "For I saw that although they [rational scientists] deal with different objects they are alike in considering nothing but the various relations or proportions that hold between these objects, and I thought it would be better to study only these proportions taken generally... Next I observed that in order to know these proportions I would need sometimes to consider them separately...this led me to think that *in order the better to consider them separately I should take them to be proportions between lines, because I didn't find anything simpler... "⁹*

Cartesian coordinate geometry was an amazing breakthrough for scientific proof and the method of logical reasoning and is still commonly used today. For instance, physicians analyzing clinical health data still *"prove"* their *"points"* by plotting data into *"lines"* drawn along a familiar x and y coordinate axis for measurement and observation on a chart or graph. Proof is still routinely, customarily, and habitually presented in this chart and graph format today in both science (and law!).

However—as Descartes himself acknowledged—his new mathematical tool had one huge and profound limitation. Data can only be plotted as points on a line of a graph if—and only if—the data can be properly quantified. However, there are some important variables of life, health, and medicine (and law!) that are not measurable that way. Unlike the anatomy of our physical bodies, for example, how can you "quantify" the qualities of the mind—its thoughts, ideas, feelings, hopes, dreams, and inspirations? How can you "prove" as a "point" the type of love and wellness that can only be felt deep in our souls?

These intangible but essential aspects of human beings were not capable of being mathematically plotted on a graph or chart. As Descartes wrote, *"[T]here is a great difference between the mind and the body...inasmuch as the body is by its very nature always divisible, while the mind is utterly indivisible."*¹⁰ Reconciling the quantifiable body with the unquantifiable mind was a huge problem for a method of reason that insisted scientists doubt and disbelieve what they could not physically measure and observe.

Remarkably, René Descartes thought he found a workable solution to this foundational quandary of science. His solution was to use the same enlightened approach of his peers—the method of Galileo, William Harvey, and so many other great minds of the early 1600s; he separated, divided, and drew ever-narrower lines. In other words, using the Enlightenment tool of sharp dissection, Descartes separated mind from matter, detached body from soul, removed *finite* from *infinite*, as if one could be disconnected and divided from the other.

His approach became known as the "mind-body duality," and his stark separation of these two realms influenced the institutions of science and medicine for centuries to come. Scientists and physicians discarded from the equation what could not be calculated and measured, like mind and soul and belief.

As the wellness movement accelerated at the end of the second millennium, these old lines of separate dualities begin to blur. We began to understand how mind, matter, body, soul, *finite*, and *infinite* are all connected together in holistic unity. Ironically, erasing these erroneous lines of the Enlightenment leads not just to greater health and wellness but to a newer and more enlightened Age of Awareness. Erasing these lines, we get closer to *truth in sciences*—the main objective of Descartes and all the other scientific stars of the Enlightenment in the 1600s and 1700s.

Science may still pretend these centuries-old lines exist. We may similarly cling to these fictional lines for purposes of convenience, convention, denial, or delusion. We may even make the lines seem real with the incredible power of our minds—for even when available data contradicts our beliefs, our incredible minds can create illusions supporting these beliefs. Clinging to our illusions, we can shunt to the side "anomalies" too inconvenient to explain, and ignore the obvious like an elephant in the room.

———

René Descartes clung to his illusions too, even as the available data told a different story.

Committed to proving his dualistic division between physical and spiritual, René Descartes made pointed arguments to prove he was right, even as problems with his separation became obvious—the need to prove you are right is a form of delusion that has no place in wellness. Descartes himself acknowledged four logical dilemmas in rationally proving his sharp separation of body from soul, mind from matter.

First, he asked, how can you prove mind, soul, spirit, God—or whatever you call these metaphysical or nonphysical forces—exists? Descartes immediately realized that these immeasurable aspects of who we are, these unquantifiable aspects of self and the universe beyond, could not be proven with his *Method of Rightly Conducting the Reason.*

Since his scientific method required hyperbolic doubt of all that could not be observed and measured, Descartes was forced to ask whether these metaphysical and nonphysical forces existed at all? Eventually, a hundred years or so after Descartes, some scientists and philosophers would deny the existence of these immeasurable forces altogether for lack of scientific proof, but surprisingly, René Descartes never did.

Indeed, for Descartes, there was no greater *truth* than these invisible, indivisible, and *infinite* forces. It was merely a logical dilemma in proving the obvious, so Descartes urged the readers of his *Discourse on the Method* to move beyond scientific reason and use their imagination instead. "Why are many people convinced that there is some difficulty in knowing God, and even in knowing what their soul is?" he asked in Part Four of his Discourse, answering: "It's because they never raise their minds above things that can be perceived by the senses; they are so used to thinking of things only in the way that is specially suited to material things…that they regard as unintelligible or unthinkable anything that they can't imagine."[11]

"I looked carefully into *what* I was," Descartes continued, and "I saw that while I could pretend that I had no body…I still couldn't pretend that I didn't exist…This taught me that I was a substance whose whole essence or nature is simply to think, and which doesn't need any *place*, or depend on any *material thing*, in order to exist."[12]

Descartes concluded that this "essence or nature" of himself was thinking, summed up in his iconic philosophy of *"I think, therefore I am."* He could not deny his glorious inner life of thoughts and feelings, though separated from his body and immeasurable. To Descartes, that inner life was beyond doubt, for "this soul that makes me what I am—is entirely distinct from the body" and the soul "is easier to know than the body, and would still be just what it is even if the body didn't exist."[13]

To those who still doubted him because this inner life lacked observable scientific proof, his belief was unwavering. "Finally, if you are still not really convinced of the existence of God and of your soul by the arguments I have presented," Descartes defiantly responded, then "I tell you this: everything else of which you may think you are more sure—such as having a body, there being stars and an earth, and the like—is less certain."[14] He knew that this leap of faith presented a quandary for believers of his scientific method of reason, but Descartes was unbowed.

"I have always stuck by my resolve not to assume any principles except the one I have just used to demonstrate the existence of God and of the soul," he said, "and not to accept anything as true unless it struck me as more open and more certain than the demonstration of the geometry [I invented]."[14] That was his final proof, but his readers might rightly ask: *How could he be so sure?*

Ironically, for René Descartes, inventor of coordinate geometry, articulator of a *Method of Reason*, seeker of *Truth in Sciences*, proof did not come from scientific measurement—but from a dream! On the night of November 10–11, 1619, while convalescing as a young soldier in the German city of Ulm—the birthplace of Albert Einstein— Descartes had a series of three visionary dreams that he openly credited as the *revelation* for his scientific method of reason.[16] It was a miraculous moment, and Descartes believed throughout his life it was brought to him by a divine spirit.

Whatever you believe was the source of his inspiration—whether divinity or imagination—what is clear is that these dreams forever changed René Descartes and the direction of his life. It is also clear that, in turn, these dreams forever changed history. The scientific method his dreams revealed became the standard for science, medicine, law, and many other areas of rational thought, all using the linear geometry of charts and graphs Descartes invented.

———

Descartes's second dilemma in separating body and soul was the question of how they came together. Despite his separation of mind and matter into different realms, he knew that somehow they still must be joined in "union, on which depends our notion of the soul's power to move the body, and the body's power to act on the soul and cause its sensations and passions."[17] In other words, there was still a connection, but where?

"[O]n carefully examining the matter," Descartes wrote, "I think I have clearly established that the part of the body in which the soul directly exercises its functions [on the body] is…a certain very small gland situated in the middle of the brain…The slightest movements on the part of this gland may alter very greatly the course of these spirits…"[18] This small gland deep in the brain was known as the *"pineal"* for its pinecone shape, and Descartes called it the *"seat of the soul."*

His ideas were not original; similar beliefs about the pineal gland were prevalent in the ancient world, in civilizations as diverse as Babylonia, Egypt, Mexico, the Orient, and the Vatican. The pineal was celebrated by ancients for its supposed ability to view the nonmaterial world through dreams, premonitions, and all manner of psychic, psychedelic, mystical, creative, soulful, and spiritual visions. It was sometimes portrayed in ancient art and writings as a third eye, a pine-coned pinnacle of rising kundalini-entwined energies, or the place where the soul rises from the body to connect with the wisdom of the *Infinite*.

This description of the pineal gland in religious, mystical, symbolic, and esoteric traditions was also found in the medical literature of the ancient world, including the treatises of Galen of Pergamon. Galen was a Greek physician who became Roman Emperor Marcus Aurelius's personal physician. A prolific medical writer whose works influenced medicine for more than fifteen hundred years, Galen's writings contained lively debates about the gland's spiritual functions. Though unsure himself about the pineal's true functions, Galen believed that spirit consists of an airy, vaporous substance that he called *"psychic pneuma."*

Even before modern scientific tools and the scientific methodology of doubt, Renaissance physicians Niccolò Massa of Italy and Andreas Vesalius of Belgium anatomically dissected the pineal and vessels connected to it, discovering that it contained bodily fluids, not the vaporous "psychic pneuma" believed by Galen. Despite this evidence to the contrary, Descartes conducted his own investigations through dissection, mostly on sheep, and concurred with Galen's ancient observations; he wrote that psychic pneuma—which Descartes renamed *"animal spirits"*—was "like a very subtle wind, or rather a very pure and vivid flame which, continually ascending in great abundance from the heart to the brain, then penetrates through the nerves into the muscles, and gives motion to all the members."[19]

New scientific tools are developed all the time, so Descartes's description of how "animal spirits" acted upon the pineal gland might have benefited from better tools of observation, like today's high-resolution microscopes.

You may be surprised to learn that these modern tools confirm the presence of "photoreceptor cells" in the pineal gland. [20] These photoreceptor cells in the pineal gland are remarkably similar to photoreceptor cells found in the eyes. If Descartes was correct and the pineal is where body connects to soul, then the presence of photoreceptor cells in the pineal begs the curious question of why it would need to capture light, since this gland is located deep within the brain, nowhere near sources of external light.

The answer might be found in the holistic way that *form predicts function*. Just as Leonardo da Vinci used this method of perception to correctly predict the vortex flows of blood in the heart's aorta and the shape of the heart's valves, understanding the form and function of the pineal gland may be as simple as realizing that our ability to *"envision"* and gain *"insight"* may depend on these photoreceptor cells. Perhaps they capture the sensations of internal light to allow internal vision in the same way the eye's photoreceptor cells capture the sensations of external light, allowing external vision.

We humans are capable of great visions of truth, insight, creativity, and imagination. Visions are associated with mystics, prophets, poets, painters, charismatic leaders, inventors, and entrepreneurs, affecting the mentally gifted as well as the mentally disturbed, but truly, all of us have internal visions. Descartes said, *"I think therefore I am,"* and thinking is a type of inner vision, even if not all our thoughts are visionary.

———

If you accept this notion of thinking as a type of internal vision, then you reach the third dilemma faced by Descartes in his strict separation of body and soul.

I know that *I think* and that *I am*—but how can I scientifically prove that *you* think or accept that *you* are? With his emphasis on scientific proof and rational doubt, René Descartes was willing to assume the *"certainty"* of his own thoughts and his own soul, but not quite as willing to assume the mind and soul of others.

It requires a leap of faith to acknowledge the mind and soul of another, since we cannot measure or observe another's mind and soul. Some people are unwilling to take that leap for others, even though they want others to acknowledge them. Sadly, it is far too easy to *objectify* others—which means denying them their thoughts, feelings, spirit, and divinity. This denial is true for humans, like the troubled teenager treated like a psychiatric case study instead of a thinking and feeling person, and this objectifying denial applies to animals, like the forest elephant harvested for its ivory tusks instead of being respected as a conscious and sentient being.

Eventually Descartes decided that all human beings have minds and souls, yet denied these immeasurable qualities to animals. Using his *Method of Rightly Conducting the Reason,* he reasoned that animals "could never use words or other signs arranged in such a manner as is competent to us in order to declare our thoughts to others."[21] In other words, Descartes denied animals a soul based on this supposed lack of language ability.

Perhaps he never bothered to look closely for communication skills in animals, or perhaps he used the wrong tools—tools of narrow separation instead of tools of holistic connection. In one apocryphal story, Descartes is said to have nailed the paws of his wife's own dog to a board, spread-eagle, and then vivisect the family pet—*dissect it while it was still alive!*—in order to "prove" that animals like his dog had no mind and no soul.[22] Whether the story is true or not, it may surprise today's readers that Descartes failed to notice the dog's willful thoughts, its pain and desire to escape the scalpel, and failed to observe the dog's loving emotion and devotion toward its human family.

As with other stories of this book, sometimes we don't perceive the obvious until someone says *"look this way."* Descartes looked long enough to see that animals move with intention before denying them a soul of their own. He reasoned animals had "animal spirits" that animated their bodies' movements and that even plants had "vegetative souls" that allowed them to turn toward sunlight, but like Linnaeus generations later, Descartes insisted that neither had a magnificent mind and soul as did humans.

In the ways of the Enlightenment, Descartes tried to solve the dilemma of whether animals and plants had souls and spirits by drawing newer and narrower lines of division and separation à la Linné. The problem in drawing these newer and narrower lines is that each line created new problems. How do you explain bodily movement in animals and plants if you deny them mind, soul, and spirit? For that matter, how do you explain motions of the human body that do not seem willed by the mind, spirit, or soul—like the physical beating of a human heart?

As Descartes looked closely at the heart and its motions, he encountered the fourth dilemma in his strict separation of body and soul. This dilemma was deeply troubling to Descartes, forcing him to openly disagree with the conclusions of his enlightened contemporary Dr. William Harvey, whom René Descartes otherwise openly admired for his devotion to the scientific method.

Dr. Harvey theorized that the heart worked like a mechanical pump, but Descartes rejected this view. In a manuscript entitled *La description du Corps Humain*, Descartes reasoned that the heart could not be an unthinking pump, believing that the movement of all human muscles was willed by mind and soul. "If we suppose that the heart beats [like a muscle] the way Harvey describes it," Descartes wrote, then "we would have to imagine some [mental] faculty causes this motion, and the nature of this faculty would be much more difficult to understand than what it [Harvey's theory] claims to explain."[23]

Descartes offered a different theory, suggesting the heart worked like a furnace by forcing circulation of the blood through the heat it generated. His furnace analogy eventually lost to Harvey's mechanical muscle pump analogy as the prevailing medical analogy for the heart, but Descartes's vigorous objections to an unthinking heart muscle, as proposed by Harvey, forced science to draw newer and narrower lines to accommodate his mistaken separation of mind and body.

"Voluntary" muscular movements like walking with our legs were eventually separated from *"involuntary"* muscular movements like the beating of our hearts, and with these newer and narrower lines of scientific separation, our hearts lost connection to our minds. The more we learn about our health and wellness, the more we realize how this line between hearts and minds is fictional too.

———

When Dr. Henry Beecher published *"The Powerful Placebo"* in 1955 in the *Journal of the American Medical Association,* one of the more surprising studies he publicized was a 1946 study by Dr. Harry Gold of Cornell University.

Gold meticulously documented a placebo cure—in about a third of all patients—for a dangerous medical condition of the heart known as *angina pectoris.* Reconnecting heart and mind did not sit well with Dr. Gold's peers, and Gold's fellow scientists and physicians immediately attacked his placebo study. They drew newer and narrower lines to try to isolate the significance of Dr. Gold's findings.

For example, these attackers claimed that "the lower the intelligence of the patient the more he is benefited by a placebo," but Dr. Beecher strongly disputed that distinction "on the basis of our own evidence."[24] Other critics said that Dr. Gold's placebo was simply "pacifying" the heart condition, rather than "benefiting" the heart medically, but Dr. Beecher also realized this newer and narrower line was ridiculous. Beecher concluded that "reasonably enough...to pacify is to benefit."[25] In other words, from the patient's perspective, healing is healing, no matter how accomplished.

Reconnecting heart and mind has profound significance for the wellness movement. Finally perceiving the holistic connection between heart and mind, we can marvel at a Tibetan monk who slows his heart-beat through mindful meditation and realize how the mind's power to *soothe our hearts* is not limited to mystical monks in a faraway land.

We can also learn how the opposite is true—how the mind's fears and anxieties can physically *damage our hearts*, leading to dangerous conditions like high blood pressure. From the patient's perspective, sickness is sickness, no matter how derived, whether from physical triggers or spiritual maladies. Indeed, you can die from an emotionally "broken heart"—though this notion was long rejected by skeptical scientists.

Just as doubting doctors attacked Dr. Gold's placebo cures for the heart, they insisted that a "broken heart" was but a popular myth, the same type of misinformation "held by the vulgar and by tradition" that Dr. William Harvey and the scientists of the Enlightenment sought to debunk. As evidence mounted in the decades of the wellness movement, though, the cynics were forced to reconsider. The American Heart Association now formally recognizes the disease of *"broken heart syndrome,"* which cardiologists have given other names, like *"stress-induced cardiomyopathy."* The disease is sometimes also called *"takotsubo cardiomyopathy"* because the damaged heart physically bulges into the shape of what researchers describe as a Japanese octopus pot or *takotsubo*.[26]

Having drawn lines sharply separating heart from mind and body from soul and zealously adhering to those lines for hundreds of years, physicians may still not be ready to honestly discuss the meaning of an emotionally-broken anatomically-bulging *takotsubo* heart. We can recite words like *"broken heart syndrome"* yet still not grasp their meaning. For instance, when the European Society of Cardiologists published a journal article on the disease of "takotsubo cardiomyopathy" in 2006, formally acknowledging this dangerous disease requiring urgent medical attention, the article gingerly sidestepped the obvious connections between heart and mind. "Many questions regarding the aetiology…of this [broken heart] syndrome remain unanswered," said these cautious cardiologists, "and further research is needed to clarify these issues."[27]

The word *aetiology* was not familiar to me, so I looked it up in a dictionary; it means *"the cause or reason"* for something. By refusing to admit that feelings and emotions can change the heart's physical shape into a bulging *takotsubo*, the European cardiologists managed to perpetuate the mistaken medical separation between heart and soul. Their unwillingness to acknowledge the "cause or reason" for the physical symptoms of the disease has profound consequences for medical treatment, for it means these physicians lose the opportunity for compassionate, empathic ways to help heal a patient's broken heart.

Physicians once fulfilled that historic function and were considered trusted advisors to lift a sagging spirit, as well as to mend a physical wound. Some medical doctors still do that, as do some nurses and other health-care workers. By offering emotional and spiritual support as part and parcel of their medical assistance, these health-care professionals acknowledge the unseen and immeasurable connections between the patient's body, mind, soul, and spirit, so as to better treat the health of the whole patient. Unfortunately, most of the health-care system and its insurers still have not followed their holistic lead.

Should health-care institutions finally move in that holistic direction, it would be an evolutionary advance of medicine toward wellness, which father of wellness Dr. Halbert Dunn would rejoice to see.

———

Halbert Dunn spoke clearly and passionately in the late 1950s about the negative health effects of this dualistic separation between mind and matter, body and soul, physical and spiritual. In his seminal article on High-Level Wellness, Dr. Dunn implored medicine and health care to reconnect these aspects of a patient, putting them back together again, for the sake of the patient's own health:

> *[W]e can longer ignore the spirit of man as a factor in our medical and health disciplines...If we are to move in the direction of high-level wellness*

for man and society, we cannot ignore the spirit of man in any discipline. In fact, the essence of the task ahead might well be to fashion a rational bridge between the biological nature of man and the spirit of man...

For most of us reared in the Western culture, a deep cleavage exists between the realm of the spirit and that of the body...This fragmentation of man into areas over which various groups [physicians, scientists, educators, psychologists, psychiatrists, motivationalists, clergy, etc.] struggle to maintain their jurisdiction appears to be nonsensical...

Harmony will result when the fact is faced that man is a physical, mental, and spiritual unity—a unity which is constantly undergoing a process of growth and adjustment within a continually changing physical, biological, social, and cultural environment...For no person can be well physically if he is sick spiritually.[28]

It is a huge mistake to see Halbert Dunn's visionary words as merely philosophical or conjectural. His sage advice bears rereading again and again as a *medical prescription* for your own health and well-being.

To most scientists and physicians of the late 1950s and to many still today, Halbert Dunn's ideas about building *"a rational bridge between the biological nature of man and the spirit of man"* made absolutely no sense whatsoever.

Dr. Dunn may have believed that what was "nonsensical" was the "fragmentation" between "the realm of the spirit and that of the body," but by the 1950s, that separation had become a settled foundation of science and medicine.

One characteristic of foundations is that they are so deeply buried that we seldom think about them anymore. We may live in a house or an apartment, appreciating its walls and windows, furnishings and appliances, but the foundation on which the building rests goes quietly unnoticed and taken for granted. Three hundred years after René

Descartes died in 1650, few scientists and physicians stopped to consider whether body and soul were connected, much less contemplate the health consequences of their mistaken separation.

Another aspect of foundations is that they support the whole load of the building—or in this case, a whole methodology of scientific and medical thinking. When a house is built upon a broken foundation, we are sure to see the building's walls crack and crumble over time. Our first reaction may be to replaster and repaint the walls, masking the symptoms of the broken foundation. Of course, this only ignores the real problem, and the walls will continue to crack and crumble until the building is placed on firmer footing. That is true too with structures of thought, sometimes described as a *worldview* or *weltanschauung*.

Worldviews can be built by foundational thinkers, great enlightened minds like René Descartes with his *Method of Rightly Conducting the Reason, and Seeking Truth in Sciences,* but those thought structures will eventually buckle and break, much like a physical building, from an erroneous foundation. That is true even as we plaster and paint a thought structure's crumbling walls, instead of fixing its foundational errors.

By the late 1950s, Dr. Halbert Dunn realized that our health-care system was broken, despite all of medicine's fantastic accomplishments and all the wonderful good it did for patients. Dr. Dunn was perceptive enough to realize that we are not just bodies—that we have minds, spirits, souls, beliefs, passions, emotions, ideas, imaginations, and inspirations, all connected together in what Dunn called *"a unity which is constantly undergoing a process of growth and adjustment."* Whatever you name these interconnected aspects of yourself and however you define them, they are not physical like your body. But as Dunn and Descartes both seemed to understand, what is invisible and immeasurable can most certainly be real and powerful.

Earlier in the 1950s, Henry Beecher wrote about *The Powerful Placebo*. If you think about it, Beecher and Dunn were really saying the same thing about a broken foundation of medical thought, though in different ways.

What is a placebo anyway? It is nothing but the power of belief, the product of imagination, an inspiring idea, or a wonder of spontaneous healing. You may define it differently than I do and you may choose to call it mind, soul, spirit, consciousness, or God, but by any name it affects your life and your health in mysterious, incredible, and miraculous ways. A placebo is powerful indeed.

Of the two doctors, Dr. Dunn was more easily ignored by the medical and health-care communities of the 1950s. His prescription for public health, published in the *American Journal of Public Health*, pointed directly at a broken foundation of nonsensical separation, but it was buried too deep beneath the surface for his colleagues to see. Halbert Dunn's message how "man is a physical, mental, and spiritual unity" and how "no person can be well physically if he is sick spiritually" was too unsettling for its day. Health care and medicine were not yet ready to "look this way"—although Dunn implored his peers to open their eyes and see for themselves.

Indeed, for some scientists of the 1950s, Dunn's notion of reintroducing spirit back into the scientific equation was *heresy*—the same type of "thought crime" for which Galileo was tried by inquisitors in 1633 and that frightened Descartes into delaying publication of his *Discourse on the Method*. The health care systems and medical institutions of the 1950s believed in mathematical precision and narrow separation, measured in dosages and defined by diagnoses. They believed that spirit had no place in medicine and health care and that its study should be left to churches, clerics, poets, philosophers, naturalists, and some said nutjobs and wackadoodles. Health care and medical institutions of the 1950s believed spirit had no consequence for health and well-being, and it would take generations more before the data proved they were wrong. Dunn's work fell into obscurity until rediscovered by a small group of physicians and professionals who kept his message alive, while it gathered the momentum of a movement over time.

Dr. Beecher was harder to ignore. He never discussed the foundational issues, the mistaken separation of body and soul. Writing in the *Journal of the American Medical Association*, he pointed to crumbling walls and physical cracks in the edifice of medicine that were easily observable and mathematically measurable. Like a good scientist, he detailed an impressive array of clinical trials, which statistically showed how placebos healed large numbers of people.

Even with his clinical data, many of Dr. Beecher's disbelieving colleagues vigorously contested his conclusions, believing there must be some error with the placebo studies. Many of these doubting physicians pretended that the data somehow did not apply to *their* patients, dismissing placebos as a curious anomaly or demeaning them as an open invitation for quackery. To others, however, this statistical evidence of a placebo response—and what it meant for medicine—could no longer be ignored.

———

Henry Beecher's pioneering article in the Journal of the American Medical Association affected the pharmaceutical industry first. The intangible and amorphous phenomenon that Beecher called a *"powerful placebo"* clearly played havoc with the mathematics of drug efficacy. As Dr. Beecher observed:

> *Many 'effective' drugs have power only a little greater than that of a placebo. To separate out even fairly great true effects above those of a placebo is manifestly difficult to impossible on the basis of clinical impression. Many a drug has been extolled on the basis of clinical impression when the only power it had was that of a placebo.*[29]

The pharmaceutical industry needed to restore faith in pharmaceuticals, based on the conclusion that "the only power" many drugs "had was that of a placebo." With the support and encouragement of governmental regulators and medical associations, the pharmaceutical industry responded with new *"double-blind"* drug trial procedures. Both physician and patient were "blinded" so that neither knew whether the patient was taking the actual drug or a dummy pill. "Double-blind" became a newer and narrower line, supposedly separating those drugs that were "effective" and "beneficial" from those drugs that were no more effective or beneficial than a placebo.

The problem was that *there are no lines when it comes to placebo*. Placebo, like mind, spirit, soul, faith, and the power of belief, is "utterly indivisible," to borrow words of Descartes.

Placebo's effect can never be truly isolated as a mathematical variable in a double-blind study, for placebo can make *even the same drug more or less* effective! If that sounds far-fetched or nonsensical, consider the 2003 findings of Dr. Fabrizio Benedetti, a neuroscientist and medical physician, who many consider the world's leading expert on placebo response.[30] Instead of comparing drugs against placebos, Dr. Benedetti and his team of researchers in Turin, Italy, tested placebo response in drugs already known to be effective medicines.

His breakthrough study focused on the popular and highly effective antianxiety medicine diazepam, better known by its trademark name Valium®—which the World Health Organization had previously declared an essential drug for every nation's medicine cabinet. Dr. Benedetti gave diazepam both to patients who knew they were taking the drug as well as to patients who did not. To their amazement, Fabrizio Benedetti and his team of researchers discovered that the *drug did not work unless patients knew they were receiving it!*

That may seem odd or unexpected, so it bears repeating. Patients did *not* benefit from the drug diazepam *unless* they knew they were receiving it. However, once they knew they were taking the powerful antianxiety medicine, then it became highly effective. What Dr.

Benedetti and his team demonstrated in this remarkable study was that belief, feeling, and thought trigger physical changes in the body, making legitimate medicines like Valium suddenly effective—or not.[31]

"The placebo effect was considered little more than a nuisance," recalled Dr. Benedetti in a 2009 interview with Steve Silberman published in Wired Magazine. *"Drug companies, physicians, and clinicians were not interested in understanding its mechanisms. They were concerned only with figuring out whether their drugs worked better [than placebo]."*[32] Dr. Benedetti went on to demonstrate how many different types of placebo effect there really can be; the placebo effect is not a "one size fits all" phenomenon and the placebo effect can cause unexpected results.

Placebos can trigger the body's own production of naturally occurring healing drug; for example, placebo has been shown to measurably increase beneficial dopamine production in Parkinson's patients. Just like placebo can interfere with drugs, making an effective drug like diazepam ineffective, drugs can interfere with placebo success too; the drug naloxone, for instance, can block the effectiveness of a placebo otherwise successfully used for pain reduction. Sometimes a drug can provide effective treatment that placebo could not, like growth hormone drugs, yet the beneficial effects of the drug can be continued even after the drug is replaced by a placebo.[33]

In other words, placebos are not the nemesis of pharmaceutical companies nor of science. Placebos can improve drug performance, as they can improve surgeries, therapies, medical outcomes, and health care itself. Since both drugs and placebo can heal, some doctors have dared to ask why not use placebo more effectively? Instead of just "struggling to increase drug effects" said Ted Kaptchuk in a 2013 interview by Cara Feinberg for Harvard Magazine, we should be "trying to increase the placebo effect."[34]

For Kaptchuk, an associate professor at Harvard Medical School, increasing placebo can enable physicians to *"transform the art of medicine into the science of care."*[85]

———

We can see the trees and still not see the forest through them. Placebo means *"I shall please"* in Latin, and caring enough about patients to try to please them—to comfort them—was once accepted by medical physicians as a tried-and-true method to help a patient feel well.

With tools of hyperbolic doubt, some physicians then began to ask whether to *"please"* a patient is also to *"benefit"* the patient. To some readers this distinction may seem ridiculous, as misplaced as the line between *"benefiting"* and *"pacifying"* that Dr. Beecher thought absurd. Pleasing, comforting, pacifying, benefiting—no matter how narrow the definition, no matter how rigid the line, what should be clear and obvious is that the simple act of *caring* actually matters to our health.

Recent studies of terminal cancer patients disseminated by the National Cancer Institute have shown how comforting and pleasing patients statistically extends their lives. It should be obvious too that caring also gives lives more *meaning* at a critical time of life. The health-care community now has a name for this approach of comforting and pleasing critically ill patients; they call it *"palliative care."* As a 2010 study in the *New England Journal of Medicine* concluded, palliative care for terminal lung cancer patients "led to significant improvements in both quality of life and mood" and also concluded that "patients receiving early palliative care had less aggressive care at the end of life [i.e., less chemotherapy, radiation, and surgery] but longer survival."[36]

There is common sense embedded in that clinical data. A warm hug or a hand held can be good medicine by itself, or it can make other good medicines work better.

As a former patient in a lung cancer ward, who still cherishes the camaraderie and life-affirming conversations with fellow lung cancer patients, I know firsthand the difference that placebos can make to one's health and wellness. That is true whether the cancer proves terminal or not. What some may call the *placebo* of pleasing and comforting helped us all feel well, inspiring deep gratitude for life, love, and the shared fellowship. I was glad to give that emotional support to my fellow patients in the cancer ward, as I saw they were glad to give that emotional support to me, even as we all were dealing with our own lung cancer conditions and our own hoped-for recoveries.

Some of my fellow lung cancer patients were lifelong tobacco cigarette smokers, though I was not, and it began to bother me how often they were chided for this history. Whether or not they were cigarette smokers, their need for nonjudgmental compassion and caring was no less significant. I was repeatedly asked that same question myself—*did you smoke cigarettes?*—and it's still the very first question most people ask me upon hearing that I had lung cancer. The question can be innocent, well-intentioned, or reflexive, but it seems to me that many people asking the question are just trying to make themselves feel better, by drawing lines to assure themselves that they are immune from a similar fate in a lung cancer ward.

In the lung cancer ward, what also became clear to me is that blaming and shaming a patient is not an effective placebo and is never a good substitute for forgiveness and compassion. Genuine caring is palpable to people and can inspire a patient's well-being, and no one should be a mere *object*, like a soulless data point in a statistical study. All patients are real *people*, with minds, spirits, emotions, thoughts, and beliefs, however varied they may be. That's not true just for lung cancer patients; it's true for everyone, whatever the condition of one's health.

There are practical lessons that medicine, its systems, institutions and professionals, can learn from placebo studies and their simple common sense. Placebos can make drugs more effective, and placebos can be good medicine with or without the drugs; indeed, unlike drugs, genuine caring is always safe to use. Drugs and placebos should not be viewed as antagonists, as if competing for medical credibility and a doctor's endorsement.

Above all, we must learn how there is great danger when drugs are used in place and instead of placebo caring, for the results of that gross medical mistake can harm the body mightily and crush the spirit tragically. *Oh my God,* how medicines administered without caring can kill!

My dear sweet niece Emily, so bright and inquisitive, with so much promise in her young life, was lost to my family—lost to a world that she lit up when she laughed—at the tender age of twenty-one. It happened suddenly and unexpectedly during the year I began writing this book, and I believe in my heart that it was the pharmaceutical drugs that psychiatrists reflexively prescribed that accelerated her suicidal thoughts and enabled her to act upon them.

Even for well-trained physicians and administratively efficient health insurers, it's too easy to forget how medicines can be poisons and how poisons can be medicines, how drugs can heal or how they can harm. It's also too easy to forget the importance of placebos and how essential placebos can be toward good medical outcomes, whatever the drug administered. Placebos begin with caring, attention, sympathy, and empathy, each of which is a healing facet of the same spirit, which is indivisible. There are no lines that can keep spirit out of the medical equation, so medicine should have never been separated from spirit.

Emily's story is a recurring one, like the story Mark Twain told about his younger brother Henry Clemens, unwittingly killed by an inattentive young physician who substituted painkilling morphine for sympathetic care. This fatal result would not have happened, said Twain, if Henry had stayed in the care of Doctor Peyton, who gave "his sympathy" to Henry and "took vigorous hold of the case."[37] Twain described Dr. Peyton as a "fine and large-hearted old physician," reminding us that the *heart* matters for medicine, though how it matters cannot be graphed as a data point on a linear chart.

Physicians prescribing psychiatric medicines to my niece Emily may have confused medicating her brain with caring for her health. Her health involved not merely her body but her spirit; as Dr. Dunn said *"no person can be well physically if he is sick spiritually."*[38] Suicide and depression are maladies of the nonphysical spirit, even when there are physical triggers, and these health crises require spiritual solutions like placebo caring.

Did Emily's physicians try to reach her spirit? Or did they mistakenly believe spirit was not part of what father of wellness Dr. Halbert Dunn called their health-care "jurisdiction"? Perhaps Emily's doctors chose to ignore her spirit as a factor in their medical protocols and procedures, choosing instead—to paraphrase Dr. Dunn—to conform to a fragmented, nonsensical system that ignored her *"physical, mental, and spiritual unity."*[39] In other words, maybe Emily's doctors confused her brain with her mind, soul, and spirit.

Maybe her doctors forgot that the brain, like the body, dies and decays, but that spirit is everlasting. Of that *truth* my heart is certain, and I pray that sweet Emily's tender spirit found the peace she could not find at the end of her young life.

———

Talking about the spirit makes many scientists uncomfortable. In medicine and health care, it's not an easy topic to discuss at all, for spirit is still the biggest, most colossal elephant in the room—a taboo topic.

Maybe talking about the spirit made Emily's doctors uncomfortable too, so instead they chose to medicate her physical brain. Historically speaking, it was not always that way. Descartes never denied the spirit, even as he separated it from the body for purposes of his method of reason for seeking truth in sciences.

When did the conversation change, removing spirit from politely acceptable scientific and medical discussions?

A hundred years after Descartes died, an influential French physician named Julien Offray de La Mettrie rejected the existence of spirit outright. In one of his books, published in 1748 as *L'homme Machine*—translated as *Man a Machine*—Dr. La Mettrie described human beings as complex physical, chemical, and biological machines and wrote that thoughts, feelings, and inspirations were mere by-products of this machine. His books were first published anonymously and were burned by readers believing them to be atheistic and immoral. When his identity was suddenly revealed, La Mettrie received death threats in France, eventually forcing him to seek asylum in German-speaking Prussia under the open-minded protection of King Frederick the Great.[40]

Dr. La Mettrie came to his conclusion by observing how the progression of his own illness affected his ideas and emotions. This led him to the belief that physical changes in the body must be responsible for nonphysical thoughts and feelings. As a physician, he also observed how the thoughts and feelings of his patients were similarly affected by other physical bodily factors, such as hunger and nourishment, old age and infirmity, sleep and insomnia, sex and pregnancy, drugs, climate, and exercise. Based on this empirical evidence, La Mettrie concluded that there was no separate thing called mind, soul, or spirit and that *"the human body is a machine which winds its own springs."*[41]

The effect of bodily conditions on a person's spirit should have been no surprise to La Mettrie. Indeed, Descartes had already written of "the body's power to act on the soul and cause its sensations and passions,"[42] and though La Mettrie vigorously studied the writings of Descartes, he may have ignored the plain meaning of that particular quotation. However, he paid critical attention to Descartes's methodology of doubt in the absence of measurable proof, and La Mettrie openly criticized Descartes and all his "Cartesian" followers for making a great "mistake" in having "taken for granted two distinct substances in man [mind and matter], as if they had seen them, and positively counted them."[43]

In other words, there was no measurable proof of spirit, said La Mettrie in *Man a Machine*, and he concluded that Descartes should have viewed humans as animals—mindless and soulless. La Mettrie's rationale for this viewpoint was sarcastic. While crediting Descartes as the "celebrated philosopher" who was "the first to prove completely that animals are pure machines," La Mettrie caustically added that "after a discovery of this importance…how can we without ingratitude fail to pardon all his [Descartes's] errors!"[44]

The worst error, according to Julien de La Mettrie, was that Descartes failed to see the similarities between animals and humans. While Descartes believed that language abilities and intelligence were unique to humans and proved the existence of a soul in humans but not in animals, La Mettrie argued that apes were capable of language and that a wide variety of other animals, from beavers to elephants, also demonstrated superior intelligence. *"If it is clear that these activities cannot be performed without intelligence,"* La Mettrie asked rhetorically, *"why refuse intelligence to these animals?"*[45]

Of course, the same exact observation can lead to opposite opinions—that's an inevitable characteristic of rationality and logic. In other words, proof of animal communication and intelligence could lead to the conclusion that humans had no souls like animals, like La Mettrie believed, or could lead to the opposite conclusion that animals had souls like humans. Dr. La Mettrie's retort was contemptuous—*"if you grant them [animals] a soul, you are lost, you fanatics!"*[46]

Truth cannot be proven with insults or sarcasm any more than it can be proven with doubt and cynicism, but seeing man as machine has practical consequences for medicine and health care.

This denial of spirit also has profound consequences for the way we see ourselves and the way we see one another. For my dear sweet niece Emily, I believe her death was due to the fatal error of the psychiatrists who treated her depression. If a patient's mind and soul lack meaning for medicine and health care, if spirit is seen as a fiction worthy of Shakespeare but not science, then physicians treat the brain as a mere anatomical organ.

There is nothing wrong with scientifically studying the physical human brain, its matter and measurements, but surely there is more that matters for mental health than just that. Our physical brains are affected by ideas, thoughts, emotions, and inspirations as surely as the rest of our bodies.

Dr. Julien de La Mettrie observed how a physical change in a body's organ, like a physical inflammation of the heart, caused a nonphysical response of emotional heartache and pain. What he failed to notice was how cause and effect was a two-way street, with thoughts and emotions causing mechanical and chemical changes in our bodies—like how emotional trauma can make the heart physically bulge into the distinctive shape of a Japanese octopus pot, indicative of *takotsubo* cardiomyopathy.

Cause and effect are unified, joining physical to spiritual, mind to matter. Even if a medical and health-care system—believing man is machine—does not recognize this dynamic connection, other institutions of science already have. Dr. Werner Heisenberg won a Nobel Prize in physics in 1932 for realizing how conscious observation affects physical outcome at subatomic levels. Heisenberg, sometimes described as a father of quantum mechanics, described the connection as the "uncertainty principle" or the "observer effect."[47] Simply stated,

German physicist Dr. Heisenberg revealed that when atomic particles are observed and measured, their path or velocity is changed by the mere act of measurement. We create uncertainty in their trajectory and momentum through our conscious observation and measurement.

Though it may seem complex, it is not a scientific abstraction confined to atoms in a laboratory—it applies on a practical level to you and me. Call it belief, placebo, mind, or soul, but whatever its name, it is the miracle of healing when a patient's spirit is genuinely touched by a doctor's caring. It is why a powerful drug like Valium® will work only if you know you are taking it and why broken bones and injured muscles best respond to the mechanics of *physical* therapy only when a patient's *spirit* is willing. Attitude affects outcome.

It is both common sense and measurable science. We can measure how a gladdened spirit causes chemical responses in the body to boost the immune system. Laughter releases neuropeptides such as endorphins, interleukins, and interferon, all of which are powerful chemicals associated with healing and well-being. The tragic mistake is medicine believing that chemical response triggered physical healing—when in fact it was a soaring spirit, uplifted by laughter, joy, and love, that began the process of healing; it was nonphysical spirit triggering chemical response.

Ignore the spirit, but force chemicals as drugs upon the body, and surprising things can happen. The chemicals can produce a grateful and healing spirit and the patient can get well, or the drugs can cause unwanted side effects or unhealthy addictions, even death. Other times, the chemicals can do nothing at all, like an unknowing dose of Valium®. As pharmaceutical labels warn, *your reactions may vary*. There is uncertainty in Heisenberg's principle because the mysteries of the connection between physical and spiritual abound.

If a gladdened spirit can be measured in chemical response, a depressed spirit can be measured in grim public health statistics—the type that alarmed America's chief public health statistician in the late 1950s. Dr. Halbert Dunn, father of wellness, warned that these statistics showed alarming increases in "chronic illness and mental disease" and "a great range of neurotic and functional illnesses, which seldom destroy life but which interfere with living a productive and full life."[48]

In the generations since Dunn, we can no longer say these neurotic and functional illnesses "seldom destroy" life. Of course, medical statistics are still plagued by a great range of neurotic and functional illnesses that interfere with a full and productive life, but suicide is now a scourge. Suicide is a wailing cry of the spirit that shreds the fabric of families throughout the world.

On the day I wrote this paragraph, in what seemed a sad synchronicity to me, Emily would have turned twenty-two. Her bright youthful spirit was robbed of its effervescence far too soon, and her tragic death haunts me still. Just a few months after my family lost Emily, American cultural icon and movie star Robin Williams shocked a nation with his own suicide. How could someone whose playful spirit uplifted the hearts and souls of so very many people leave us feeling so heartbroken, so empty? A few years before, I lost my warm and brilliant friend Greg Giraldo, a former Skadden Arps legal colleague turned Comedy Central Channel roastmaster; Greg died of a drug overdose, and though it may have been unintentional, it was a suicidal loss that still gives me chills.

The grim public health statistics of suicide are also seen too in all-too-familiar shooting massacres in America, that turn schools, offices, theaters and shopping malls into morgues. It is a pox on the spirit, a derangement of the mind and soul, that ends in the recurring pattern of a hail of bullets and the shooter's own anticipated death. These illogical events make no sense and leave our spirits in painful sorrow and grief as an icy wind whips through our collective hearts.

This is not just about mourning in America. In the decades after the start of the third millennium, the whole world witnesses the ceaseless spectacle of young adults detonating themselves as suicide bombs of mass terror. Each death causes reverberating waves of horror and anguish. Soldiers are sent into battle to combat such suicidal terrorism, and the tragic result is too often that the soldier takes his or her own life when the mission ends, distraught from the fog of war and its frightful memories. These are more than statistics, for these deaths affect us all, casting a pall without regard to lines or borders, for spirit knows no lines or borders.

Yet some still cannot see the spirit that is plainly there at the root of it all. Can our doctors and nurses see it? Can the health care system with its business mandates and its insurance protocols? Can our scientists and public health statisticians see it? Can our businesses and governments? How many more sweet young adults like Emily must die before we all see the *truth* of the vital spirit within us all, and admit how the life force commonly called "spirit" connects us all together indivisibly, like trees connected together in a forest?

What more proof do we need—the investigation of a Royal Scientific Commission?

Chapter 12

BE SPIRITED

A Royal Scientific Commission was convened in 1784 at the request of French King Louis XVI. The mission of the commission was to scientifically investigate a popular Parisian physician, who claimed that a mysterious invisible universal force was at the heart of good health and natural healing.

Their findings were published on August 11, 1784. Looking back at the report of these Royal Scientific Commissioners, it can be seen as a fitting culmination of the Age of Enlightenment, the historical period that most historians say began in 1600 and lasted for about two hundred years. The report's findings can also be seen as the Enlightenment's enduring influence on medical science, which continued for hundreds more years to come.

Indeed, in 2010, at the start of a new millennium, ever-enthusiastic believers in the Enlightenment's method of reason republished an English translation of the official report of these Royal Scientific Commissioners. These staunch believers in Descartes's methodology of doubt for seeking truth in sciences were members of the Skeptics Society and by their own account were inspired to republish the report by the words of a popular scientific writer, Stephen Jay Gould. Gould called the 1784 royal report "an enduring testimony to the power and beauty of reason" and "a key document in the history of human reason" that should be "rescued from its current obscurity."[1]

Actually, the historic scientific inquiry of 1784 never really fell into cultural obscurity, for it is still remembered in the common English language by the word *mesmerize*. Like the word itself, the commission's investigation captivated popular imagination—in the way Galileo's Inquisition once did and as great trials of history often still do. It was spellbinding spectacle, this Royal Scientific investigation, mesmerizing Paris with its hearings and testimony and experiments, all designed to uncover the *truth*.

The Royal Scientific Commissioners were celebrity scientists and included Benjamin Franklin, the famous inventor and an American Founding Father, residing in Paris as the new nation's first ambassador to France. It also included a bevy of famous French scientists, among them Antoine-Laurent de Lavoisier, sometimes known as the father of modern chemistry, who is believed to be the primary author of the royal report; Jean Sylvain Bailly, a celebrated astronomer who correctly predicted the appearance of Halley's comet and became the first modern mayor of Paris; and Joseph-Ignace Guillotin, a prominent French physician whose last name later became synonymous with a device for execution by beheading.

This superstar scientific commission was convened to investigate the controversial claims of a German physician named Franz Anton Mesmer. By the time the commissioners convened in 1784, Dr. Mesmer's reputation as a miraculous healer had grown large in Paris. His enthusiastic patients included the king's own wife, Queen Marie Antoinette.

The Royal Scientific Commission examined case studies of patients and acknowledged Dr. Mesmer's many medical successes. In the words of the official report, it was apparent that some patients treated by Mesmer's methods became "fully recovered" after treatments, including those stricken with "grave" diseases where "ordinary medicine" had proved "ineffective."[2]

The commissioners, however, were not interested in Dr. Mesmer's impressive record of cures. They were commissioned by King Louis solely to investigate the "reason" behind Mesmer's medicine—its "mechanism of action," to use a scientific phrase. Their job was to prove or disprove the invisible universal force that Mesmer claimed made his health-care treatments so safe and effective.

To accomplish that analysis, the Royal Scientific Commissioners used the tools of the Enlightenment, its *Method of Reason*.

———

Franz Anton Mesmer claimed his methods of medicine worked because of a force he called "animal magnetism"; this force was the "Universal Agent"[3] that animated our human bodies, he said, and it was the healing force used by nature herself:

> Thus we have seen, in all ages, maladies which become worse or better, with or without the help of Medicine, in accordance with different systems, and by the most discordant methods. These considerations convince me that there exists in Nature one universally acting principle which, independently of ourselves, operates in and through what we vaguely attribute to Art, Chance and Nature.[4]

In reaching this conclusion, Dr. Mesmer compared the way a sailor's compass needle used the force of mineral magnetism for navigation to the way medicine could use the force of animal magnetism to restore good health, balance, and function:

> A non-magnetized needle, when set in motion, will only take a determined direction by chance or hazard. A magnetized needle will, after various oscillations proportional to the impulse and magnetism received, will recover its initial position and remain there...Thus the harmony of organic [human] bodies, when once interfered with, goes through the uncertainties of

[disease and dysfunction until] brought back and determined by the Universal Agent.[5]

The "nature and action of ANIMAL MAGNETISM" said Mesmer could be better understood with this "analogy" to a mineral magnet in other ways too.[6] The invisible forces of animal magnetism and mineral magnetism both were sensitive to "flux and reflux"[7] both with "existent opposite poles" which exhibited "properties of attraction and repulsion."[8]

Despite these useful analogies to a sailor's mineral magnet, Mesmer cautioned against "the mistake of confusing animal magnetism with that of mineral magnetism"[9] and stressed that animal magnetism had unique scientific properties of its own. He described how animal magnetism flowed like "universal fluid which is so continuous as to be without vacuum,"[10] and believed this universal magnetic "fluid penetrated everything and could be stored up and concentrated, like the electric fluid."[11]

Many of his medical techniques were based on the concentration and release of animal magnetism in order to restore healthy movement of magnetic flows through the human body, much like a battery releases stored electricity to flow into a circuit. At first, Dr. Mesmer developed therapeutic techniques using mineral magnets and electric currents in order to direct healthy "animal" magnetic flows in the body, but eventually he decided to use the more natural force of animal magnetism itself. Dr. Mesmer developed a medical device he called the "*baquet*"—it looked like a bathtub with iron rods and ropes attached—and he said it transmitted animal magnetism and directed its flow.[12] Mesmer also developed other therapeutic techniques that if observed today might seem to resemble modern hypnosis, tree hugging, faith healing with laying on of hands, hand-holding support group sessions, consumption of magnetized water, mild electroshock therapy, and Freudian trances to plumb the unconscious mind.

Because animal magnetism was a universal fluid, it could be transmitted from one body to another—that principle applied to any body or every body. In other words, magnetism could be transferred from one "human body"[13] to another—like between a physician and his or her patient. Mesmer himself described how he "transferred animal magnetism to [one male patient] by taking his hands" and how he brought about "convulsive movements."[14] Convulsions were one very dramatic aspect of the transmission of this universal magnetism, but Mesmer described many others; the magnetic force could "be excited, changed, destroyed or reinforced, and even the properties of attraction and repulsion can be observed" and "existent opposite poles may also be distinguished."[15]

Universal magnetism was not only transmitted and received by the human body, Mesmer said, but by any "animate body"—all of which bodies undergo a type of "ebb and flow...intensification and remission...alternating effects similar to those endured by the sea...the animal body being subjected to the same action..."[16] Because this magnetism Mesmer described was universal, its ebb and flow applied to not just to humans and living creatures, but to "heavenly bodies and of the earth."[17] The natural ebb and flow "explained by this magnetism" caused "the cyclical changes which we observe in sex, and in a general way, those changes which physicians have observed during the course of an illness."[18] By helping direct these ebbs and flows of animal magnetism in humans, Dr. Mesmer claimed he could induce tides of magnetic waves that coursed through sickened bodies, adding more magnetic fluid when lacking and dislodging it when stuck, to help heal his patients.

Many of these healed patients confirmed their experiences with Dr. Mesmer, who had "many fans and followers, including persons of note. But not everyone was impressed" as one prominent university historical library, examining about seventy-five publications from 1784 (the year the Royal Scientific Commission investigated Dr. Mesmer) explained.[19] Some of Mesmer's theories were difficult for enlightened scientists, following their method of reason.[20]

For instance, Franz Mesmer's notion of the universality of magnetism—applying to human and animal bodies as well as to celestial and heavenly bodies—seemed to rationalize the ancient and controversial practice of astrology. In fact, the influence of these celestial forces upon the human body was the very subject of Mesmer's doctoral dissertation in medicine at the University of Vienna, entitled *"Dissertatio physico-medica de planetarum influx"*—which has been translated as "Medical Dissertation on the Influence of Planets on the Human Body."[21] It became the first and most basic principal of Mesmer, who said: *"There exists an allied and reciprocal influence between the Heavenly Bodies, the Earth and those Bodies which are animated.'*[22] In other words, Mesmer argued for the influence at great distances of these planets upon human health:

"According to the familiar principles of universal attraction, ascertained by observations which teach us how the planets mutually affect one another in their orbits, how the sun and moon cause and control the ocean tides on our globe, and in the atmosphere, I asserted that those spheres also exert a direct action on all the parts that go to make up animate bodies, in particular on the nervous system, by an all-penetrating [magnetic] fluid."[23]

Proving this medical astrology seemed farfetched in an Age of Enlightenment, but even more troubling for rational scientists of 1784 was Mesmer's claim that the force was "incomparably subtle"[24] and how this magnetic "flow…subtle and rare, penetrates all bodies without a loss in activity."[25] Of all the many qualities and characteristics of animal magnetism identified by Dr. Mesmer, this one would be his undoing before the Royal Scientific Commission, because animal magnetism's subtlety made it impossible to observe and measure with the scientific tools of 1784. Even Galileo needed the tools of a telescope to observe and measure—and thereby prove—the *truth*.

"I am aware that my thesis will present difficulties," Mesmer argued to his critics, "but these difficulties cannot be overcome by [the method of] reason alone, but must have the assistance of experience to be successful." Even without tools to detect this magnetic force, Mesmer said his experience healing patients taught him this force was real. "Experience alone will scatter the clouds and shed light on this important Truth: Nature provides a universal means of healing and the preserving of the human being."[26]

————

The Royal Scientific Commission strongly disagreed. Using their *Method of Reason* and its tools of hyperbolic doubt, Mesmer's experience was to be disbelieved—there could be no *truth in sciences* without measurable and observable physical proof.[27]

Back then, all those centuries ago in 1784, the commissioners could find no scientific proof. In their report, the commission explained how Mesmer's "magnetic fluid escapes detection by the senses." It was "neither luminescent nor visible," so animal magnetism could not be seen, and it was "without taste or smell" as well. It could not be heard since "it spreads noiselessly," and "sense of touch" gave no "warning of its presence" so "if it exists in us & around us, it does so in an absolutely undetectable manner." Though a mineral magnet could at least be verified by the way it visibly attracted or repelled iron, Mesmer's animal magnetism "does not manifest itself visibly as does the attraction of a [mineral] magnet."[28]

Mesmer and his supporters, including Charles d'Eslon, protested and reminded the Royal Scientific Commission of the many medical case studies of amazing cures and recovery. The commission was not convinced, rhetorically asking in their report, "But could not a natural occurrence alone have been responsible for this recovery?"[29] Their historic report reminded how miraculous cures can be effected by "Nature alone & without the help of medical treatment"[30]—an opinion that Mesmer himself shared.

Unlike Mesmer, however, the Royal Scientific Commission did not explore the deeper question of how nature alone can make us well *without* the help of medical treatment. Nor did they ask why nature's own powers to heal might be *helped* by Mesmer's therapeutic techniques. These profound questions—questions that Helen Keller's teacher, Miss Sullivan, called "unfathomable mysteries" that "perplex and confuse all minds"—were not the concern of these Royal Commissioners.

The scientific commissioners had neither the time nor the energy to devote to such profound and perplexing questions and they said so themselves. "The treatment of diseases," they concluded, "can only furnish results that are always uncertain & often misleading; this uncertainty could not be evaded, & all cause of illusion offset, except by the infinity of cures, & perhaps the experience of a few centuries." The commissioners could not wait a few centuries for answers nor analyze the infinity of these cures. They needed to reach their royal decision with the data and scientific means available in 1784. "The purpose & importance of the Commission requires means more prompt," they explained, which meant that the "Commissioners have had to confine themselves to purely physical proofs."[31]

Without physical proof of animal magnetism, the Royal Commissioners could only offer a simple, dismissive explanation to account for Mesmer's many medical successes. They "concluded that for many [patients] the imagination plays a necessary role in the effects attributed to animal magnetism."[32]

Imagination! The commission's report described a series of sixteen experiments that tested its awesome powers, and concluded that imagination can "make one feel pain, heat, even a substantial amount of heat in all parts of the body" and "that the imagination on its own can produce various sensations."[33] Like early critics of the placebo effect, the commissioners also unfairly concluded that women and unintelligent patients were especially susceptible to this "chimerical" force of "imagination."[34] In the final analysis of their royal report, the commission's headline conclusion was that "Imagination does everything, magnetism is worthless."[35]

Looking back today, centuries later, it was the type of "shallow answer" that Miss Sullivan said educators give to children when they ask profound questions, so that "they are quieted by such answers." Saying that remarkable results could be caused by imagination begs the bigger question of *"What is the imagination?"*[36] How does imagination arise, and what explains its potent potential to heal?

Although these questions were not answered in their 1784 royal report, the commissioners nonetheless recognized how *imagination requires belief*. Analyzing Dr. Mesmer's many medical case histories "permitted the Commissioners to observe that magnetism has seemed to be worthless for those patients who submitted to it with a measure of incredulity."[37] In other words, Dr. Mesmer's treatments did not work without the patient's belief—a finding that foreshadowed Dr. Benedetti's placebo studies in 2003 that even effective medicines like Valium® did not work unless patients believed they were receiving the drug.

If belief is needed to activate a therapy or a drug, some might see the therapy or drug as invalid—yet others would encourage belief as a basis for miraculous medical cures. Mesmer's protégé Charles d'Eslon argued to the commissioners in 1784 that if diseases and infirmities could be cured with animal magnetism—even if it was nothing more than imagination—than medicine should embrace the powers of magnetism; d'Eslon "remarked to the Commissioners that the imagination directed in this way toward the relief of human suffering, would be a great blessing in the practice of Medicine."[38]

The commissioners emphatically disagreed with d'Eslon's assessment, stressing how the power of the imagination—especially in Mesmer's group therapy sessions—could do real harm. "But the imagination is this terrible, active power that produces the great effects one observes with astonishment in the group treatment. These effects are astonishing in the eyes of everyone, while the cause is obscure & hidden."[39] The commissioners compared imagination in these group support settings to "dangerous upsets [that] may only be used in Medicine the way poisons are."[40]

Is imagination poison, or is it medicine? Is it a terrible upset or a great blessing? Either way, the commission warned that the power of the imagination in Dr. Mesmer's magnetic therapy treatments was seductive and that its "effects have captivated men esteemed for their merit, their knowledge, & even genius." The commission pointedly chided the number of "persons who are educated, enlightened" and "even a great number of Physicians" who "have been taken in."[41]

The implication of the commission's report—though never stated explicitly—was that if Mesmer's claims of animal magnetism could not be proven scientifically with the method of reason, then Mesmer was a fraud, nothing more than a quack doctor fooling the public into parting with their money, offering false hopes of cure to desperate people. "The Commissioners have therefore concluded that not only the processes of a particular practice but the processes of magnetism in general could in the long run become disastrous."[42] With that stark conclusion of the French Royal Scientific Commission in 1784, Mesmer's reputation was ruined in France.[43]

Disgraced, Dr. Franz Anton Mesmer fled Paris to seek refuge in more tolerant environments of the German-speaking countryside, just like Dr. Julien de La Mettrie a generation or so earlier in 1748. Ironically, while La Mettrie was forced from France for denying the spirit and seeing *man as machine*, Mesmer was exiled for saying that it was magnetic spirit that kept the human machine alive and well.

———

One of the recurring themes of this book is that the way you look at *truth*—the questions you ask, the approach you take, the tools you use—can determine what you see, and how you perceive *truth*.

Try asking different questions. In the story of Franz Anton Mesmer, the *truth* might appear to be that he was discredited by a Royal Scientific Commission and forced to flee France in disgrace. Even centuries later, when *Skeptics Magazine* republished the commission's report, it was prefaced by introductory words of Stephen Jay Gould that it should be "reprinted by organizations dedicated to the unmasking of quackery and the defense of rational thought."[44]

Quackery! Irrationality! For Dr. Mesmer, whose formal education included a doctorate in medicine from the prestigious University of Vienna, those harsh indignities could have been emotionally devastating. Shame can shatter the immune system, leading to diseases and dysfunctions, or depress the spirit to the point of suicide—look how many suicides today arise from humiliations like teenage bullying, insensitive social media posts, and the disappointment of expectations. From that perspective it is easy to imagine a *truth* of history that revolves around Mesmer's disgrace as a doctor—a physician labeled "worthless" by a Royal Scientific Commission.

However, the *truth* seemed far different than that for Dr. Mesmer himself—perhaps because he asked different questions about the meaning of the event in his own life's journey. Moving beyond the obvious disappointment, Mesmer found refuge in a breathtakingly beautiful lake region at the foot of the Alps, where international lines between German, Swiss, and Austrian borders became blurred. It was a place where wine from the Rhine Valley flowed freely, and where by all accounts Mesmer lived a healthy and productive life, his thriving medical practice still firmly focused on the power of animal magnetism—or if you prefer, the power of *imagination*.

Indeed, look even closer, and the real *truth* of Mesmer's story may be that the forced exile actually saved his life. Mesmer fled Paris in 1785, in time to escape the bloody French Revolution that began in 1788. Like most great revolutions, the one in France began with a spark of *imagination*, resonating as if magnetically from mind to mind, but its inspirational democratic ideals soon turned murderous. By 1793, many of Mesmer's investigators—including King Louis, Queen Marie Antoinette, Commissioner Jean Sylvain Bailly, and Commissioner Antoine-Laurent de Lavoisier, who likely wrote the commission's damning report—were each publicly beheaded by guillotine in a macabre spectacle of public vengeance known historically as the "Reign of Terror."

The Royal Scientific Commissioners had warned the royals about the danger of public imagination—their report's final concluding sentence said that "group treatments in which the means of magnetism will be used, can in the long run have only disastrous effects"[45]—but the decapitated commissioners could not have imagined the cruel irony of their own words.

Irony can be cruel, but it also can be funny, like the way the guillotine device used for these public executions was named for a commissioner who opposed capital punishment in any form. Dr. Joseph-Ignace Guillotin was a Parisian physician who disapproved of executions, but who also insisted that if beheadings were to be done, they should be done swiftly, efficiently, and painlessly. Contrasting beheading with a dull axe or a slow sword—the execution tools often used at the time—Commissioner Guillotin said of the new execution invention, "I strike off your head in the twinkling of an eye, and you never feel it."[46] He meant his words humanely, as a man of medicine, but people laughed and they laughed, even singing popular songs to mock him, and the murderous machine soon became known as the *guillotine*.

Like all great ironies, the humor comes from the *truth* it reveals. What made Dr. Guillotin's words so absurdly funny was the notion that a beheading device could kill *humanely*, as if humans were soulless objects for slaughter! Eyewitnesses to execution by guillotine describe severed heads rolling around on the executioner's platform, still consciously witnessing their own body's decapitation with open eyes. The grotesque terror in those still-twinkling eyes of the victims may not have been scientifically measurable, but it was palpable and unforgettable, shocking and nauseating the conscience of the gathered crowd—and humane spirits everywhere—in reverberating waves of horror. When *truth* is denied, the irony can be cruel indeed. No matter what Commissioner Guillotin claimed, there is no proper way to cut a man's head off—it is inhumane however you devise it.

There is cruel irony too that denying the *imagination* of others can spark their *imagination* against you. That is precisely what the Royal Commission's words of condemnation against Mesmer did, sparking the spirit of revolution against their scientific tyranny. With fiery zeal, one of the French Revolution's great revolutionaries, Jacques Pierre Brissot de Warville, condemned the Royal Scientific Commission's report and the resulting exile of Dr. Franz Anton Mesmer:

> To accept that despots, aristocrats or electors are supposed to certify genius by their seal of approval, is to violate the nature of things, the freedom of the human mind. It would conspire against public opinion which alone has the right to crown genius. It would be to introduce a revolting despotism, to make a tyrant of each elector and slaves of all the other scientists.[47]

This revolutionary oratory was spoken while Brissot (known popularly in France as "*de Warville*") was leader of the Girondist war party. It remains a cautionary lesson to government regulators in our own day—those who permit with their seal of approval only a certain brand of medicine or a certain theory of science. In my own career of wellness ventures, I have witnessed many amazing breakthrough technologies rejected by regulators simply because they don't conform to conventional scientific views or because they fall outside inflexible legal definitions. *Who has the right to crown genius?*

For uncrowned health-care geniuses of today, rejected by the institutions of medicine though hugely popular with patients, that might mean persevering without regulatory approvals, medical licenses, or even insurance payments. I have seen my own wonderful acupuncturist and her capable assistant fight for insurance reimbursement despite their cost-effective and impressive results, because their medical treatment is outside the mainstream.

Narrow-minded institutional bias is not new or unusual. Rogue Australian physicians believed that a simple bacterial infection could be causing stomach ulcers; they were geniuses, yet insulted and vilified by their peers for years until finally winning a Nobel Prize. A Funky Polish chemist believed vitamin deficiencies caused diseases like beriberi; he was a genius too, whose approach to medical science saved millions of lives in generations to follow yet the Nobel Prize committee snubbed him altogether. Committees make mistakes too, like all of us do; wellness requires we forgive their trespasses too.

Doubters and disbelievers can delight in their own intolerance. They can speak of justice, though unable to perceive truth, can commit injustices. They can force exiled separation, ridiculing ideas and defaming with words like "quack"—as *Skeptics Magazine* labeled Mesmer—but forget how beliefs cannot be banished, they can only be changed. Sometimes, they can gather in dangerous mobs to avenge their supposed victims, yet stay blind to their own reckless villainy. Each time, their intolerance begets intolerance, and their violence begets violence.

The attitudes we project have a real effect on others, and are often projected back at us. Think of the power of resonance that makes the wineglass vibrate sympathetically from the singer's voice from clear across the room. Consider how commissioners who forcefully condemned popular imagination were ironically beheaded by it. Some call that the law of attraction, others call it karma, you may say you reap what you sow, but any way you say it, the point of view you vigorously oppose can energize another's *truth*.

The revolutionist Jacques Brissot was called "de Warville" for his vengeful beliefs, and he was guillotined in a Reign of Terror. Mesmer's investigators and Brissot's executioners each believed in the *truth* of their own vengeance. However, the real *truth* is that wellness requires an altogether different approach to *truth*.

The real *truth* of wellness is that vengeance can never make us well, for only forgiveness and reconciliation can bring true healing. Even wise military men understand that to defend is to attack. Of course, a vigorous defense and readiness for attack may be necessary, but being defensive truly hurts your own health as well as your adversary's. That is why the World Health Organization declared in solemn words of constitutional principle that living in a state of war—even a just and necessary war against Nazis—takes its toll on our collective health.

If you live in a personal state of war, constantly attacking and defending, your wellness may mean taking a new approach to life. That new approach may be as simple as a story of peace to tell yourself and tell others, but it might help you witness a new *truth*—a *truth* far truer than what you believed before.

———

During his final years in exile, by all historical accounts, Dr. Franz Anton Mesmer never sought vengeance, nor did he dream longingly of defending and avenging wrongs done to him in France. Mesmer continued to believe he could help heal his patients with animal magnetism and continued to believe in the *truth* of his scientific ideas. He knew that his *truth* did not depend on the opinions and judgments of others.

As a man of medicine, Dr. Mesmer probably understood how vengeance was not good for the health of his patients nor his own health. One 1920s biographer, R.B. Ince, wrote of this final chapter of Mesmer's life in exile that "those who knew Mesmer testified to his goodness of heart; he gave the same care to the poor as to the rich; and being of service was his greatest pleasure."[48]

The data may be anecdotal, but Franz Mesmer's caring, charitable, and generous approach to life seems smart for health and wellness today too. Mesmer lived for thirty more years after he fled Paris, passing peacefully in 1815 at eighty-one years of age. By contrast, Julien de La Mettrie died just three short years after he fled France, only forty-one years of age. Though it may also be anecdotal, La Mettrie's years in exile are described in most historical accounts as embittered, angry, narcissistic, or hedonistic—the cause of an early death for a man who led a soulless existence, denying both his own spirit and the spirits of others.

There is another story told by several Mesmer biographers that I find charming in a mesmerizing sort of way. It is a story about the importance of honoring our spirits and souls. It is a story of how being spirited in daily life truly matters to health and wellness.

Mesmer had a pet canary that lived in an open cage in his bedroom. Like many humans and their animal pets, Mesmer and his canary were quite fond of each other. Mesmer would gently wake the bird or put it to sleep with a light stroke of a loving hand, and the canary would gently wake Mesmer too. Early each morning the bird would fly out of its cage and softly perch on Mesmer's head, delighting Dr. Mesmer as he awoke with its beautiful birdsong until Mesmer arose from his bed. The two were like old friends sharing a song of the morning.

The canary seemed to enjoy Mesmer's songs too. Mesmer was a musician as well as a physician, and he believed that music can healthily move the animal magnetism within us—the way you may believe that rock and roll, hip-hop, jazz, funk, folk, pop, punk, opera, country, classical, blues, or whatever your favorite music healthily moves the spirit within *you*—so music became part of Mesmer's medical protocols for relaxing and rejuvenating patients during their therapeutic treatments. Mesmer especially enjoyed improvising on a musical instrument known as a glass armonica.

In yet another irony that reveals a deeper *truth*, the glass armonica was invented by Benjamin Franklin, the Royal Scientific Commissioner in whose French residence the commission convened because of Franklin's poor health at the time. The deeper *truth* of this historical irony may be how Mesmer chose to live his life, seeking peace not vengeance. A man embittered like La Mettrie might have spitefully quit playing Franklin's musical instrument, forever associating it with his harshest critics. Mesmer, however, lived his life in spirit not spite; despite his personal disappointments with Franklin and the commission, Mesmer joyfully played on, entertaining the canary, patients, friends, and himself with Franklin's glass armonica for fifty years, until the day he died.

On that day, according to Mesmer's friend and fellow physician Justinus Kerner, the old doctor died smiling in his sleep, but the canary never smiled again. As Kerner told the story, "Next morning Mesmer lay as though he were still alive, but never again did the canary bird fly on to his head to wake him. It ate no more and sang no more and soon it was found dead in its cage."[49]

Back then, centuries ago, there were no little birdie MRI's nor other sophisticated scientific tools to prove the canary's death from an emotionally broken heart—yet the story still resonates with the *truth* of its meaning. The story resonates because it speaks to the spirit within us, a spirit that connects us all together—people and pets, friends and lovers, family and community, an elephant and the forest, even strangers all somehow linked, inexplicably but undeniably, intertwined as if in a butterfly effect.

Does the story become more "true" with scientific measurement of the canary's broken heart?

———

Dr. Mesmer described the spirit as subtly magnetic, with properties different than mineral magnets. He said this "animal" magnetism had a musical and rhythmic nature, with fluid dynamics like tides and waves ebbing and flowing through human bodies and all living things. He said it connected us to one another and to the heavens above. He said that this magnetic force had powers to heal, which could be demonstrated by medical case study.

He was not the first to say all that, nor was he was the last. Dr. Mesmer just had the opportunity to prove his theories before a Royal Scientific Commission convened as judge and jury in 1784. Unfortunately for his case, the scientific tools back then could not prove what Mesmer described. It was as if Galileo, with all his great intellect, had no telescope for observation. In 1784, the subtle magnetic fields of our bodies and all living things could not be seen, heard, smelled, tasted, nor touched; they could not be measured nor detected by laboratory apparatus of the times. As proof Mesmer could point only to his experience and his medical cases and give the analogy of a mineral magnet.

Mesmer asked for our intuition and our sense of the obvious—the sense many have that there is something more, an energetic force that gives us health, joy, love, light, and life itself until it mysteriously passes from our physical body in death and returns to God. The Royal Scientific Commission could not accept that proposition; they said that without observable and measurable proof, there could be no subtle magnetic force, only the immeasurable powers of *imagination* and *nature* herself.

The funny thing way back then was that none of this discussion was new to science.

Sir Isaac Newton, pillar of the scientific community and the popular icon of enlightened thinking, said much the same thing in the final analysis of his *Philosophiae Naturalis Principia Mathematica*. The *Principia* is considered by many experts to be the most influential treatise ever published on the laws of physics. In it, Newton concluded that this magnetic *Spirit* was subtle but undeniable: *"And now we might add something concerning a certain most subtle Spirit which pervades and lies hid in all gross bodies,"* said Sir Isaac, believing this hidden subtle Spirit was how *"sensation is excited, and the members of animal bodies move at the command of the will, namely, by the vibrations of this Spirit, mutually propagated along the solid filaments of the nerves."*[50]

Though this Spirit was obvious to Sir Isaac, Newton also knew that *"these are things that cannot be explained in few words, nor are we furnished with that sufficiency of experiments which is required to an accurate determination and demonstration of the laws by which this electric and elastic Spirit operates."*[51] Newton's words inspired Mesmer's doctoral thesis, which hypothesized that the spirit was more magnetic and fluid, than electric and elastic.

Both Newton and Mesmer somehow reached similar conclusions, though both lacked tools of measurement and sufficiency of experiments. Instead, both men used tools of intuition, deduction, osmosis, or *imagination*, to borrow the word of the Royal Scientific Commission—although such tools were not seen then or now as sufficient for scientific proof. Ironically, as years passed and decades turned to centuries, it would be the tremendous power of *imagination*—with new scientists inventing new tools and devising new experiments to measure subtle hidden electromagnetic forces—that would set the *truth* free for all who care to look.

If that sounds strange to you, then it might be helpful to think of the *truth* of an innocent man falsely accused and imprisoned until the tools of modern DNA forensics set his body free from jail. The *truth* will set you free too, as you begin to see how newer tools of science finally prove this magnetic, fluid, electric, elastic spirit.

———

True understanding often starts with the heart, in life as in science.

The breakthrough scientific tool for understanding our electromagnetic nature was the EKG or electrocardiogram. Dutch physician Willem

Einthoven developed the EKG in 1903, inspired to do so by his desire to hear the acoustic sounds and rhythms of the heart more clearly—to listen to the heart's musical essence, as Mesmer might say. The device graphically mapped and measured the heart's subtle but strong bioenergetic signals, and Dr. Einthoven revealed how these electromagnetic waves and currents were indivisibly connected to the heart's beats and melodies.

Heart often radiates to head, and Dr. Einthoven then discovered electromagnetics at work in the mechanism of the eyes. In 1924, the same year that Dr. Einthoven won the Nobel Prize for his invention of the EKG, a German physician named Hans Berger invented an EEG or electroencephalography tool that began to map and measure the electromagnetic signals of the brain itself.

This EEG device revealed the brain's waves and currents, for the first time recording their length and frequency. What Hans Berger also discovered was how these EEG brain signals revealed types and characteristics of mental activity hidden in the brain—how states of consciousness were connected to the electromagnetics of the brain! Distinguishing between different forms of these brain waves, Dr. Berger and his followers began to give them names from the Greek alphabet—*alpha* waves associated with relaxation, *beta* waves that accelerated with physical and mental activity, *delta* waves appearing in sleep, *theta* waves associated with meditation, and so forth.

These Greek alphabet patterns were but generalities, for the waves and currents observed by Berger were neither uniform nor consistent. Like the waves on the ocean and the currents in a river, the flows varied over time and were each unique. These flows hid subtle complexities that reflected the conditions of consciousness and the qualities of thought and emotion.

There was so much to learn about the meaning of these electric and elastic signals, Hans Berger realized—they were like hidden vibrations of the mind recorded as squiggles on an EEG chart. Dr. Berger pored over these charts in the 1920s and 1930s, motivated to learn all their hidden meanings. "Is it possible," he wrote in his diary, "that I might fulfill the plan I have cherished for over twenty years and even still, to create a kind of brain mirror!"[52]

His cherished plan was a story of inspiration, dating back to a life-changing event while Hans Berger was still a young man in the German military. In the recurring and self-similar patterns of history, Berger's story is reminiscent of the story of another young soldier stationed in Germany and the mystical and extrasensory experience that inspired the young René Descartes to scientific greatness.

On a spring morning in 1892, as a nineteen-year-old soldier stationed near the German city of Würzberg, Hans Berger was thrown from his horse directly into the path of oncoming heavy artillery traffic. By all accounts, he should have died instantly, but the artillery battery suddenly stopped, and young Hans miraculously survived the terrifying accident without serious injuries. What was truly remarkable about the story was not that he survived, but that his sister—from hundreds of miles away—had an ominous sense something horrible had happened to her brother that very morning.

In a technological era long before today's near-instantaneous communications, she pleaded with their father to find out if Hans was all right. Later that day, young Hans received a telegraph message from his family inquiring of his health—having never received a telegraph message before—and he was deeply moved by the inexplicable psychic forces of his sister's telepathic cognition. Years later, Dr. Berger recounted that "It was a case of spontaneous telepathy in which at a time of mortal danger, and as I contemplated certain death, I transmitted my thoughts, while my sister, who was particularly close to me, acted as the receiver."[53]

To some, stories like these are irrational—the product of a fertile *imagination* or wishful coincidence. And yet, these stories are not uncommon.

Throughout recorded history, many mothers have claimed to know when their sons had fallen on a foreign battlefield, describing a queasy feeling deep inside, as if an invisible thread between the two had been cut. I had a similar experience in my own early adult life, of a lover who woke me in the middle of the night to tell me a terrifying dream that her grandmother had just died suddenly, and then, the very next morning, though hundreds of miles away, finding out her dream had been true. As I can attest, the experience can leave a deep and lasting appreciation of the unfathomable capabilities of the mind and affect your view of what is real and rational.

You can believe these stories or not, but for a young Hans Berger, what is clear is that the event provided the inspiration to learn the scientific *truth* about how minds and spirits communicate and connect together. Inspired to learn more, young Hans changed his academic focus and committed himself to the study of medicine, psychology, and neurology. In time, he would invent the EEG and scientifically prove that the brain produces electromagnetic signals that are connected to the mind's thoughts, feelings, and consciousness.

Though the EEG could not provide all of the answers to unravel the mystery of the telepathic communication between young Hans and his sister, it was a fantastic first step in that direction for Dr. Berger. It was also a great advance in the history of ideas, which led humanity one step closer to scientifically understanding our true spiritual nature.

———

Ideas are never isolated. They are released into the world by their creators and, like little magnets, are attracted to similar ideas or repelled by dissimilar ideas.

Some ideas gain instant acceptance but fade with the fashions of the times. Other ideas may be strongly opposed by the prevalent opinions of others. If grounded in *truth*, however, even strongly opposed ideas seem to survive, though they can wait patiently in exile for years or centuries or longer, sometimes becoming an enormous elephant in the room, until we can no longer dismiss or ignore the idea's essential *truth*.

When Dr. Berger released his ideas, they were not well received by his medical peers. Most of his fellow German-speaking psychiatrists and neurologists during the 1930s were focused on other important questions about the brain. In the fashions of the day, these doctors were busily tracing the mind's many functions to specific anatomical locations in the physical brain. In effect, Dr. Berger asked his colleagues to look at electromagnetic forces that brought unity to the whole of the brain, asking them to see the transcendence beyond localized brain functions. Their response was to mock Berger as "a naive amateur and an outsider"; in the words of medical historian David Millett, Hans Berger became "an easy target of criticism among prominent German physiologists."[54]

Sure enough, the 1930s were trying times for Hans Berger—but that was true for many people living under the rise and rule of the Nazi government. It is not difficult to imagine the unwanted attention Dr. Berger received from the cruel and manipulative Nazis, who were busily co-opting the technology of many leading German scientists. Governments around the world were already using the skin's electromagnetic signals for military purposes like polygraph lie detector interrogations, and Berger's electromagnetic brain breakthroughs had potential for much more sinister military purposes.

One can only imagine Berger's distress at seeing his life's work, born of inspiration in the grace of his teenage brush with mortality, diverted by Nazis toward their evil ends. Hans Berger's torment may have also included the conscientious regret of his own complicity. With military credentials and a history of continued service to the institutions of the German government, Dr. Berger had become part of the Nazi system, whether he liked it or not.[55]

These stresses affected Berger's health in the way that an internal environment of conflict always does. He developed persistent skin infections, and his heart physically weakened. By 1941, the same year that the Nazis bombed Buckingham Palace in London and expanded their extermination camps in Auschwitz, Hans Berger fell into a deep, dark depression. On June 1, 1941, he committed suicide by hanging himself.

During his lifetime, Hans Berger never received the recognition of his peers that he so rightly deserved. He never knew the profound impact his ideas and invention held for our health and wellness. Even today, as I write this, we are only slowly beginning to recognize the meaning of our brain's subtle electromagnetic signals and how they resonate with our thoughts, activities, motions, emotions, soul, and spirit, each vibration reflecting an indivisible aspect of our flowing streams of consciousness.

Today's psychiatrists and neurologists may utilize the EEG in their medical practices and may even accept Dr. Berger's idea that the brain's electromagnetism can be measured and observed like "a kind of brain mirror." However, that does not mean these doctors appreciate the true meaning of Berger's ideas, and they may still disbelieve how the brain's electromagnetic signals—Berger's EEG measured some but not all of these signals—could explain his sister's telepathy all those years ago.

These medical professionals may not see these subtle signals as evidence of a subtly magnetic spirit, nor recognize how these signals connect us to the universe and to one another. They may even reject the notion that spirit is the essence of *who we are*. Some psychiatrists and neurologists still do not understand—but some do. Some doctors, divining *truth*, use spirit's healing energies to help restore good health and wellness for their patients. That is as true today as it was in Berger's own day.

Although Dr. Berger's ideas were rejected by most of his medical peers, there was at least one other prominent German-speaking psychiatrist and neurologist in the 1930s who used the spirit's life-giving powers to treat his patients. Sadly, Hans Berger never had the opportunity to meet this like-minded peer, for Dr. Viktor Frankl might well have saved Berger's life, providing a skilled psychiatric physician's healing light to dispel the darkness of Berger's suicidal despair.

———

Dr. Frankl specialized in the treatment of depression in his hometown of Vienna, Austria.

In the 1930s he established a "suicide pavilion" at a local psychiatric hospital, with innovative prevention programs that tended to tens of thousands of patients. In another visionary project, Dr. Frankl offered teenage high school students free psychiatric counseling at report card time, raising their spirits and saving countless young lives from depression or worse. With these proven successes, Viktor Frankl's reputation began to grow from Austria into Germany, and he was soon invited to visit Berlin by the famous (and later infamous) Dr. Wilhelm Reich, a protégé of the even more famous Dr. Sigmund Freud. Dr. Frankl's approach—which he called "logotherapy" and considered a type of "existential analysis"—was to help his patients discover the beautiful meaning and purpose of their lives, in order to dissuade them from suicide.

Unfortunately for Hans Berger, by the late 1930s, as Berger fell into his deep depression that spiraled toward suicide, Viktor Frankl could no longer help him. By then, Dr. Frankl could no longer help patients even in his hometown of Vienna—for in 1938, Nazi troops marched into Austria and annexed its German-speaking people into Hitler's murderous Third Reich, and began systematically separating and removing Austrian citizens of Jewish heritage like Frankl and his family. By 1942, the Frankls were forcibly taken from their home in Vienna and deported from one concentration camp to another, eventually reaching the Auschwitz death camp in Poland.

Viktor Frankl's wife, mother, father, and brother all died in Auschwitz or other Nazi concentration camps. Perhaps it was luck or perhaps he used his own existential methods, but either way Viktor Frankl survived. Forced into slave labor, Frankl was eventually reassigned by his Nazi captors to work as a physician and psychologist for fellow prisoners in the death camps, until April 27, 1945, when Frankl was physically liberated by American troops, just days before Germany's unconditional surrender in the Second World War on May 7th.

Soon afterward, in 1946, Dr. Frankl became famous worldwide with the publication in German of his book *Trotzdem Ja zum Leben sagen—Ein Psychologe erlebt das Konzentrationslager (Saying Yes to Life in Spite of Everything—A Psychiatrist's Experience in the Concentration Camp)*. The book was renamed for English-speaking readers as *Man's Search for Meaning*. The new title blurred lines of commercial publishing genres and transformed a psychology text into a bestselling inspirational classic, still read and admired today.

It was indeed inspirational! However, as the original German title suggests, Frankl wrote the book from the perspective of a neurologist and psychiatrist. His focus on health care and medicine was of course not surprising—Dr. Frankl was a prominent physician, who received his doctoral degree in medicine at the prestigious University of Vienna, and was well-schooled in the illustrious medical traditions of Vienna, Austria. This Viennese medical heritage connected Viktor Frankl to Franz Mesmer's magnetic healing, Sigmund Freud's hypnotherapy and psychoanalysis[56], Alfred Adler's inferiority complex, Carl Jung's synchronicity and collective unconscious, Wilhelm Reich's orgone energy, Rudolf Steiner's and Ita Wegman's anthroposophical natural medicine, and Abraham Maslow's self-actualization.

Even the notion of a psychosomatic disease, which some of my childhood doctors speculated was the cause of my stomachaches, can be traced to this Viennese medical tradition. The father of psychosomatic medicine, Georg Groddeck, was a young German physician who courted the older and better known Sigmund Freud in letters. Freud became mentor to Groddeck, helping him publish his manuscripts, but in the way that teacher and student can be indivisibly connected, each man inspired the other. Freud marveled at Groddeck's insights into self-analysis and the *it* and credited Groddeck in Freud's now-famous concept of *ego*, *id*, and *superego* as observable and medically treatable aspects of the human mind.[57]

Clearly, the medical institutions of Vienna, Austria were willing to inquire into mysterious forces that could not be easily explained—but could not be easily denied either. Doctors educated in these traditions were willing to blur illusory lines between science, nature, spirituality, religion, philosophy, psychology, personality, consciousness, and metaphysics, developing theories and therapies in order to heal patients and help make them well. Sometimes Viennese physicians drew lessons of healing from even the cruelest and most depraved sides of humanity (Reich and Freud, for instance, both studied sexual depravity to learn lessons about human diseases and dysfunctions). Frankl applied the same approach to learning from his Nazi ordeal.

"[I]n the concentration camps," Dr. Frankl observed, *"we witnessed how faced with the identical situation, one man degenerated while another attained virtual saintliness."*[58] Frankl asked how some people could achieve such profound wellness in this caustic environment, while others became physically debilitated and died from the hopelessness. The difference, he said, was whether the person found a way to affirm meaning and purpose in his or her life, despite the experience. *"He who has a 'why' to live, can bear with almost any 'how,'"* Frankl wrote, quoting German philosopher Friedrich Nietzsche[59], explaining how *"I can see in these words a motto which holds true for any psychotherapy."*[60]

In other words, at its heart, *Man's Search for Meaning* was not merely about Frankl's experience in the Holocaust, but the importance of attitude for good health and wellness. *"[E]ven the helpless victim of a hopeless situation, facing a fate he cannot change, may rise above himself, may grow beyond himself, and by so doing change himself. He may turn a personal tragedy into a triumph.*"[61] Some may call that the power of placebo or belief, others may say it is about choosing to live your life in spirit no matter what the circumstances, but whatever you call it, Dr. Frankl believed it had medical meaning:

> "[I]n the final analysis it becomes clear that the sort of person the [concentration camp] prisoner became was the result of an inner decision, and not the result of camp influences alone. Fundamentally, therefore, any man can, even under such circumstances, decide what shall become of him—mentally and spiritually. He may retain his human dignity even in a concentration camp... It is this spiritual freedom— which cannot be taken away—that makes life meaningful and purposeful."[62]

———

Viktor Frankl realized that some fellow physicians cringed at the use of the word *spirit* in a scientific and medical context, yet Dr. Frankl insisted that it was spirit that played the central role in our health and wellness.

In another medical book entitled *The Doctor and the Soul*, which Frankl first published in 1946, he commented that *"terms such as 'soul' and 'spirit' are loaded with so many distinctly religious connotations that, at least in the eyes of the scientifically minded psychiatrist and/or psychologist, the title more often than not works as a deterrent."* Frankl urged those physicians to see religion in its broader context, *"that is, in the widest possible sense of the word, namely, religion as an expression of man's search for ultimate meaning."*[63]

"The spiritual dimension cannot be ignored," Dr. Frankl emphasized, *"for it is what makes us human."*[64] Viktor Frankl wisely warned of the health consequences of separating our body from our spirit. *"Just consider the mass neurotic syndrome so pervasive in the young generation,"* he said, in words reminiscent of father of wellness Dr. Dunn; *"there is ample empirical*

evidence," Frankl continued, *"that the three facets of this syndrome—depression, aggression, addiction—are due to what is called...the existential vacuum, a feeling of emptiness and meaninglessness."*[65]

For health care to be effective, Viktor Frankl continued, it must ultimately form *"a picture of man in his wholeness—which includes the spiritual dimension."* He urged that we adopt medical therapy that *"not only recognizes man's spirit, but actually starts from it."*[66]

Generations after Dr. Frankl taught that valuable medical lesson about spirit and wholeness, an extraordinary lesson learned as a physician in Nazi concentration camps, have our health care institutions yet accepted and applied his wisdom? Or do physicians and scientists still cringe at the very use of the word *spirit?* The true answer is sad and unfortunate for too many patients with urgent health crises, like my dear niece Emily.

Too many physicians and psychiatrists today still believe spirit is something properly confined to religious study, and still quibble over its religious connotations. Too many continue to deny its importance to medical science, rejecting the spirits of their patients and perhaps their own. Clinging to their measurable points of proof, refusing to blur their narrow lines of separation, these doubting doctors can be emphatic in their lack of empathy and their dry and coldly rational analytics. These scientific naysayers believe that everything real can be plotted mathematically on a Cartesian coordinate geometry chart and graph using their scientific *method of reason.*

Their faith and reliance in the geometry of points and lines is woefully misplaced.

———

What has become abundantly clear in the accelerating wellness movement, all these many years after the health lessons taught by Nazis and

World War II, is how science needs a new geometry—a new mathematics that leads us towards wellness.

Science needs a way to measure and prove the transcendence of our spirits and better understand our selves and our universe—a new mathematical system to better explain how *everything is connected to everything else*. In the same way that the linear geometry of Descartes built a foundation for a method of rational thinking, propelling an Age of Enlightenment that accelerated in the 1600s, today's science needs a new geometry to become the foundation of a new method of holistic connected thinking to advance our new Age of Awareness.

You may doubt that any geometry could ever explain our transcendent spirit or describe what some call soul, consciousness, mind, thoughts, feelings, God, or the Great Beyond. These may seem like fuzzy religious, philosophical, spiritual, or abstract concepts, not capable of being measured and described with the formal language of mathematics.

But a new mathematics is needed to explain much more than that—everything we see all around us in *nature*, here on Earth and in the cosmos beyond, requires a new geometry too, because linear geometry with its Cartesian methods of point-by-point scientific analysis cannot explain such ubiquitous shapes and forms. If that notion seems strange, consider the wise words of the late great mathematician and Yale professor Benoît B. Mandelbrot, who asked:

> *Why is geometry often described as 'cold' and 'dry'? One reason lies in its inability to describe the shape of a cloud, a mountain, a coastline, or a tree. Clouds are not spheres, mountains are not cones, coastlines are not circles, and bark is not smooth, nor does lightning travel in a straight line.*[67]

These simple words appear in the introduction of Mandelbrot's seminal work *The Fractal Geometry of Nature*, published in 1982. Until he developed his revolutionary new type of geometry, mathematics was unable—or perhaps unwilling—to measure the familiar forms and forces of nature. Poets, not mathematicians, were entrusted to explain the soft puffiness of a cloud, the spiraling majesty of a mountain, the craggy beauty of a coastline, the lovely wonder of a tree's bark and branches.

Though these natural images and contours are profoundly pleasing and deeply inspirational to our human senses, they cannot be understood using the geometry of points, lines, and three-dimensional shapes created with points and lines. Nor can linear geometry describe the natural forces of electromagnetic energy, like lightning flashing through the sky. It should be no surprise, then, that linear geometry also cannot measure the transcendent spirit radiating through your heart.

———

Throughout history some mathematicians tried—but failed—to measure and describe the common forms and forces of nature.

The ancient Greek Euclid is considered the father of geometry, and his theorems and formulas became the foundation on which Descartes built his Cartesian coordinate geometry system. Yet Euclid ultimately called these familiar shapes "formless" and "amorphous," realizing the stark inadequacies of his Euclidean geometry to analyze natural things like trees and mountains. A few courageous mathematicians tried after Euclid—brilliant luminaries like Fibonacci and Johannes Kepler—but until Mandelbrot's *The Fractal Geometry of Nature*, all of *nature* seemed unmeasurable to those who think in points and lines.

If mathematics is a universal language, as is so often said, it must apply to recognizable objects and everyday experiences. It should explain the universe around us, the shapes of clouds and coastlines, the movements of stars and stardust. How to describe these forms and forces of *nature* seems an obvious question—the type of innocent inquiry an inquisitive child might ask drawing a cloud in a coloring book, while asking why the sky is blue.

As miracle worker Miss Anne Sullivan said, *"Children ask profound questions, but they often receive shallow answers, or, to speak more correctly, they are quieted by such answers."* The lonely silence born of shallow answers helps explain why a question as glaringly obvious as the geometry of nature could be ignored for so long. As Mandelbrot himself realized, *"a question that had long asked itself without response tends to be abandoned to children."*[68]

Most mathematicians were content to let children ponder these shapes of *nature*, instead of looking more closely at them for clues. Mathematicians, said Mandelbrot, had *"increasingly chosen to flee from nature by devising theories unrelated to anything we can feel or see."*[69] Mathematical careers were devoted to convoluted abstractions of linear thinking, as profoundly obvious questions about the nature of our universe went unasked and unanswered. It was as if all of *nature* became a mathematical anomaly, shunted aside from serious academic inquiry.

It is difficult to see forms and forces of *nature* for what they are if we only see with lines. Perhaps Benoît Mandelbrot persisted in his quest to discover the geometry of nature because he learned as a child how lines can be hateful illusions, wrongfully used to justify pernicious points. In 1936, as an eleven-year-old boy, he fled with his family from Poland to Paris, trying to escape the lines that Nazis used to cruelly separate Jews like him. As the world went to war and Paris fell to Nazis, young Benoît lived life on the lam, running and hiding in France, spurring a lifelong fascination with maps and geography.

Like most refugees, he dreamed of distant shores. The inspirational coastline of Britain was just across a narrow channel of water from Normandy, free from the German conquerors of France and the European continent, but it might as well have been an ocean away. It was accessible, however, with *imagination*. As Mandelbrot visualized the coastline's features, he noticed its roughness, and he wondered how something so irregular and linearly uneven could be so distinctive, instantly recognizable, and beautiful. He asked how an aspiring young mathematician like himself could measure and describe it.

Never quieted by the shallow answers he received, his quest took him on a journey as jagged yet familiar as a seacoast. Looking back at the end of his long life, Benoît B. Mandelbrot said, *"If you take the beginning and the end, I have had a conventional career. But it was not a straight line between the beginning and the end. It was a very crooked line."*[70] His career may have been as craggy as a coast, but it birthed a new geometry that proved that *nature*—like life itself—does not move in straight lines and cannot be measured that way.

———

Nature, as B. B. Mandelbrot discovered, can be measured and described. Not in points and lines, as we are accustomed to think, but in patterns and degrees.

Mandelbrot's mathematical insights first gained scientific attention with an article he published in the prestigious journal *Science* in 1967. It was entitled *"How Long Is the Coast of Britain? Statistical Self-Similarity and the Fractal Dimension,"* and it showed how a natural coastline, though rough and irregular, had self-similar patterns that could be statistically measured.

His brilliant insights would change the way we see the universe and ourselves, but Mandelbrot was not the first mathematician to notice *nature* had prevalent patterns. Thousands of years before, the ancient Greek Euclid, father of linear geometry, described one recurring natural pattern he called the *"golden ratio"* or *"divine proportion."* Since then, artists have used the ratio for its calming aesthetics and architects for its pleasing design; Leonardo da Vinci's iconic drawing of *"Vitruvian*

Man" is based on it too. Scientists too have observed its proportional patterns in the motion of planets, the arrangement of petals of flowers, the branching of tree limbs and blood veins, the spirals of galaxies and hurricanes, and the geometry of snowflakes and crystals, to name but a few examples.

You do not need to be a mathematician nor scientist to recognize recurring patterns throughout nature. Even to a child, the shape of clouds, mountains, and lightning are all instantly identifiable—though they defy mathematical description with Euclid's linear geometry. Mandelbrot said most mathematicians of his generation no longer cared about these natural patterns, and he spoke frankly about how measuring Britain's coastline in the journal *Science* was a practical way to begin a conversation anew. "It was intended to be a 'Trojan' Horse," he wrote, "allowing a bit of mathematical esoterica to 'infiltrate' surreptitiously hence near-painlessly, the investigation of the messiness of raw nature."[71]

A Trojan horse indeed! Measuring the distance between two points along a coastline seems such an innocent and irresistible inquiry, with all the allure of the place where land meets sea. The question can trigger our innate wanderlust for discovery or some intuitive sense that answering its riddle can put a deeply meaningful *truth* within reach. We fear the answer complex yet longingly hope the solution simple.

You might think you could draw a straight line between points on the coast to obtain its "length," but that method does not take into account the bending and twisting shape of the coast as it juts into the sea and recedes back from it. There can be bays and inlets, bluffs and dunes, so truly, the coast is not a line. In his *Science* journal article, Benoît Mandelbrot said a "coastline" is better described as a type of "geographical curve"[72] between two points. Some geographical curves are rougher, rockier, and more rugged than others—he said the west coast of Britain is "one of the most irregular in the world"[73]—but no coastline in the world is perfectly smooth. The natural roughness of a seacoast "is in marked contrast with the ordinary behavior of smooth curves," Mandelbrot wrote, "which are endowed with a well-defined length."[74]

In other words, in contrast to smooth and measurable curves, "[t]he concept of 'length' is usually meaningless for geographical curves" like a rough coastline; its curves "are so involved in their detail that their lengths are often infinite or more accurately, undefinable."[75] This became known as the *"coastline paradox,"* described by British mathematician and peace activist Lewis Fry Richardson in 1961. Most mathematicians thought the coastline paradox was illogical or anomalous, but not B. B. Mandelbrot, whose 1967 *Science* journal article began with L. F. Richardson's empirical observations about coastlines.

To understand how much this coastline paradox matters, think of its consequences for cartographers mapping the British coastline during the Second World War. "[A]s even finer features [of the coast] are taken into account," explained Mandelbrot, "the total measured length increases."[76] How can you map (and defend in wartime) a coastline whose length increases the more details you observe? The paradox might seem odd, but it's as simple as the difference in perspective in seeing the seacoast from high above in an airplane or traversing its rocky outcroppings, sandy shores, and tide pools on foot.

Since the coast is not a curved line with measurable length, answering the deceptively simple question of *"How long is the coast of Britain?"* required more than Euclidean linear geometric analysis. "Quantities other than length are therefore needed," Mandelbrot realized, concluding he needed some *nonlinear* quantity to "discriminate between various degrees of complication" in measuring the coast's curve.[77]

Mandelbrot found these *"degrees of complication"* in the familiar patterns of the coast—its characteristic sandy peninsulas, rocky promontories, cliffs, spits, and stretches of land extending and retreating from the sea. These recurring features are "statistically 'self-similar,' meaning that each portion can be considered a reduced-scale image of the whole," Mandelbrot said. "In that case, the degree of complication can be described by a quantity…that has many properties of a 'dimension,' though it is fractional."[78]

It may sound difficult to understand at first, but it is really simple. Picture in your mind the shape of clouds. Though no two clouds are identical, their shapes are self-similar—which is why they are recognizable as clouds. Mandelbrot realized that most self-similar patterns in *nature* were like clouds—each one "fractured" in some degree or dimension from one another. Exactly "identical" self-similar forms are rare indeed, although Mandelbrot observed in his 1967 *Science* article how "crystals are one exception"[79] since crystals can be exact duplicate copies of one another when found in *nature* or when replicated in a science laboratory.

Years later Benoît Mandelbrot would give other common examples of self-similarity.

In a TED® talk he gave in 2010, before he died later that year at the age of eighty-five, Mandelbrot illustrated the concept with the florets of a cauliflower. "Now why do I show a cauliflower, a very ordinary and ancient vegetable?" he asked, displaying its familiar image for the audience on a big overhead screen as he chuckled warmly with good nature. If you cut the florets of the cauliflower with a knife "again and again and again," Mandelbrot explained, each time "you get a smaller cauliflower." Since antiquity, he reminded his audience, we have known that some objects, like cauliflowers, have self-similar shapes at every scale, "the peculiar property that *each part is like the whole—but smaller.*"[80]

It was a fascinating fun fact for Mandelbrot and his audience, more reminiscent of the ancient art of mandalas (strikingly self-similar to his own name!) than to linear geometry—but what did it really mean on a practical human level? After all, knowledge does not imply the wisdom to apply that knowledge usefully. *"Now, what did humanity do with that?"* he asked starkly, professorially, staring directly at his TED® audience for an answer.

Before anyone could respond, Benoît Mandelbrot answered his own question. *"Very, very little,"* he said, his words slow, somber, deadpan, until an impish grin formed on his playful face. The audience got the joke and joined in the hearty laughter, appreciating the self-deprecating humor of a mathematical genius, a pioneering legend who appeared on the stage as a kindly old man, whose wisdom came from deep painful lessons learned in his own rough but rewarding life.

Disbelieving peers had disapproved of his ideas, misunderstanding and belittling Benoît, before finally appreciating him in his old age for his brilliant insights, at least to some small fractured degree. "Roughness is part of human life,"[81] Mandelbrot told his audience, hinting at the experience of what it was like to be an eighty-five-year-old self-described "scientific maverick"[82] resisted and opposed by authorities and institutions.

Mandelbrot looked directly at the audience again, and without a word, the same joke—*"very, very little"*—seemed to take on a new scale about the importance of laughing at ourselves and our foolish egos, his own included. The humor seemed a painful recognition of how much we still must learn—all of us—and how our limitations are always measured by our willingness to try. As the laughter subsided, Mandelbrot began seriously and excitedly answering the question he had first asked, showing his audience the practical and useful applications of what humanity has begun to do with the mathematical knowledge of self-similar patterns and their fractal degrees.

On the big display screen, the next slide of his presentation showed a picture of an actual human lung, revealing its intricate branching shape, with bigger branches of the lung turning into smaller ones, smaller branches turning into even smaller ones, and so forth, the pattern reminiscent of trees, rivers, veins, and lightning. As I watched the video on YouTube, my own heart jumped a beat with anticipation, thinking how a cancerous lobe of my own lung had been removed by surgeons years before. "The volume of a lung is very small," Mandelbrot explained, *"but what about the area of lung?"*[83]

The medical experts had "enormous disagreements" about the answer to that question, Mandelbrot said, with some anatomists speculating the lung's area was five times greater than other anatomists. Since the lung's function depends on the surface *"area"* over which air is breathed and absorbed—not the linearly calculable *"volume"* of lung tissue—it seemed an obvious question, profoundly important for respiratory health and medicine. Yet, lacking the geometry to calculate the area of a lung's branching shapes, doctors did not have a clue how to answer such a simple and obvious question.

The audience was engaged, finding it astounding that medicine did not yet understand such basic information about the physical structure and geometry of the lungs. *"Surprisingly enough, amazingly enough,"* Mandelbrot continued, his now gleeful voice raised an octave, "the [medical] anatomists had a very poor idea of the structure of the lung until very recently, and I think that my mathematics, surprisingly enough, have been of great help to the surgeons studying lung illnesses and also kidney illness—all these branching systems for which there was no geometry."[84] He beamed with pride at the accomplishment, knowing he had made a real difference in people's lives and health.

"So I found myself, in other words, constructing a geometry for things that had no geometry," he concluded. "And a surprising aspect of it is that very often, the rules of this geometry are extremely short," with simple mathematical formulas that are repeated *"again, again, again, the same repetition"*[85] to create familiar images, like clouds and coastlines, the branches of a tree or a lung. Mandelbrot showed the audience how an image of a cloud could be generated by a computer based upon a simple mathematical formula for the pattern, with the pattern's formula repeated over and over by a degree of roughness commonly found in nature for clouds.

It was a new geometry that could be applied to many, many things—the shapes of *nature*, the patterns of music, the behavior of stock markets, the paradox of a dark night sky, and your health and wellness too. *"Wonders spring from simple rules,"* Benoît B. Mandelbrot said, concluding his TED® talk, holding up a crooked finger with creased skin to emphasize the point, *"which are repeated without end."*[86]

———

In 1982, when *The Fractal Geometry of Nature* was first published, I graduated college from Brown University in Providence, Rhode Island, winning the award that year for best honors history thesis.

My thesis advisor, Professor Gordon S. Wood, had an incredible mind, with a gentle nature and a sharp wit. Many years later, Gordon Wood became a National Humanities Medal Winner and was popularized by the bar scene of the Academy Award-winning movie *Good Will Hunting.* In that bar scene, a South Boston townie (played by actor Matt Damon), with a rough upbringing and a photographic memory, wins the affection of a beautiful woman (actress Minnie Driver) by intellectually deflating an arrogant Harvard history graduate student (actor Scott William Winters) for unoriginally *"regurgitating Gordon Wood."*

For me, the irony of the scene was that Gordon Wood and my other wonderful history professors, like William G. (*"Bill"*) McLaughlin and John L. (*"Jack"*) Thomas, always encouraged students to think originally and creatively for themselves. From their great mentoring minds, I learned how history was *never ever* a cold and dry "regurgitation" of facts and events, but rather the confluence of powerful ideas and ideals, colliding and coalescing in historically significant ways (like in the American Revolution, which was Gordon Wood's particular historical focus).

I learned from these history professors how ideas and ideals can be found in literature, art, architecture, politics, military conflicts, economics, science, law, religion, nature, pop culture, and many other facets of everyday life and academic study. I learned too how these ideas and ideals could reflect the beliefs, values, symbols, and thought structures of the times in which people lived. This type of learning requires interdisciplinary and open-minded thought, and it was not limited to Brown's history department—it was strongly encouraged by most of the Brown University faculty and by the Brown curriculum itself.

Perhaps this holistic approach to education and learning was one reason why Benoît Mandelbrot's book became instantly popular on the Brown campus. My friend Rich Nourie, who majored in psychology and music, with broad interests in many other subjects, was the first to tell me about the book. Soon after, my friend Jodi Green, who concentrated in computer science (and went on to lead the Microsoft® team that first created the word-processing program with which I wrote this book on an Apple® MacBook Pro computer), showed me examples of computer-generated fractal animation and told me how Mandelbrot himself developed some of the software as a research fellow at IBM. This was many years before personal computers were common, and I found the colorful, evolving fractal geometric shapes that Jodi showed me on the university's computer terminals to be wonderfully artistic, evocative, and mesmerizing.

You did not need to be a mathematician to appreciate the beautiful patterns and ideas of Benoît Mandelbrot's book.

I took no math classes at Brown—in fact, I stayed far away from the subject, scared off much earlier in my education before ever reaching calculus. In looking back, perhaps I was frightened by the complex equations that Mandelbrot called a "gallery of monsters" and "pathological" in his introduction to *The Fractal Geometry of Nature*. Mandelbrot said this mathematics was "akin" to "cubist painting" and "atonal music." Some may like those styles of music and art, but personally, I like my music with tone and melody, and I like my art with feeling and beauty—I may not know why, but I know it is so. Similarly, the complex linear mathematics that Mandelbrot described as a "gallery of monsters" never seemed useful or relevant to my own life experience, so I stayed far away from the subject.

But in 1982, as a senior at Brown University, for inexplicable reasons, Mandelbrot's *The Fractal Geometry of Nature* resonated with me. Its mathematically derived computer visuals were art for my eyes, and its keen understanding of patterns and degrees was like music soothing my soul.

I was not scared away by the notion of reading a book on geometry either. The subject had intrigued me when I studied it as a thirteen-year-old freshman at Spackenkill High School in Poughkeepsie, New York; Euclidean geometry seemed useful and relevant to me back then, perhaps because it helped explain the common shapes of our manmade environment. Linear geometry had also taught me a valuable lesson about the importance of visualizing forms, structures, and simple solutions, though for reasons that had nothing to do with Euclid, Descartes, nor their mathematics—it was a life lesson that came with an indelible memory, courtesy of the New York State Regents Examination.

I cannot remember a single question from that statewide geometry exam, but I still vividly recall the feeling of terror as I discovered—*moments to go, clock ticking on the wall*—that I had misread the test's instructions and still needed to solve an entire set of problems, with multiple parts. When I discovered my mistake, I was nearly out of time, and in that moment of realization, I panicked. I knew that each difficult problem required sufficient time to solve, point-by-point, line-by-line, with careful measurement and intricate calculation. I no longer had time to be methodical and plodding, as science and mathematics often require, and I remember feeling abject fear, realizing how I could now fail the final exam.

All at once, that realization crushed some value I held dear—a value cherished by many American middle-class parents and their daughters and sons like me—the hope of a good college education as an essential step toward a brighter future. I remember thinking that the consequences of my careless stupidity in not reading directions on a Regents Examination might shatter my own American dream; that in a split second of time, this dream could be gone and lost forever. Of course, my fear was grossly exaggerated, and besides, all fear is of our own making—even when triggered by an external event—but those were painful lessons I would learn much later in my life. At that moment, though, as a thirteen-year-old public high school freshman taking a State geometry final exam, the fear had my full and undivided attention.

I quickly looked at the remaining geometry problems I still needed to solve, and in the brief instant of time I had available to me before the test came to a close—*put your pencils down!*—I hurriedly wrote down my final answers, simply and speedily, hoping for partial credit for the mathematical proofs I offered. Afterward, the exam over, I was crestfallen and confided in the geometry teacher, Mr. Pantaleo, what had just happened.

Joseph Pantaleo was a good teacher, a caring middle-aged man with curly brown hair who told funny stories, though the class mostly laughed at the white chalk marks all over his jacket and tie from leaning against the chalkboard that he filled with equations. I thought it funny myself but was mostly amused how he pretended not to notice—yet seemed in on the joke. *Don't take yourself too seriously*, I think he wanted us to understand. When our Regents' geometry exam came back a couple of weeks later after being graded, Mr. Pantaleo explained to the class that it was a very difficult test and we should not be disappointed by our grades. He seemed to look directly at me as he prepared the class for the bad news, and my heart sank.

He also announced that one person in the class had received a perfect grade of 100 percent. I remember a smug, arrogant classmate shooting me a look of pride and expectation that it was he, as if a *fait accompli*. As Mr. Pantaleo returned the graded exams to each student, handing them one by one as he walked about the classroom, to my great jaw-dropping surprise, it was my test that received the 100 percent grade. Of course I was delighted in that moment, but in time I realized that what was most important was not the grade, but the many lessons the experience taught me.

It showed me how visualizing a solution to complicated problems can take but an instant of time, and how that instant can be an eternity. The experience emphasized how insight can be immediate and how sometimes we confuse and confound our insights with plodding logic and labored analysis. It showed me the importance of calmly seizing the moment and doing your best, persevering no matter what the circumstances. Of course, never again did I forget to carefully read directions on an exam. Maybe most of all, I learned how fear can seize your attention and force you to take notice of some event immediately, but that what you do in that frightful moment of clarity is then up to you.

———

The Fractal Geometry of Nature did not just gain my attention and the attention of other Brown University students. This unusual casebook on mathematics gained the attention of open-minded people in all walks of life and became an international best seller.

Despite its success with mainstream readers, however, the book irked many professional mathematicians and scientific institutions. They could not argue with its proofs, yet they treated Mandelbrot with hostility and disdain, labeling him as unconventional and insufficiently rigorous, which was to say *nonlinear*. This unkind treatment seemed to bother Benoît, as it would disturb most humans at some level, and he spoke out publicly and privately against his critics.

The more Mandelbrot pushed his peers for the recognition and respect justly due to him—*feeling appreciated and loved makes us all feel well!*—the more his colleagues pushed back.[87] They mocked and criticized him for the ego of his accomplishments, and then they marginalized his fractal geometry as a psychedelic sideshow of freakish computer imagery.

In other words, Benoît B. Mandelbrot experienced the same recurring historical pattern of institutional resistance, followed by evolving acceptance of his revolutionary scientific advances. His experience was self-similar, in fractured degrees, to the same pattern described by Thomas Kuhn in *The Structure of Scientific Revolutions*. Like other natural fractal patterns, the "rules" of this recurring historical pattern are "extremely short," though when repeated *"again, again, again, the same repetition"* can create a cloud or a coastline—or a historical movement like wellness.

The same succinct historical pattern of revolution, resistance, and evolution can be seen in the lives of other scientific pioneers of the wellness movement, some of whose stories have been told earlier, though in varying fractal degrees of roughness. For example, Benoît Mandelbrot's description of himself as an "outsider" and a "scientific maverick" is reminiscent of the same pattern experienced by Hans Berger, the inventor of the EEG brain wave scanner. As the story was earlier told, Berger eventually committed suicide at the age of sixty-eight, his spirit crushed by the weight of institutional ignominy and by the ridicule and ostracism of his peers.

Fortunately for science and for us all, Mandelbrot persevered despite the criticism. In the decades that followed his mathematical breakthrough measuring the coastline of Britain in the prestigious journal *Science* in 1967, and his popular success with the publication of *The Fractal Geometry of Nature* in 1982, he was not warmly welcomed into the mainstream of the mathematical community. Not until 1999, at the turn of a new millennium, was Benoît B. Mandelbrot finally given tenure as a mathematics professor at Yale University. Already seventy-five years old, with a lifetime of mathematical innovation, his faculty appointment was a long time in coming.

By the time Mandelbrot died in 2010 at the age of eighty-five, his mathematical ideas had been applied to medicine, finance, geology, astronomy, engineering, law, art, music, and many other fields of study; in each discipline, we are now able to understand how self-similar patterns recur in degrees and how they scale to *infinity*. Despite the many applications of Mandelbrot's ideas, and despite the visionary work of other pattern-theorists (like Brown University Professors Ulf Grenander and his protégé David Mumford, a Fields Medal winner and Macarthur "genius grant" fellow), we have scarcely begun to understand the impact and meaning of *The Fractal Geometry of Nature*, because our minds still cling mistakenly to the same old lines of linear thought patterns.

Changing our minds and developing new patterns of perception is measured in fractured degrees too. Evolution of thought can be slow and gradual, so barely perceptible we may not realize it at first, or new patterns of thinking can be rapid and seem revolutionary.

———

Whether we realize it or not, we have only just begun to use the geometry of *nature* for holistic thinking in a wide variety of human pursuits.

Nature does not design based on straight lines, and neither should we, but linear thinking has dominated since the Age of Enlightenment, so we cling to its same old recurring patterns of thought. Linear thinking can surely be useful—in writing a book, running a business, composing a song, presenting a legal case, or improving health, all examples to which I can personally attest the utility of linear thinking—as it helps organize thoughts and then orient them in a focused direction.

By itself, though, linear thinking has stark limitations. In my own experience, it lacks the spark of inspiration and the wisdom of understanding found in holistic thinking, so linear thought alone can create outcomes that often badly miss their mark. Sometimes, logical processes by themselves ignore simple common sense—just look at America's health-care system today!

By the early 2000s, health-care administration in America became a check-the-box system of classifications, categories, and codes, worthy of Linné. Line-by-line protocols determine not only medical treatment, but insurance payments and processing. This system—euphemistically described as "managed care"—allows no place for holistic thinking, nor does it assist physicians in caring for their patients.

As if to viscerally remind me of the rigid and unnatural nature of lines and check-boxes, while I was writing this passage I needed to navigate a telephone messaging system to try to make an appointment with my physician. It is now a comically familiar feature of customer service in health care, like many other enterprises relying solely on "rational" linear logic, but I had to press buttons to choose the best of bad choices (*"enter '1' if you…"*), input information for the privilege of continuing the automation (*"enter the last five digits of…"*), listen to useless advertisements (*"did you know we now offer…"*), and so forth, all the while waiting for someone who could actually help me. As I waited, I amused myself thinking how this automated check-the-box linear process could not be good for one's health, except perhaps to encourage patience in patients.

When I finally reached a human, I politely explained how I needed to speak with my *"primary care provider"*—a term given meaning in the rigid check-box system because insurance companies today can disallow care for new medical issues like mine unless originating with a "primary care" physician. The customer service representative asked if I was calling about a medical emergency; *I said I hoped not!* but that my lung surgeon at Memorial Sloan-Kettering Hospital had specifically asked me to follow up with my primary care physician on a potential medical issue my surgeon detected. To be precise, my surgeon asked me to follow up with my *"family physician,"* but that phrase seemed quaint and oddly outdated in an age of automated answering systems and line-by-line managed-care insurance protocols.

The customer service representative told me I could not make an appointment with my doctor for another two months because I was not having a medical emergency, but what bothered me most was that I could not even *speak* to my physician in the interim. The system of linear inflexibility disallowed that commonsense communication option, though that's what I asked to do. I knew too that the woman providing this poor customer service had a mind, heart, and spirit, just as I did, but she was not permitted to use those human aspects of herself to do her job. Her humanity had been sacrificed for linear logic and check-box efficiency by a "practice management" system typical of managed care.

I remained calm throughout the conversation, but I imagined the effect of this inhuman treatment on a patient worried sick about a medical issue. It was clear to me that the placebo of *"pleasing"* or *"comforting"* a patient—an essential part of health care—never figured into the managed-care equation. In other words, erroneous linear thinking had replaced the natural connection between people so essential for good health and wellness.

———

What connects us together is not a straight line. What connects *everything to everything else* is not a straight line either.

Mandelbrot's *The Fractal Geometry of Nature* provides the proof for this fuzzy holistic connection, for within its natural geometry of patterns and degrees is a way to understand how spirit connects us to one another, subtly and magnetically, and how it connects each of us to the *infinite*. Within its fractal mathematics is a way to understand the power and influence of our minds, hearts, and souls and how self-similar thoughts and emotions join us together.

It may still seem strange and unscientific to you, but Mandelbrot's mathematics allows a place for God, angels, karma, prayer, telepathy, and other inexplicable forces, to which we give different names and which may forever be beyond the grasp of our imperfect human understanding. It explains how we humans are a part of *nature* and how we can connect to our better natures. Its natural geometry requires us to acknowledge the divinity in one another, no matter how dim or shadowy the light may sometimes seem.

If these words have no meaning for you, if they sound like irrational babble or nonlinear fuzzy-speak, then think about the significance of *The Fractal Geometry of Nature* another way—think of it as the mathematics that proves Franz Anton Mesmer's case if the French Royal Scientific Commission could be reconvened anew. If I were representing Dr. Mesmer in his defense today—as his attorney—I'd show how Mandelbrot's math supports Mesmer's medical claim that *"there exists in Nature one universally acting principle which, independently of ourselves, operates in and through what we vaguely attribute to Art, Chance and Nature."*[88]

Whether Art, Chance, or Nature (pay heed all you Royal Scientific Commissioners!), it is obvious that Mandelbrot's mathematics creates beautiful *art*, that its "self-similarity methods are a potent tool in the study of *chance* phenomena,"[89] and that it is a fractal geometry of *nature*. Today, the word commonly used to vaguely describe this "universally acting principle" is *"placebo"*—the current favorite word for physicians, government regulators, and pharmaceutical companies to describe spontaneous healing that they don't quite understand—but it is the same phenomenon. Indeed, whether you call it *art, chance, nature, placebo,* or even *"imagination"* (the vague term used by the Royal Scientific Commissioners), whatever name you give this miracle of healing, Dr. Mesmer would say the force behind the cure is always *magnetic*.

What if this magnetic healing force had a self-similar shape, like lightning, that could be scientifically observed and mathematically measured? Though Mesmer did not claim to see this animal magnetism with his naked eye, he described its shape as *"fluid"* and said it *"underwent a kind of ebb and flow."* This recurring pattern, like the waves and tides of the ocean, is reminiscent of the self-similar shapes observed by Hans Berger after his invention of the EEG in the 1930s. These self-similar shapes allowed Berger to identify alpha waves, beta waves, and so forth, which though different in fractal degrees indicated recurring states of mind and consciousness.

Dr. Berger's EEG measured the brain's *electrical* waves and then correlated them with certain mental and emotional states—but what Berger's EEG device could not observe were the *magnetic fields* that always surround electric flows. For those magnetic measurements, our story cannot stop with Hans Berger and his invention of the EEG in the 1930s. Observing and measuring these natural magnetic fields in the human body required newer tools, developed by newer teams of scientists.

One of the first teams were American electrical engineers Gerhard Baule and Richard McFee, from Syracuse University in upstate New York. In 1962 they recorded the magnetic field of a human heart for the first time, creating a magnetocardiogram, or MCG. Though their early recording was very noisy, its crude magnetic measurements were valid, and later teams built on Baule and McFee's pioneering research.

The scientific breakthrough came a few years later in Boston, in 1969, when Dr. David Cohen, who pioneered MEG (magneto-encephalography), teamed up with Dr. James Zimmerman, the lead inventor of SQUID (superconducting quantum interference device). Dr. Edgar Edelsack, a commanding officer of the US Navy who supervised research grants for both men, facilitated their meeting. Ed Edelsack is sometimes described as a collaborator, and sometimes not, but regardless, he certainly deserves credit for his visionary intuition that these two men, who grew up nearby on the Great Plains (Cohen in Winnipeg, Manitoba, and Zimmerman in Landry, South Dakota), would accomplish great things together.

The historic collaboration of these two physicists from the North American heartland began with the heart too. Years later, David

Cohen told the story how "Jim [Zimmerman] arrived near the end of December [1969]" at Cohen's MEG laboratory at the Massachusetts Institute of Technology in Cambridge. "It took a few days to set up his system in the room, and for Jim to tune the SQUID. Finally, we were ready to look at the easiest biomagnetic signal: the signal from the human heart...Jim stripped down to his shorts, and it was **his** heart that we first looked at. The resulting MCG [magnetocardiogram] signal exceeded my best expectations. It was as clear as a conventional ECG [electrocardiogram], and several orders of magnitude better than the MCG from [earlier technologies like Baule and McFee]... Although I didn't realize it," Cohen concluded, "a new era had arrived in biomagnetism."[90]

The journal *Science* later described that moment in 1969 as the *"birth"* of biomagnetism.[91] Zimmerman's SQUID quieted the omnipresent magnetic background noise, boosting the MEG's sensitivity, so Cohen's MEG could measure and observe the magnetic fields of parts of the body with greater precision than ever before.

From the milestone of a biomagnetic heart, Cohen and Zimmerman would become the first to measure and observe the biomagnetic fields of the head. MEG/SQUID is now used to measure changes in the patterns of the brain's magnetic field, observing the unmistakable magnetic relationship to the mind's thoughts, feelings, sensory perceptions, memory, language, and many other functions and dysfunctions.

Hans Berger would have surely delighted in the MEG/SQUID, because it provides an even better "brain mirror" (to use Berger's phrase) than his EEG. Indeed, Dr. Berger would have intuitively understood how the projection of a magnetic field from his own mind explained his sister's telepathy—how she could sense Hans's fear and anguish as a nineteen-year-old soldier after a near-fatal accident all those years ago. It makes sense, since MEG/SQUID detects magnetic fields from brain activities as they are projected *outward*, hurled into the airspace outside our skull, skin, and physical body.

This bears repeating—for one of the revolutionary features of MEG/SQUID is that it detects brain activity from physically *outside* the body. This feature makes it attractive for medical purposes, because other technologies (like MRIs, implanted electrodes, CT scans, and PET scans) measure what occurs *inside* the brain, but need needles, probes, chemical trackers, or electromagnetic signals sent invasively *into* the physical brain. MEG/SQUID does not—it measures brain activities in the airspace outside the skull.

The ability to measure projected magnetic fields from the outside of the physical body applies to other anatomical parts besides the brain. Dr. David Cohen used the device to measure magnetic fields projected from the lungs, and Dr. Jim Zimmerman measured the pulsing magnetic fields projected from the hands of healers.[92] Los Alamos National Laboratory has also used MEG/SQUID to detect previously undetectable fetal arrhythmias from the magnetic fields projected outward by a baby's heart in the womb.[92]

Science and its institutions once scoffed at the notion of a biomagnetic field extending *outside* the physical body, which contained detailed information about our medical condition and our mental state. The ancient idea of a spiritual *"aura"* around us, an energetic field containing information about our thoughts and feelings, our health and well-being, was routinely mocked as mysticism and pseudoscientific quackery.[94] Then again, Dr. Berger was once considered a "naive amateur" for boldly suggesting that the brain produces transcendent electromagnetic wave signals that correspond to states of consciousness, thought, emotion, and physical activity.

———

At the dawn of a new millennium, MEG/SQUID technology is still in its infancy, primarily because the magnetic fields from a single human brain are so very subtle and therefore so very difficult to detect.

The magnetic fields projected by your brain are much weaker, for example, than the magnetic fields projected by the Earth. To measure a single brain's magnetic field, it must be shielded and isolated from other magnetic fields—which is the very purpose of the SQUID portion of the MEG/SQUID device.

Whether we realize it or not, we are all immersed in a sea of subtle invisible magnetism. These magnetic fields surround us constantly, coming from Earth, from other humans, animals, plants, and living things, from motors, machines, computers, and phones, from mountains, clouds, trees, lightning, galaxies, and other forms of *nature*.

A fish swimming in the ocean may not realize it is immersed in water nor comprehend how vital the water is to the fish's own existence. This is true too with the sea of magnetism, in which we all live and breathe every single day, from birth to death. Whether we realize it or not, we are never apart from this invisible ubiquitous ocean of magnetic currents—far more prevalent than the oxygen in the air we breathe.

Chapter 13

BEYOND MEASURE

To truly appreciate the magnitude of all this magnetism and begin to comprehend its miraculous meaning, we should realize that invisible magnetic fields extend beyond our physical bodies, beyond our planet Earth, beyond our solar system and galaxy, to the cosmos beyond that, into deepest space.

In 2010, the same year Benoît Mandelbrot died, astrophysics researchers concluded that *"universal ubiquitous magnetic fields"* permeate the most remote *"primordial"* areas of space and date back to the very origins of the universe. It was a major discovery in the history of science by Professors Shin'ichiro Ando and Alexander Kusenko, physicists affiliated with Caltech, UCLA, and the University of Tokyo.[1] Their groundbreaking research was funded by the US Department of Energy, Japan's Society for the Promotion of Science, and the space agency NASA. Their cooperative effort is a shining example of how former enemies in a world war can connect in unity and harmony to find common wonder in the universe we all share.

The origins of all this magnetism in the cosmos remain a great big scientific anomaly today. It is a giant mystery waiting to be solved that may challenge the *big bang* theory that currently prevails among scientists to explain the origins of the universe. *What is the meaning of all this magnetism?*

The fact that magnetism is always in the background—*universal* and *ubiquitous*—may obscure its true meaning. Water has real meaning to a fish, even if the fish doesn't realize it is fully immersed, taking for granted the very life-giving liquid in which it moves and breathes.

Magnetism might be like background music to which we stopped paying attention. If some of these magnetic fields contain patterns of thought and emotion projected outward beyond our physical bodies—as MEG/SQUID devices have scientifically confirmed—then we may still be capable of perceiving their faint signals if only we try. Like adjusting the frequency on an FM radio dial to find a favorite music station, maybe we need to tune in better. That might be a wonderful metaphor to help understand the telepathy of EEG inventor Hans Berger's sister after his near-fatal accident.

Though the signal may be subtle, it is possible to tune in from even great distances. The strength of a magnetic field lessens over distance, but the field never really stops, for unlike a point or a line, magnetic fields are neither static nor fixed and extend endlessly into space. This is not mere metaphor, though, for it describes the scientific property of all known magnetic fields.

Magnetic fields and their forces truly have no start and no end—there are "no sources nor sinks," as are characteristic of electric currents. Some magnetic fields loop around and back again, while others extend into *infinity*. These properties of a magnetic field are scientifically described in Gauss's law for magnetism and based on the mathematics of Carl Friedrich Gauss (1777–1855) and James Clerk Maxwell (1831–1879), two giants in the scientific history of electromagnetism. Carl Gauss was historically known as the "Prince of Mathematicians,"[2] and Albert Einstein said of James Maxwell that "[t]he special theory of relativity owes its origins to Maxwell's equations of the electromagnetic field."[3]

Magnetic fields seem to leap and dance, zigging and zagging in intricate patterns that are instantly familiar—like the way iron filings arrange themselves on a piece of paper held above a child's toy magnet, with some curving around while others stretch outward at the poles. Along the way, magnetic fields are attracted and repulsed by other magnetic fields, which change their direction and trajectory, like invisible currents in an ocean. This pattern is true when a child's toy magnet encounters another toy magnet and is true for the magnetic projections of our thoughts and feelings.

As these universal and ubiquitous magnetic fields expand endlessly into space, colliding and coalescing, flowing like currents in an invisible ocean, recent mathematical equations and physics experiments have revealed they create beautiful self-similar fractal patterns. Physicists call one such pattern of a magnetic field's expansion "Hofstadter's butterfly"[4] because its gorgeous shape resembles a butterfly, its wings extended in flight, with "each part" in Mandelbrot's words, "like the whole—but smaller."[5]

Some expanding magnetic fields may seem like butterflies, some may appear as branches or clouds as if thought bubbles above our heads, but all magnetic fields are simply sublime in the fractal complexity of their exquisite self-similar shapes. In other words, the mathematics of magnetic fields are like mountains, coastlines, lightning, galaxies, and other forms of nature, all best explained by Mandelbrot's *The Fractal Geometry of Nature*—not by the lines and points of Cartesian coordinate geometry, nor the charts and graphs which science reflexively requires as *"proof."*

———

None of this knowledge about magnetism was known when the French Royal Scientific Commission rejected Dr. Mesmer's medical claims—calling them "worthless"—so on that basis alone, Franz Anton Mesmer deserves a new trial.

The commission should not be blamed for their decision, though, for back in 1784 there were very few tools to measure magnetism.

Their best tool was a compass, invented by the Chinese thousands of years earlier, used for feng shui as well as magnetic navigation. By the time of the Royal Scientific Commission, this magnetic compass tool had become common among Arab and European mariners at sea.

Back in 1784, the commissioners also understood how magnetic forces mutually attract and repel. They knew Earth had a magnetic field too, having studied the scientific treatise of an English medical doctor named William Gilbert, personal physician to Queen Elizabeth, who in 1600 published a classic of early Enlightenment thinking, translated from Latin as *On the Magnet and Magnetic Bodies, and on That Great Magnet the Earth.*

The French scientific investigators of 1784, American Benjamin Franklin among them, certainly did not understand that magnetism is "universal" and "ubiquitous," extending into "primordial" areas of remotest space, nor did these celebrity scientists realize how magnetism was found in forms of *nature* like clouds, mountains, lightning, and galaxies. They probably never contemplated the shape of a magnetic field either, although perhaps they knew how iron filings formed irregular but familiarly recurring patterns on a paper held above a mineral magnet. The Royal Commissioners certainly had no idea about principles of magnetic resonance, as used in the development of the MRI.

To put their limited knowledge about magnetism into perspective, the Royal Scientific Commissioners did not even understand how *electricity* was connected to *magnetism*. Perhaps the closest any of the commissioners came to understanding electricity was the brilliant polymath and electrical pioneer "Doctor" Franklin (as he preferred to be known after receiving his honorary doctorate in science from Oxford University in England in 1762). Benjamin Franklin's scientific fame spread worldwide in 1752 after he published a detailed scientific experiment about flying a kite with a key in a thunderstorm, with sufficient insulation for the kite-flyer, to collect the electrical charge in a Leyden jar, thereby demonstrating the electrical nature of lightning.

Some say Franklin never flew a kite with a key assisted by his son in a storm, as the story goes, but whether truth or myth, his ideas inspired scientists worldwide. Unfortunately, an experiment to capture lightning in a bottle has considerable risk, and it killed Russian scientist and fellow electrical pioneer Georg Wilhelm Richmann in Saint Petersburg a year later, in 1753. In France, Thomas-François Dalibard, replicated Benjamin Franklin's experiment, and then corresponded and collaborated with Doctor Franklin on other electrical experiments. Inspiration certainly knows no boundaries.

Despite all of Doctor Franklin's incredible scientific accomplishments, the discovery linking electricity to magnetism did not occur until 1820, when the Danish scientist Hans Christian Ørsted noticed how a compass needle was magnetically moved by an electric battery. Although Ørsted is popularly credited for the scientific discovery, some say an Italian lawyer named Gian Domenico Romagnosi learned the link between electricity and magnetism more than a decade earlier. Either way, Franklin and the French Royal Scientific Commission knew very little about magnetism when they condemned Mesmer in 1784.

———

Knowledge does not always imply *understanding*, nor does it mean the ability to *apply* the knowledge usefully or practically.

On a practical level, for instance, patents are not awarded in the American legal system merely for advancing knowledge; patents must show how knowledge is newly applied—that some *utility* arises from the application of the knowledge. Indeed, US patent law requires some understanding how knowledge has been previously applied by others, and to get a patent, there must be innovation beyond the obvious—a *"flash of creative genius,"* in the words of the US Supreme Court[6], though the legal standard for defining inspiration and imagination continues to evolve.

In other words, *even if* the Royal Scientific Commissioners of 1784 knew electricity has a magnetic aspect and *even if* they knew the human body uses electrical signals (which, arguably, they may have, since Italian bioelectricity pioneer Luigi Galvani demonstrated in the 1780s how electricity made a frog's muscles twitch and jump), then there is *still no guarantee* the Royal Commissioners would have understood magnetic forces exist in the human body. Knowledge of two separate things does not mean the wisdom to apply them—you still need to *"put two and two together,"* to use an old math idiom.

Human beings have known that lightning contains electricity since at least Benjamin Franklin's time, and have known that electricity creates magnetism since at least Ørsted's discovery of 1820 (or Romagnosi earlier), but knowledge of these two things does not imply their useful and practical application. *"Now, what did humanity do with that?"* is the question Mandelbrot had asked, before humorously answering *"Very, very little"*—reminding us how difficult it can be to grasp the obvious. For example, although we have known about lightning and electricity since Ben Franklin's time, archaeologists remained puzzled by magnetic "anomalies" commonly found on their dig sites until 2004, when archaeo-physicists David Maki and Geoffrey Jones finally put two and two together, realizing these anomalies were the remnants of a lightning strike's powerful magnetic fields.[7] The explanation proved simple and obvious, well within our grasp of understanding and application, yet it was ignored and overlooked.

Even today, our understanding of common magnetism may be rather limited, though it is a *universal* and *ubiquitous* force. When my son Jason was in fifth grade (a long time ago—he has since graduated from law school), I recall how his science textbook shallowly described the force of *"magnetism"* as *"having the property of a magnet"*—as if that tautology of circular logic could have any real meaning! Surely magnetism may be complex and mysterious, but where in its definition is the transcendent simplicity sufficient for fifth-grade understanding?

This is not just about magnetism or other complex subjects of science. Our need for transcendent simplicity applies to basic questions about life, health, and healing essential to a book on the heart of wellness.

Some obvious questions about life, health, and healing—questions so simple a fifth grader might ask them—go unanswered and go unasked by most scientists even today.

Learning how the powerful force of gravity pulls us down to Earth, a budding fifth-grade scientist might ask, *"How can life spring up and defy gravity?"* Learning how a baby grows from a single cell, a fifth-grade future physician might wonder, *"How do all the specialized body parts know how to grow in the right places?"* Maybe you asked curious questions too— essential to your own health and wellness—when you were a child like *"How does my body heal?"* when you saw your playground scrapes and bruises get better and disappear. Or with childhood innocence, maybe you asked basic questions about life itself, like *"What does it mean to be alive?"* or *"What does it mean to be dead?"*

If you think about it, these questions still remain at the heart of wellness. How can you be well if you let gravity pull you down? How can you be well if you stop growing, stop healing, or stop living?

Somewhere along the way, most of us stopped asking these simple questions, quieted by the shallow answers we received, eventually abandoning them to children. Most scientists and physicians stopped asking these questions too, or to speak more correctly, they have yet to answer them. These simple questions—so essential to health and wellness—were shunted aside as scientific anomalies, much like mathematicians looked at the anomalous shapes of *nature* and archaeologists looked at anomalous *magnetism* on dig sites.

Is life itself really just an anomaly? Saying that we have not yet solved the unfathomable mysteries of life should not be an excuse to abandon its essential questions.

———

If the scientific approach of the Enlightenment has not done a particularly good job answering these simple questions about health and wellness despite centuries of trying, maybe it is time for science to acknowledge that too much time is being spent narrowly dividing and linearly separating, instead of seeking wholeness and indivisible unity.

One thing is for sure: *scientists have already collected quite a lot of data!* Mark Twain offered my favorite view of this phenomenon, seeing how scientists can gather facts without realizing what they mean:

> *That is the way of the scientist. He will spend thirty years in building up a mountain range of facts with the intent to prove a certain theory; then he is so happy with his achievement that as a rule he overlooks the main chief fact of all—that all his accumulation proves an entirely different thing.*[8]

Of course, Twain's insight is not limited to scientists, for overlooking *"the main chief fact of all"* afflicts us all from time to time—like silly me failing to see my eyeglasses when they are on the nose of my face! Though it might make me an object of ridicule, I think it is fun (and healing!) to laugh at myself, so long as it helps me realize what was plainly there all along.

"The hardest thing to see is what is in front of your eyes," Johann Wolfgang von Goethe is said to have said. Goethe was a philosopher and lawyer, best known for his classic play *Faust*, the tragic story of a man who lost his soul in a deal with the devil. His cautionary tale reminds us how our spirit is far more important to our well-being than the material and worldly things we may covet. Goethe lived from 1749 to 1832, during the time of Mesmer and the French Royal Scientific Commission,

and in *Faust* he wrote how even educated men and women, with their reductionist logic of separation, can fail to see the obvious: *"When scholars study a thing, they strive to kill it first, if it's alive; then they have the parts and they've lost the whole, for the link that's missing was the living soul."*[9]

One of the recurring themes of this book is how often scientists *"overlook"* what Twain called *"the main chief fact of all"*—and then ridicule those who see the truth more clearly than they do. By recognizing this recurring pattern in scientists, as in us all, we can gently question what others fail to see, and reveal truth. It is but a simple error in perception; as Goethe wrote in Faust, *"A man sees in the world what he carries in his heart."*[10] Search your own heart for the beliefs you carry, and ask yourself how it affects your perception of truth.

So many scientific stories have been told in this book how truth can be cruelly mocked, only to be revealed later as true. In the 1930s, you may recall, Dr. Hans Berger was ridiculed as *"a naive amateur"* for finding transcendent brain signals with his EEG, those waves and currents that rose above the localized brain function studied by his scientific peers. His peers all had access to the same *"mountain range of facts"* (which thankfully physicians and scientists share through journals and publications), yet *"so happy"* with their theories and achievements were these German-speaking neurologists and psychiatrists of the 1930s, they missed the obvious and mocked Berger for seeing it.

If you believe Berger's story is an exception to a rule, and not the patterned rule itself, remember that recurring patterns repeat at every scale. All you need to do is zoom in. Consider the big bang theory of the origins of the universe, still prevailing among scientists at the start of a new millennium. The theory is so widely popular today that it is the name of one of America's longtime favorite television comedy shows.

Zoom in, however, and you'll see that the mountain range of accumulated facts do not fully explain nor prove this big bang theory. So *"intent to prove a certain theory"* are big-bang scientists today that they have created exciting new concepts like *"dark matter"* and *"dark energy"* and *"magnetic monopoles"*—all to prove their theory works.

However, these exciting new concepts while imagined have not been observed in the mountain range of facts—nor in nature. Indeed, if all you have is a fifth-grade understanding of magnetic fields, the imagined concept of a *"magnetic monopole"*—a magnet with one pole— is especially amusing, because every magnet observed in nature has two poles, sometimes called "north" and "south" like the poles of a globe.

In nature even these two poles of a magnet are not fixed by *"monopole"* points and *"monopole"* lines; each pole moves about fluidly, as if spinning and dancing, and the two poles can suddenly reverse, like dance partners do. The poles seem pulled by the dynamic fields of the magnetic field, which move in loops and circles around the magnet and then sometimes fly off to *infinity*. This pattern is true for all known magnets and in all observed magnetic fields—except of course the magnetic monopoles that exist in the imagination of scientists *"intent to prove"* their theory of a big bang.

Should these imaginative scientists be believed? Remember how a French Royal Scientific Commission would not accept Mesmer's theory of animal magnetism because it had never been observed. Without measurable proof, said the commissioners, Mesmer's theory was *worthless*, nothing more than mere *imagination*. Whether you call that a double standard, whether you believe in a big bang or accept Mesmer's magnetism—or neither or both—it does not matter for this book.

All that matters is connecting the dots in a mountain range of data collected by scientists to help you answer simple questions about life, health, and healing essential to your wellness.

One obvious data point if you're finally ready to connect the dots—and this is true even if you believe *man* is *machine* à la La Mettrie—is that the human machine uses electromagnetic energy in its operation. Although that fact was not proven to La Mettrie in 1748 or to a Royal Scientific Commission in 1784, with new scientific tools like EKGs, EEGs, and MEGs, it is now indisputable scientific *truth*.

The *meaning* of these electromagnetic forces within our bodies is less clear to scientists, with some skeptics still insisting that electromagnetism is the mere by-product of chemical or other physical reactions. Look closer at these electromagnetic energies, though, and what becomes apparent is that these forces represent something far more fundamental to health, healing, and life itself.

You do not need to take my word on that.

However, you do need to *carefully choose those scientists whom you believe.* Choose scientists daring to ask questions so simple that a fifth grader might naively have asked them. Choose scientists willing to persevere in their attempt to answer these innocent but essential questions despite the ridicule of their conformist colleagues. I believe we owe these courageous scientists our unswerving gratitude, for it is they who discover *truth in sciences.* They inspire us—at least they inspire me—which is one reason why I wrote this book and have included so many of their stories.

Many other heroic scientific stories were not included, forgotten or obscured by the fashions of historical recollection. Perhaps they will once again be remembered and celebrated after the *truth* of their discoveries is revealed—for that seems to be a recurring pattern of history too.

You may have heard of Nikola Tesla, a Serbian born in Croatia in 1856, who died an American in New York City in 1943. When it comes to the scientific understanding of electromagnetism, Tesla may be the greatest genius the world has ever known. Among the many inventions he pioneered are the alternating current motor and generator system that powers the electric grids of today—think of Tesla every time you plug into an electrical outlet on a wall—as well as remote controls and wireless devices, fluorescent bulbs, electromagnetic coils, bladeless turbines, X-rays (before Röntgen), and radio (before Marconi), just to name a few of Nikola Tesla's many inventions.

Despite Tesla's incredible insights and audacious accomplishments, he was ridiculed by the institutions of science for generations, and nearly forgotten by history. Sometimes described as the quintessential "mad" scientist, his very name was used as the villain of an early *Superman* movie. Some of his inventions were misunderstood and remain beyond today's scientific comprehension, while other patents of his were ignored, denying him credit (and royalties) for inventions still used every day. Government regulators banned other Tesla inventions as medical quackery, like violet-ray devices sparked by low-current high-voltage Tesla coils. By the time of his death, Tesla was fashionably condemned by scientific peers and press, and he died alone and in relative poverty in New York City at the age of eighty-six, his most cherished friends—Mark Twain among them—having passed long before him, his papers and notes confiscated by federal authorities.

Thankfully, some people seek science for its *truth*, not its fashion. Today, public opinion has once again crowned Tesla's genius. He is honored in history, culture, literature, technology, and commerce, including a popular American high-tech electric car and battery company that now proudly bears his name.

Nikola Tesla is a reminder how the influence of ideas can change over time. Though not included as one of Dr. Schlesinger's *"Ten Most Influential People of the Second Millennium"*—Tesla's contemporary Albert Einstein was number six on the list—his star has risen in a new millennium. The Internet website *Listverse* put Tesla as number three on its *"Top Ten Scientists"* list, behind only Einstein and Newton.

335

That is deeply gratifying to me personally, for Nikola Tesla has long been a source of inspiration. The essence of this inspiration, like lightning, cannot be captured in a bottle, so it is difficult for me to explain in words how incredible his influence has been in my life. What I can say with certainty, however, is that joining with Tesla in spirit led me on a wonderful journey of wellness discovery and eventually to write this book.

———

Nikola Tesla is not the only visionary nearly forgotten by history, a scientific pioneer somehow ahead of his time awaiting rediscovery by future generations.

For a book on wellness, few scientific pioneers are more deserving of rediscovery than Harold Saxton Burr. Dr. Burr had impeccable scientific credentials, a chaired professor of neuroanatomy at Yale University School of Medicine in New Haven, Connecticut, with the holistic approach of a Renaissance man whose landscape paintings and abstract artwork were exhibited in his lifetime. Not surprisingly, Burr took what he learned in one discipline and applied it to other fields of study.

In the 1920s and 1930s, about the same time Hans Berger began studying electromagnetic brain signals in Germany with the new EEG tool he invented, Harold Burr began measuring electromagnetic signals too, but with a hundred year old tool known as a *voltmeter*. Invented by Frenchman André-Marie Ampère in 1824, more than a generation after Mesmer's investigation by a French Royal Scientific Commission, it measures "voltage," which, simply explained, is the "potential" of an electrical circuit, the difference in charge that makes electricity flow from one point to another—like the way water flows from where pressure is highest to where pressure is lowest. Like many tools, the voltmeter was honed by succeeding generations of scientists and engineers, and Harold Burr helped refine the voltmeter still further so it could measure the *electrical potentials within living biological beings*.

First, Dr. Burr measured fertilized salamander eggs, observing the development of their nervous systems as eggs grew from conception into embryos. He discovered how, remarkably, the salamander's head always grew at the point of maximum voltage and how its tail always grew at the point of lowest voltage. Observing how bioelectrical potentials oriented the growth and formation of the salamander's brain and spinal cord, Dr. Burr retested his observations on the fertilized eggs of other species, like frogs and chickens. The results were always the same, suggesting an answer to the innocent but unanswered fifth-grade question *"How do all the specialized body parts know to grow in the right places?"*

More research followed. More discoveries, more data, more dots to connect, and Harold Saxton Burr's research began to answer more naive but anomalous grade-school questions, like *"How does the body heal?"* In 1938, Burr tackled that topic directly in an article titled "Bioelectric Correlates of Wound Healing" in the *Yale Journal of Biological Medicine*. Asking still more questions with his voltmeter, Burr learned how electromagnetic changes predicted the onset of cancer in mice long before cancer cells could be physically detected. He saw how electromagnetic changes preceded cycles of life, like ovulation in female patients. His research led him to study both mice and men, along with cottonseeds, maple trees, rhesus monkeys, frogs, goldfish, slime molds, and other life-forms, publishing ninety-three scientific papers in prestigious peer-reviewed journals.[11]

Always cautious and methodical, Dr. Burr concluded how *"a living organism possesses not only many small fields but a single large field,"* which he began to call the *"L-field."* He wrote how this invisible field *"may be bound up with the dynamic wholeness of a living system."*[12] Harold Burr's voltmeter observations mirrored Hans Berger's EEG discoveries that the dynamic wholeness of the brain produced electrical signals that transcended and connected localized brain functions.

Dr. Burr described this single large field as a *"blueprint"* or *"organizing principle"* for anatomical development and for life itself. Of course, Harold Saxton Burr had but a single measuring tool, so his data was limited. To understand what he could not prove with his voltmeter, Dr. Burr used the analogy of a mineral magnet—like Dr. Mesmer did for the Royal Scientific Commission. Once again, Burr's description was so easy a fifth-grader could understand:

> [I]f iron filings are scattered on a card held over a magnet they will arrange themselves in the pattern of the "lines of force" of the magnet's field. And if the filings are thrown away and fresh ones scattered on the card, the new filings will assume the same pattern as the old.[13]

The same pattern as the old! It may sound unbelievable, but knowing nature has a fractal geometry, why would the idea of recurring patterns be different for iron filings than for human cells? Why would it be any different for trees, clouds, mountains, lightning, or galaxies, all organized by the same ubiquitous forces of an electromagnetic field? *The same pattern as the old!* That's exactly what Burr believed from his voltmeter experiments, though Burr lacked scientific tools like MEG/SQUIDs and lacked the mathematics of Mandelbrot to explain the shape of electromagnetic fields in living things:

> *Something like this [pattern of iron filings over a magnetic field]… happens in the human body. Its molecules and cells are constantly being torn apart and rebuilt with fresh material from the food we eat. But, thanks to the controlling L-fields, the new molecules and cells are rebuilt as before and arrange themselves in the same pattern as the old ones…Now the mystery has been solved, the electro-dynamic field of the body serves as a matrix or mould, which preserves the "shape" or arrangement of any material poured into it, however often the material may be changed.*[14]

A matrix or mould that preserves the shape! It was an amazingly simple theory that explained so many unanswered questions of medicine. But the science seemed strange in Burr's time and the mathematics was absent, so Burr's ideas did not gain traction among most of his medical peers. Like Berger and Mandelbrot, he was ridiculed and resisted.

Even today, generations after Harold Saxton Burr's death in 1973, that's still true. As I write these words, the popular Internet encyclopedia Wikipedia dismissively says of Dr. Burr: *"His theory has been rejected by most scientists."*[15] In decades after death, Tesla overcame the backward biases of his peers, and I know Burr someday will too—when science is finally liberated from the lines blinding it from truth.

———

In the 1930s and 1940s, while Harold Burr was busy measuring biological functions with his voltmeter in America, Benoît Mandelbrot—the man whose mathematics could prove Burr's theories—was awaiting liberation of a different sort. In those years, Mandelbrot was a young boy fleeing from Poland, first escaping to Paris with his family, then forced into hiding while the Nazis occupied France.

Liberation is such a simple idea, but it is seldom easy. It can demand the unwavering commitment to *truth* of courageous men and women. It can require brave soldiers landing on a blood-soaked beach in Normandy under heavy artillery fire in the deadly D-day invasion of the Second World War to forcibly free France from a German occupation. Soldiers like my father in-law Martin Lifschultz, who lied about his age and enlisted at seventeen in the US Army, a boy soldier first landing in Normandy, then continuing on to the Battle of the Bulge, and eventually helping liberate prisoners of the deadly Buchenwald concentration camp from their Nazi captors.[16]

Marty Lifschultz learned the high costs of freedom firsthand, receiving purple hearts and many other medals and ribbons for his wartime valor. He continued his military service, eventually retiring as a full colonel in the army's reserves. Though seldom talking about his wartime experiences, he proudly continued giving speeches in uniform on memorial and veterans holidays. Fifty years later, he returned to Normandy as a guest of the French government, honored for serving the cause of *truth* in the liberation of France.

This liberation of France and her people was not merely from German occupation, but more profoundly, from Nazi ways of thinking. Liberation from false patterns of thinking does not come easy either—even when the patterns are as malicious and destructive as those of Hitler and his henchmen.

Like all other natural geometric forms, thoughts have self-similar patterns, so changing recurring ways of thinking *first requires that you see the pattern*. Only by seeing the same old errors of a wrongful and harmful pattern of thought can you begin to adopt new patterns more closely aligned with the *truth*. Adopting new patterns may involve painful and difficult adjustments to the values, beliefs, habits, and foundations of the old thought pattern, but change can be liberating.

Transformations in thinking often come gradually, one small step at a time, in fractal increments. Indeed, our collective understanding of *truth* changes only as more and more people, in fractions of the whole of humanity, become willing to fracture their own patterns of thought and see things a bit differently. As Mandelbrot explained, sometimes fractal changes are rougher and sometimes smoother, and the line toward change is never straight, for it zigs and zags, in patterns and degrees. We don't often describe our ways of thinking as having a geometry but the same patterns that apply to other forms of *nature* apply to our thoughts and our branches of knowledge. These shapes apply to our lives.

In the brief story of Colonel Martin Lifschultz's life, for instance, is a pattern that seems instantly familiar to many of his World War II generation. Coming home from the war, he continued his education with a veteran's scholarship provided by the US government; he married, raised a family, and grew a small business, yet he never lost his commitment to freedom or forgot the importance of fighting for just causes. Perhaps there are variations between Marty's life and many others of his generation—that's the fractal part—yet the story of the colonel's life seems like the story of so many others of his era.

The next part of Lifschultz's story may also have a self-similar ring to readers of this book. He died at age eighty from a fatal reaction to a medicine named *thalidomide*, prescribed by his own doctors as chemo-therapy to treat a bone marrow cancer known as multiple myeloma. The cancer had been slowly growing inside of him for many years already, but Marty had been living a relatively healthy and comfortable life, with aches and pains to be sure. Unaware of the disease, the dangerous bone marrow cancer might have killed the colonel eventually, unless of course something else did.

His doctors diagnosed the bone marrow cancer after Marty complained of stiffness and discomfort during his long daily walks. From that diagnosis his doctors reacted like many doctors of their generation. They thought of themselves as generals in battle, waging war against a disease, instead of considering the wholeness of Marty's life.

A good soldier, Martin Lifschultz never questioned his diagnosis nor the aggressive treatment his physicians prescribed. He believed in them, trusting them to vanquish the disease and help free his body of the cancer, as Marty had once freed subjugated peoples from Nazi tyranny so long ago as a boy soldier.

Tough and tenacious, Colonel Lifschultz expected his liberation from cancer to be a difficult battle, but never suspected that his very first dose of chemotherapy would send him into a coma from which he would never recover, dying months later in a hospital tethered to life-support machinery.

If the name of the drug *thalidomide* sounds vaguely familiar, it may be because its manufacturer apologized in 2012 for causing birth defects in more than ten thousand babies. Ranging in severity from infant death to the flipper-like limbs that became a familiar deformity among babies born in the early 1960s (when my wife Jane and I were both born), the drug manufacturer's apology came fifty years after thalidomide was recalled in 1961 as a medicine to treat a common symptom of pregnancy. Thankfully, thalidomide was never given to my wife's mother, Nancy, to treat "morning sickness" while she was pregnant with Jane, but it resurfaced decades later as a chemotherapy medicine for her father Marty's multiple myeloma cancer.

Physicians pushing pharmaceuticals is a recurring pattern in need of more fractal change. If we expect today's doctors to do *"good and wholesome things,"* then—like the oath that influential Enlightenment physician Dr. William Harvey swore in the early 1600s—they must give their *"best advice"* to patients *"without any affection or respect to be had to the apothecary."*[18] In other words, their concern should be for the patient's well-being, not the drug company's profits.

Today some physicians would seek better medical options than *thalidomide* for the colonel and his cancer. These holistic-thinking physicians might have asked Marty about his routines, caring enough to find ways to help him preserve the desires and dignity of his daily life. Their *"best advice"* could have been as simple as prescribing a new pair of sneakers and a slower pace for the walks and exercise regimens he so loved (often to a John Philip Sousa marching band). As wellness-oriented physicians, they might have guided Marty through mild medicines, made them stronger as his needs progressed, to ease the pain of his aching bones and calm his physical discomforts.

A skeptical physician who sees health as *"merely the absence of disease"* might say that sounds naïve. Believing that the purpose of medicine is to wage war against diseases, they might laugh out loud at the suggestion of a new pair of sneakers instead of chemotherapy. Best-selling author and Boston-based surgeon Atul Gawande, a professor at Harvard Medical School, might have thought that too until he began to look closely at the colossal failure of medicine for folks like Colonel Lifschultz. He asked simple questions about how the systems and institutions of medicine treat ordinary people as they grow older, their health declining toward death—as sooner or later befalls us all. In his book *Being Mortal*, Dr. Gawande concludes:

We've been wrong about what our job is in medicine. We think our job is to ensure health and survival. But really it is larger than that. It is to enable well-being. And well-being is about the reasons one wishes to be alive. Those reasons matter not just at the end of life, or when debility comes, but all along the way. Whenever serious sickness or injury strikes and your body or mind breaks down, the vital questions are the same: What is your understanding of the situation and its potential outcomes? What are your fears and what are your hopes? What are the trade-offs you are willing to make and not willing to make? And what is the course of action that best serves this understanding?[19]

In reaching his bold conclusion about the need to change patterns of medical care, Dr. Gawande encountered patients with terminal cancers, dangerous heart conditions, and all manner and types of deadly diseases and debilitating infirmities. He discovered that focusing on a person's wellness—instead of merely seeking diagnosis and treatment for their disease—transforms medical protocols and, with that, medical outcomes.

That wellness-oriented approach is not the way most physicians are trained in medical school, including highly skilled surgeons like Atul Gawande himself, so first and foremost, it requires a *change of thinking*.

Dr. Gawande told a story of a medical consultation he witnessed, with the patient's permission, between an eighty-five-year-old woman with multiple medical maladies and the chief geriatrician in his hospital. "It seemed to me that, with just a forty-minute visit," Gawande wrote, the examining physician Dr. Juergen Bludau "needed to triage by zeroing in on either the most potentially life-threatening problem (the possible [colon cancer] metastasis) or the problem that bothered her the most (the back pain). But this was evidently not what he thought. He asked almost nothing about either issue. Instead, he spent much of the exam looking at her feet."[20]

As geriatrician Bludau later explained to surgeon Gawande, the patient's feet affected the quality of her life in ways that her other ailments did not; her feet were the cause of falls, statistically the most likely threat to her well-being, as well as a signal of dangerous side effects from her prescription drugs. *"The job of any doctor, Bludau later told me,"* said Gawande, *"is to support quality of life, by which he meant two things: as much freedom from the ravages of disease as possible and retention of enough function for active engagement in the world."*[21]

"Most doctors," Dr. Bludau explained to Dr. Gawande, instead *"treat disease and figure that the rest will take care of itself."*[22] *"Most doctors"* are not unskilled nor ill-intentioned, but they might be the type of physician who reflexively prescribes thalidomide chemotherapy to an eighty-year-old colonel, who had been unknowingly living with his disease for many years already, trying to enjoy the remaining balance of a long and fulfilling life.

In other words, *"most doctors"* still ignore their patient's spirit as the starting place for medical therapy and marginalize the placebo of pleasing a patient. Within the legal system, medical malpractice is judged against the current standards of the medical community, so if *"most doctors"* treat patients a certain way—like surgery for a bacterial stomach ulcer, or thalidomide for an elderly multiple myeloma patient—then we still consider that to be acceptably competent medical care.

What is urgently needed, then, is to change the beliefs of *"most doctors"* and not accept medical protocols because most think the same way. You need courage and commitment to liberate yourself from recurring ways of mistaken thinking.

———

If *"most scientists"* today, as Wikipedia said, reject the theory of Dr. Harold Saxton Burr—refusing to consider how an electromagnetic *"matrix"* preserves the shape of the body and provides the biological basis for healing—then are *"most scientists"* to be believed?

It is easy to confuse belief with *truth*, which leads to a bigger and more profound question. The question may be uncomfortable, requiring you to engage in self-searching honesty: *How would you react if you found out that your own beliefs were untrue?*

Would you deny the *truth*, stubbornly refusing to question your mistaken beliefs? Or would you try to undo your misplaced beliefs, gently correcting them and then aligning new beliefs with the *truth*? Perhaps your answer depends on the "type" of wrongful beliefs— whether it was a trivial belief that you discovered was incorrect or some deeply entrenched foundational belief that supported your entire thought structure.

Each of us may answer the question differently, but perhaps we can all follow the admirable example of Wikipedia, as an online encyclopedia committed to the evolution of knowledge and the pursuit of true wisdom. Wikipedia was of great help to me in my research for this book, and I am sincerely grateful to Wikipedia for that assistance, yet from time to time I found gross errors and prejudices in their online articles. This was especially true in biographies about wellness pioneers, many of whom were unfairly disparaged with empty epithets like *"pseudoscience"* and *"quackery"* and other invective ad hominem attacks.

Fortunately for the sake of *truth*, Wikipedia invites its community of users to correct their errors by asking them to dig a little deeper, to find new references and challenge the biases of old assumptions. In the course of years of diligent research for this book and previous projects, I watched the ongoing and evolving process of how errors were corrected by Wikipedia's readers, even as other errors remained. To my delight, I watched how ideas and ideals evolved in plain sight on the Internet.[23]

Just like Wikipedia allows its users to self-correct their errors, you can do that too. Dig deeper within your self to gently self-correct your own mistaken beliefs. Forgive your own errors, and don't be hard on yourself, for as the poet Alexander Pope wrote: *"To err is human; to forgive, divine."* Start by self-correcting self-limiting beliefs that mistakenly deny your *infinite* spirit. Its magnetic force is what connects you to *truth*.

———

If Wikipedia is correct that *"most scientists"* reject the bioenergetic matrix research of Dr. Harold Saxton Burr, it is also true that *"some scientists"* believe otherwise. Though their beliefs may differ, those scientists outside the mainstream can be just as committed as their conventional-thinking peers to seeking *truth in sciences*, with both groups of scientists diligently using the same *method of reason*.

Dr. Burr began his voltmeter research with a simple salamander. As many children know, if an ordinary salamander loses a limb, it grows a new one. If you've ever wondered about the miracle of playground scrapes and bruises healing, now imagine if you could shed a badly wounded arm or leg, and then grow a brand-new one in its place. This phenomenon of healing is truly worthy of wonder by fifth graders!

How does the salamander replace its lost limb? Dr. Robert O. Becker, a physician and a chief orthopedic surgeon who served in the US Army Medical Corps, bravely resumed Dr. Harold Saxton Burr's research into the salamander and its matrix of electromagnetic fields. To some, it may seem the stuff of science fiction, but Becker expanded on Burr's observation how voltage orients the growth and formation of a salamander's brain and spinal cord beginning in the salamander's fertilized egg.

Bob Becker began measuring electromagnetic signals as the salamander's limb was wounded and as it healed. His measurements showed how the salamander's wounds triggered electromagnetic signals that regulated and directed the healing process, eventually replacing the lost limb. From foundational research on salamanders, Becker applied his findings to humans, daring to ask the simple question of how healing happens, to ask the type of obvious questions long abandoned to children.

He was no ordinary scientist. A pioneering research professor at Upstate Medical Center in Syracuse, New York, in 1995 Dr. Becker demonstrated the first adult case of human fingertip regeneration, photographing and patenting some of his innovative techniques. His medical specialty was orthopedics—human bones and skeletal structures—and Bob Becker understood how bones like some crystals are *piezoelectric*, which means they generate electromagnetic signals when stressed. They become stressed during exercise and during injury, and he saw how these stresses trigger natural healing processes. Applying his knowledge, Dr. Becker invented revolutionary electromagnetic devices to help heal difficult bone fractures.

Just as most scientists rejected Burr's breakthroughs generations before, most scientists ignore Becker's brilliance too. Finding out your beliefs are untrue can be a humbling experience, even for most scientists. It is often easier to deny the *truth* than to correct mistaken beliefs, when correcting those beliefs requires a simple change in perception exposing a new worldview.

Fresh new perspectives create both a challenge as well as an opportunity, as Dr. Becker seemed to intuitively recognize in the introduction to his seminal 1985 book *"The Body Electric: Electromagnetism and the Foundation of Life,"* cowritten with Gary Selden:

I believe these discoveries presage a revolution in biology and medicine. One day they may enable the physician to control and stimulate healing at will. I believe this new knowledge will also turn medicine in the direction of greater humility, for we should see that whatever we achieve pales before the self-healing power latent in all organisms...I hope this realization will

*make medicine no less a science, yet more of an art again. Only then can
it deliver its promised freedom from disease.*[24]

Over time, more courageous scientists add their own scientific data
to the growing mountain range of facts already proving how healing is an electromagnetic phenomenon in all life-forms, not just
salamanders and humans. Sea urchins, for instance—the focus of
a 2008 article published in the *Journal of Medical and Biological Sciences*
by Lisanne D'Andrea-Winslow, Don Johnson, and Amy Novitski of
the University of Northwestern in St. Paul, Minnesota. These scientific pioneers proudly proclaimed how "To our knowledge, this study
represents the first report of bioelectromagnetic energy treatment
having an effect on immune cell activation and wound healing in an
invertebrate species."[25] Like many of these scholarly articles, the 2008
invertebrate study contained a detailed research bibliography, showing
that the phenomenon of bioenergetic healing is widely known and
studied—there is a mountain range of data available to all who are
willing to look.

———

As science begins to connect the dots in all this data, it is still easy to
miss the meaning of all the magnetism.

How can electromagnetism trigger healing, as Becker believed?
How can it order the arrangement of the cells in our bodies, as Burr
supposed? As these pioneering scientists looked closer, it became
obvious that this magnetism is a vital life force.

This belief in a life force was shared by many ancient civilizations. Known by "chi" to Chinese, "prana" to Hindus, "pneuma" to
Greeks, and "mana" to Polynesians. Among the many tribes of Native
American Indians, who also shared this belief, it was loosely translated as the "Great Spirit." I find that description resonant and reminiscent of Cyrus Edwin Dallin's magnificent and enduring sculptural

masterpiece *"Appeal to the Great Spirit,"* which depicts a Native American man on horseback, arms outstretched and looking upward, beseeching the heavens for guidance and assistance.

Of course, there are many other names for this life force across many other cultures and religions worldwide, including Christianity, Judaism, and Islam. Many ancient healing practices were based on applying this life force, and many of these healing traditions remain popular today in alternative and integrative medical practices ranging from acupuncture, homeopathy, therapeutic touch massage, reiki, qi gong, faith healing, prayer, yoga, to meditation.

Even if *"most scientists"* and the mainstream medical systems are not yet willing to look at this life force, *"some scientists"* throughout history have painstakingly studied the phenomenon. For example, Germany's Dr. Hans Driesch at the turn of the twentieth century and England's Dr. Rupert Sheldrake at the turn of the twenty-first, both men rigorous in their scientific methods, described the life force as a type of "morphogenetic field"—a description not unlike Harold Burr's "L-field."

We can give the same thing different names or describe it differently, but its name or description does not change its true nature. French philosopher Henri Bergson called it *"élan vital"* or vital energy in his book *Creative Evolution*, winning the Nobel Prize for Literature in 1927 (for what the Nobel Committee called his "rich and vitalizing ideas"). Though "most scientists" today still mock these ideas under a broad epithet of "vitalism" (which Wikipedia dismissively labels a "discredited scientific hypothesis"[26] in 2016), some say the notion of an invisible energy that gives life and health, a force for miracles and healing, is simple common sense.

In fact, the more you look at this subtly magnetic vital life force energy, whatever name you give it, what becomes apparent is that it explains many of life's greatest mysteries. You may be accustomed to believing that some of life's simple questions are but philosophical riddles that can never truly be answered, like *"How can life spring up and defy gravity?"* Yet some believe these questions can be answered the more you look at the science behind natural electromagnetic forces.

———

Legend says that Sir Isaac Newton came to fame contemplating the motion of an apple falling to Earth, discovering the force of gravity in the process. Hundreds of years later, in the pristine wooded mountains of Austria, an inquisitive forester named Viktor Schauberger quipped, *"I think it would have been much better if Newton had contemplated how the apple got up there in the first place."*[27]

Viktor Schauberger revered *nature*, and he believed that the force that allowed the apple tree to grow from the ground, opposing the gravitational pull of the apple to Earth, was a type of natural levitation. In the 1930s Viktor Schauberger designed, engineered, and built log flumes that he claimed applied these natural levitating forces for better forestry management. His flumes had practical purposes, transporting the densest of harvested trees—physically lifting the logs that would otherwise sink to the bottom of a river—across great distances in only shallow waters.

Schauberger claimed that the spinning, spiraling waters in his log flumes released what he called "dipolar" vital energetic forces and said these forces "levitated" the logs to allow their movement. He said he was harnessing the same powerful force that *nature* used, comparing the scientific mechanism behind his revolutionary log flumes to the imploding vortex of a tornado.[28]

The very notion of levitation—defying the force of gravity— seemed laughable to scientists of the 1930s hearing of Schauberger's inventions. Though he received several patents for these inventions[29], most scientific experts mocked him. Instead of being evaluated on the merits of his ideas, Schauberger was criticized for his lack of scientific education and formal training.

Schauberger was defiant, believing like Twain that you should never let schooling get in the way of your education. He said *science* should not stifle man's intuitive intelligence, and he said that a university classroom could not teach the incredible secrets of *nature* herself. Schauberger pointed to an ordinary trout hovering effortlessly in place in a stream's swift-moving waters, somehow staying still against the strong current until the fish decides to dart upstream in a flash. Viktor Schauberger said it was natural levitation at work in the beauty of the forest and its life-giving rivers, and knew that his harshest critics could not offer an alternative scientific explanation for the trout's motion.[30]

Levitation might seem an amusingly bizarre notion to you too, absent proof that uses the scientific method of reason. If so, then consider how scientists in this new millennium have proven how levitation is *real*.

Andre Geim and Michael Berry won an "Ig Nobel" Prize in 2000 for levitating a live frog using the physics of water's now well-known *"diamagnetic"* properties. The experiment was described as *"the physics of flying frogs"* or *"levitation without meditation"* in its Ig Nobel honors[31]— a somewhat sarcastic award parodying the Nobel Prize to "honor achievements that first make people laugh, and then make them think."[32]

Laugh if you want—*it is good for your health!*—but it really ought to make you think. Viktor Schauberger may have lacked formal education, but Sir Andre Geim and Sir Michael Berry are highly credentialed physicists exploring the physical properties of water. These men are not naive amateurs; both were crowned geniuses in Britain for their many scientific accomplishments. Berry was knighted in 1996, years before the flying frog experiment, and the Russian-born Geim was knighted in 2010, the same year Sir Andre won a *real* Nobel Prize, along with colleague Sir Konstantin Novoselov, for discovering the physics of graphene and the material's remarkable quantum properties.

Whether frogs fly with "diamagnetic" energy or logs levitate with a "dipolar" life force, once again, the dots of data are already there—available for all to see and study in a mountain range of scientific facts. Even if "most scientists" are not willing to look, it is still up to *you* to connect these dots together to find the *truth*.

Even against a tide of hostile and disapproving beliefs, *truth* can prevail. It prevails because *truth* is true and because brave souls seek the *truth* for the liberation it brings. So connect the dots together as if your wellness depends on it, for it surely does.

————

If you are still looking for the dots, maybe you should *look for the connection* instead.

Truly, the connection is where *truth* is found, not in the dots. Indeed, once you find the connection, the dots may then appear, as if by magic.

That may sound laughably strange, according to a *method of reason*. We expect careful doctors to gather symptoms and statistics before connecting their dots of data into diagnosis for medical treatment. Using the same *method of reason*, we also expect diligent lawyers to gather evidence before connecting their points of proof into conclusions of guilt or innocence. The method is logical and rational, and it is especially helpful to avoid a rush to false medical diagnosis or false legal judgment. In the final analysis, though, this method of reason works only when—and if—it finds the *truth*.

Without finding *truth*, the method of reason does not work, and the result can be a health misdiagnosis, a miscarriage of justice, or some other costly error that happens when you focus on the wrong dots or misconnect them into illusory lines. Sometimes, as experience teaches, rationality can lead to conclusions that lack common sense, so reason must always resonate with *truth*; otherwise, the rational conclusion rings false.

Sometimes rationality's errors go undetected for years or longer, in the way misinformed medical doctors mistreated my grandfather's stomach ulcer with surgery, the way my own childhood stomachaches were thought to be diverticulitis or psychosomatic instead of a dairy allergy, or the way my niece's suicide may have been caused by psychiatric mistreatment—though that *truth* may never be known.

Other times, *really* good doctors—or *really* good lawyers, judges, scientists, managers, administrators, and other rational thinkers—somehow manage to avoid the errors of purely rational thinking, knowing how their logical conclusions must still ring true in the final analysis. Seeking *truth in sciences* and its *method of reason*, these *really* good thinkers know at some deep, intuitive, or unspoken level of understanding that science must still connect resonantly with spirit.[33] Their views may be ridiculed by disbelieving peers, as in so many stories of this book, but as Einstein famously said: *"Great spirits have always encountered violent resistance from mediocre minds."*

Knowing that *truth*, these *really* good thinkers fill themselves with flowing spirit, facilitating a connection to what rings true in their hearts and minds. Truly, our greatest scientists have always realized that insight, invention, inspiration, imagination, and the light of understanding are found in the *connection*—not the dots!

Sir Michael Berry, the esteemed and witty physicist of flying frogs, quipped on his Internet blog that *"my contribution to particle physics"* is naming the *"elementary particle of sudden understanding."*[34] He gave the particle the funny name *"clariton,"* based on his observation that *"any scientist will recognize the 'Aha!' moment when this particle is created."*[35] In the clarity of that *Aha!* moment, the connection is revealed, and dots can then be easily gathered. Eventually, the *Aha!* idea seems obvious and simple. As Sir Michael said, *"how sad that a clariton is sometimes less than astonishing, well known to those who know well, a mere claritino.'*[86] Be well, Sir Michael, for you know well.

History's greatest scientists and inventors know well what Sir Michael meant too. The sudden connection of an *Aha!* moment—that soon seems an obvious truth—is the same way that Nikola Tesla described his invention of the electromagnetic induction motor in 1882.

"The idea came like a flash of lightning and in an instant the truth was revealed,'[87] Tesla explained; in that miraculous moment, while on a walk with a friend in a park in Budapest contemplating words from Goethe's *Faust,* Tesla said the *"images I saw were wonderfully sharp and clear.'*[88] Immediately following that *Aha!* moment, according to Tesla, he *"drew with a stick in the sand"* a diagram at the heart of his sudden insight, and just *"six years later"* he drew the exact same diagram, filling in more dots of detail, for a lecture he presented to the American Institute of Electrical Engineers in New York.[39] That lecture of 1888 for *"a new system of alternate current motors and transformers'*[40] changed history, marking the beginning of the "plug-in-wall" power generation systems and industrial institutions we know today and which we now see as obvious. For Tesla, then, it began with a connection—not a dot.

Albert Einstein spoke of the same *Aha!* experience. In 1905, he imagined a clock keeping time on a building and how time would appear if he moved away from the building in a streetcar traveling at the speed of light. *"A storm broke loose in my mind,"* Einstein recalled, and *"suddenly I understood where the key to the problem lay.'*[41] With that flash of insight, he wrote his famous paper on special relativity. It was an *Aha!* connection, but it still lacked the dots of proof, so Einstein boldly invited the world's astronomers to observe and measure the light during the next solar eclipse, predicting how the light would bend based on his principles of relativity. Most mocked Einstein, but finally his friend Finlay Freundlich, an astronomer and fellow scientist, took up the costly challenge in 1914. Freundlich found a wealthy German industrialist from the Krupp family to finance his scientific expedition to the peninsula of Crimea, deep in the Black Sea, where the next solar eclipse was best observed and measured.

It might have been the right place, but it must have been the wrong time. World War I broke out, and Freundlich was captured in Crimea by Russian soldiers, unmoved by his story about being a German astronomer searching for answers of physics in remote observation sites. Finlay Freundlich spent part of the war in a Russian prison, having wasted his investor's money and the opportunity to advance physics with his scientific measurements. It just didn't seem fair; however, in the way that suffering can disguise greater blessings, the wartime experience may have prepared Freundlich for a greater ordeal later in life, though he didn't know that then. All Finlay and his friend Einstein knew at that moment, in 1914, was how tiresome it can be waiting for a dot to appear, even after you've made the connection. Indeed, without patience and gratitude, waiting can be the hardest part, and even then, the dot may not appear as you wish.

Five long years later, in 1919, Sir Arthur Eddington of Britain organized a rival expedition to the island of Príncipe in the Gulf of Guinea off the coast of West Central Africa to observe another rare solar eclipse. There, he captured the measurement that eluded Freundlich in Crimea, and became the first scientist to find the dot that proved Einstein's theory. Following his astronomical victory, Eddington wrote a treatise that popularized a new *truth in sciences* among English speakers, which Eddington entitled *Mathematical Theory of Relativity*. Albert Einstein himself said that Sir Arthur's book was *"the finest presentation of the subject in any language,"*[42] and it helped transform our notions of space and time.

We value and appreciate when Eddington measured the dot of data in 1919 and also when Einstein made the connection of insight in 1905, for both are historic scientific moments of discovery. Of the two, though, most people would say the *truly transformative* moment was when Einstein found the *Aha!* connection—more than a decade before a dot was visible.

———

The moment you connect to *truth* is always transformative.

You don't need to be an Einstein to know these moments of sudden clarity and connection. The moment might be experienced as a personal insight that heals a damaged relationship or as a patentable invention that solves a problem of commerce; the moment can be a beautiful inspiration that propels your purpose forward or a reflective realization that restores your inner peace. Though great and small, all of these moments are miracles, because they all transform lives through their connection to *truth*.

Sometimes these moments transform slowly. Over a period of time, as my friend Andy Kadison likes to say, *moments can become movements*. At other times, a moment can transform us so completely and all at once, shining its light of truth so bright that, as "miracle worker" Anne Sullivan said of her student Helen Keller, *"behold, all things are changed!"*[43]

In 1905, *Aha!* connections seemed to happen all at once for Einstein. There were so many moments of sudden illumination that year that it is popularly known as Einstein's *"Miracle Year"*—some call it the *"Annus Mirabilis"* in the custom of Latinizing even miracles to conform to scientific naming conventions. There was Einstein's *Aha!* moment of special relativity between time and space, his famous *Aha!* equation of $E = MC^2$ linking energy to matter and the speed of light, and his *Aha!* insight how subatomic photon particles explained the photoelectric effect. He wrote breakthrough scientific papers on each of these three topics in 1905.

Einstein had one more *Aha!* moment that year, and it is this fourth insight which is at the beating heart of wellness, because of its miraculous potential for personal transformation and healing. This insight will help draw this final chapter of the book to a close shortly, but before revealing Einstein's fourth *Annus Mirabilis* connection, it is important to remember that Einstein did not win a Nobel Prize for this breakthrough discovery of wellness. This *Aha!* connection remains obscure and largely misunderstood even today. Indeed, as seen elsewhere in this book, sometimes even the most important insights do not win prizes nor receive awards. Sometimes, deserving ideas go unacknowledged or are recognized only slowly over time.

You may be surprised to learn that even Einstein did not win a Nobel Prize for his famous formula on matter and energy nor for his brilliant revelations about the relativity of time, and that he received his first and only Nobel Prize for his scientific paper on photons and photo-electricity. He won the 1921 Nobel Prize for Physics—which appropriately was awarded in *1922!*[4] I thought that funny, not because of the odd quirk in the Nobel rules that permit awards to be reserved for the future, but because of the comic irony how even Einstein's award can bend notions of time's relativity. Like Einstein in 1921, your award might have already been given, but maybe not yet been announced.

Time's relativity is important for your wellness because it reminds you that time is not confined to the speed of light. When you connect to *truth*, time is no longer measurable by a clock on a wall. How do you measure the interval of time of an *Aha!* moment or quantify the depth of its meaning? In these moments of profound connection, time seems magically suspended, as if it could expand into eternity.

That feeling of *infinite* expansion applies not just for *Aha!* moments of scientific insight and invention, but for any connection to spirit and its transformative *truths*. To see that's true, think how you experience moments of love, passion, peace, beauty, music, caring, compassion, creativity, or conscience. Think how you experience moments of freedom, forgiveness, laughter, joy, justice, redemption, empathy, or wellness. *Each of these aspects of truth is like the facets of a diamond*, as my friend Don Schreiber likes to say, sparkling individually yet connected together in glorious unity.

Truly connecting to all of these wonderful spiritual *truths* can change how you experience time, enabling miracles in your life and allowing the dots to move into place for you. Dots moving into place through spiritual connection may seem unscientific, but it is not unlike the way magnetic fields invisibly organize iron filings on a piece of paper.

You may recall how Harold Saxton Burr said "molecules and cells" arrange themselves into place oriented by the "electro-dynamic field of the body" that "serves as a matrix."[45] Dr. Burr eventually realized that these electromagnetic fields are not limited to our molecules and cells but extend beyond our bodies throughout the universe. *"The Universe… is organized and maintained by a… dynamic field capable of determining the position and movement of all charged particles,"*[46] he wrote many decades before NASA-funded scientists confirmed that the "universal ubiquitous" magnetic field extended into the most remote areas of deep space. *"Since you and I are components of the field of the Universe,"* Harold Burr concluded, *"we are all tied together in the same bundle of field properties. None of us can ever be independent of the universal field or of our own individual fields."*[47]

Shortly before his death in 1973, Harold Saxton Burr published two books with science-meets-spirituality themes, entitled *Blueprint for Immortality: The Electric Patterns of Life* and *The Fields of Life: Our Links to the Universe*. However, these books were not quack pseudoscience, for they were based on Dr. Burr's voltmeter experiments carefully conducted and reported at Yale University's School of Medicine *"for nearly half a century"* under *"rigorously controlled experimental conditions"* that *"met with no contradictions."*[48] In other words, a lifetime devoted to science and medicine convinced Dr. Burr that science was truly intertwined with spirit, part of the same connected whole. Harold Saxton Burr's startling conclusion was that *"We are part of a designed whole which is not chaos but organized."*[49] He realized that *"the Universe has meaning and so have we. Though we do not understand it, the meaning is there."*[50]

By aligning ourselves with this field of spiritual connection, Burr believed we could find that meaning for ourselves. He saw a chance to rethink our understanding of the laws of science and physics, for *"if we can accept that there is...one overall field, to which all humanity is subject,"* then *"there is no longer"* need to separate *"one law for the material and another for the spiritual."* Dr. Burr believed this alignment applied to the laws of society too, for "even the laws devised by lawyers, which ostensibly reflect the 'conscience' of the community, may one day be brought into closer relation with the laws of Nature as that 'conscience' becomes less confused and variable."[51]

Science and its laws, like all the other laws of humankind, cannot be separated from spirit, for humanity is born of spirit. Spirit does not undermine humankind, nor does spirit undermine science. *It is spirit that enables science and guides science in the right direction.* Indeed, a thought system in which science is disconnected from spirit is truly terrifying, as it can threaten humanity with death and destruction.

More than a decade before the Austrian Archduke Franz Ferdinand was assassinated in Sarajevo, triggering the start of the First World War, it was apparent to Mark Twain that humanity was on the eve of annihilation. Twain wrote from a hotel in Vienna, Austria, to his scientist friend Nikola Tesla back in New York, describing a conversation *"in the hotel"* with *"some interested men discussing means to persuade the nations to...disarm."* Twain wrote that *"I advised them...to invite the great inventors to contrive something against which fleets and armies would be helpless, and thus make war thenceforth impossible."* Twain urged Tesla to use his scientific knowledge *"to introduce into the earth permanent peace and disarmament in a practical and mandatory way."*[52]

Nikola Tesla, who had already been criticized in the press for his earlier experiments with a deadly "death ray" invention (the supposed basis for the "star wars" technologies of the future) apparently took Twain's letter to heart and in 1905 Tesla wrote a visionary article in an electrical engineering journal that dreamed how his latest invention, *"the transmission of electrical energy without wires,"* could be *"a means for furthering peace."*[53] The year 1905 may have been a miracle year for Albert Einstein that transformed modern physics and 1905 may have been the year in which Dr. Robert Koch won a Nobel Prize for the "germ theory" of disease, which became a foundation of modern medicine, but in some ways, Tesla's own 1905 vision—of wireless energy transmission as a means of furthering peace—deeply transformed the entire direction of humanity. As ordinary people joined together electromagnetically regardless of physical distance, wireless technology changed our perception of how interconnected and interdependent we truly are.

The story of how Twain and Tesla searched for lasting peace through science also reminds us that the scariest part of science is not its technology but its separation from spirit. Scientific technology can be used for purposes of terror or for purposes of peace, but the only difference between the two is the intangible intentions of *spirit*. The story reminds us how spirit must always direct the progress of science; truly, *science* must never be separated from con*science!*

You may recall the story how the powerful technologies of Hans Berger, the German inventor of the EEG brain scanner, nearly came into the hands of the Nazis. Berger seemed crushed by the weight of his own conscience, and some say committed suicide instead of cooperating with evil intent. The Nazis tried to co-opt the levitating implosion technologies of Viktor Schauberger too, after some of Schauberger's patents caught the eye of the Führer's henchmen. Immediately pressed into service by the Nazi military machine, Schauberger took an altogether different approach than Berger. Clever and calculating in his conscientious resistance, Schauberger is said to have sabotaged his own scientific experiments, slyly appeasing the Führer with proof of his technology's great power, yet intentionally denying Hitler functional military devices.

All truly great scientists understand the paramount need to connect science to conscience and to connect science to other shining spiritual *truths*. The Nobel Prize was named for Alfred Nobel, who made a vast fortune by inventing dynamite and manufacturing mass weapons of war and destruction. When Alfred Nobel read his own obituary—a newspaper mistakenly believed Alfred had died instead of his brother Ludvig and described Alfred Nobel as a *"Merchant of Death"*[54]—he asked deep spiritual questions about his life's purpose and meaning. As a result of this epiphany, Alfred Nobel established his annual prize to encourage *"those who, during the preceding year, shall have conferred the greatest benefit on mankind"* including *"champions of peace."*[55]

It is a huge mistake for science to see itself limited to only a skeptical *method of reason*, unhinged from more meaningful *truths* that come through connection to spirit. We may mistakenly assume all scientists are cold and rational, drawing their conclusions from points of proof deduced in straight lines of logic, yet truly great scientists have always understood that science can never be disconnected from spirit.

My favorite part of the story of Finlay Freundlich and Sir Arthur Eddington, the two astronomers racing to prove or disprove Einstein's theory of relativity in the observation of a solar eclipse, is the part that resonates with the spirit of kindness and love. Historians who see history as a system of points and lines, where there are only winners and losers, say Sir Arthur won and got the fame and fortune that came with the discovery of an important dot of data, while poor Finlay lost with his internment in a Russian prison at the outbreak of the First World War. A few of these historians have even wrongly accused Eddington of mishandling astronomical data to advance Eddington's own career; knowing that Freundlich was planning his next solar eclipse expedition, they allege Eddington's ill intent was to beat his scientific rival in the race to prove relativity.[56]

To me, the real *truth* of history is that Finlay Freundlich survived his time in a Russian prison, learning valuable lessons from his wartime experience that benefited him decades later during Hitler's rise to power. As Hitler's armies advanced throughout Europe, Freundlich and his Jewish wife fled, always just a few steps ahead of the Nazis, until finally reaching a dead end as the Germans advanced on tolerant Holland—where diary writer Anne Frank famously hid from Nazis until the young teen was discovered and deported to Auschwitz, dying there as a slave laborer. To me, the real *truth* of the story was how Eddington helped Freundlich escape from Holland with his family in the nick of time, zealously advocating on Freundlich's behalf until finally securing a professorship in astronomy for his friend Finlay at the prestigious University of St. Andrews in Scotland. Freundlich stayed at this post for nearly twenty years, long past the end of the war, popularly beloved by the students of St. Andrews as *"Herr Professor"* until university administrators adhering to rigid policy lines foolishly forced Freundlich into retirement.[57]

We can exaggerate a scientific rivalry in the pursuit of science, but like sportsmanship in the pursuit of sports, it is the spiritual conduct of fairness and graciousness that truly matters. Kindness and love, like in the story of Eddington and Freundlich, are fondly remembered miracles not measurable by a clock on a wall. Their *truths* transform lives in ways we may never truly understand, but we all can surely appreciate.

Of course, there are many ways of interpreting history, but the story of Sir Arthur Eddington's kindness and love should not be surprising for an intensely spiritual man who wrote—more than a decade before he helped Finlay Freundlich find refuge from Nazis in 1939— how *"we recognize a spiritual world alongside a physical world"* and how *"we all know there are regions of the human spirit untrammelled by the world of physics.'*[58] This aspect of Eddington's self was consistent with someone who declared himself a *"conscientious objector"* in 1918, a year before finding the dot of data in 1919 that made him famous for proving Einstein's relativity.[59] Eddington's spirituality may have had its roots in his Quaker upbringing, as some historians believe, but it flourished based on his direct observational experience. *"Mind is the first and most direct thing in our experience"* wrote Eddington, for *"all else is remote inference."*[50] Eddington's conclusion mirrored the observation of René Descartes, who established the foundational methods of scientific rational thinking, yet never denied his own spiritual consciousness, staunchly believing *"I think therefore I am."*

Eddington saw spirit as the paramount force of the universe, which made science itself possible. In his 1927 book *The Nature of the Physical World,* he wrote how scientific inquiry derives from what he called the *"mind-stuff"*[51] of spirit, since *"the pursuit of science springs from a striving which the mind is impelled to follow… the light beckons ahead and the purpose surging in our nature responds."*[52] Eddington's insight is essential to science, for it compels scientists to be more than merely logical or physical—successful scientists must be spirited! Eddington's insight applies to you and me too, for when the light beckons us ahead, we must respond with the surging purpose of our own nature. So be spirited—it will make you feel well.

The foundational importance of spirit for scientists may sound fantastical, yet it is observable and plainly obvious, if you are willing to look. Spend a moment considering some of our most accomplished scientists, and how the light beckons them too.

Consider Sir Andre Geim and Sir Michael Berry, who magnetically levitated frogs to usher in a new millennium in 2000. Through the Internet and its multimedia-rich resources, we can now glimpse the light beckoning their spirit. The World Wide Web has made it easier than ever before for historians to see the twinkles in their eyes and the smiles on their faces, those subtle but undeniable cues and manners that tell us, in Leonardo da Vinci's words, the *"intention"* of their *"soul."*[53]

The Internet makes it plain to see how both Geim and Berry relentlessly pursued *truth in sciences* in the competitive and highly politicized

atmosphere of systems and institutions, yet how each refused to sacrifice the highest and best side of their *self*—their *spirit!* Too often,
mediocre institutional systems draw narrow lines that stifle spirit (the
way some short-sighted university administrators forced Freundlich
into retirement), but great spirits like Sir Andre and Sir Michael do not
suffer such foolish limitations gladly. Both men seem to understand
how their prodigious scientific accomplishments spring from their
good humor, humility, honesty, curiosity, creativity, courage, kindness,
authenticity, and other attributes of great spirits.

For instance, Berry's Internet blog revealed Sir Michael's honest
humility, openly admitting in a discussion of the 2000 Ig Nobel Prize
how *"The flying frog was [my friend] Andrey Geim's experiment."* Berry also
brought his spirit of collaborative creativity to the project, daring to
imagine how *"in principle, a person could be magnetically levitated too—like
frogs, we are mostly water."* Sir Michael's spirit of selfless courage was
obvious as well; though no frogs were hurt in the experiment, he logically observed that *"of course nobody can be sure"* whether human levitation *"would be a harmful or painful experience,"* but *"[n]evertheless, I would
enthusiastically volunteer to be the first."*[64]

Sir Michael Berry's selfless courage volunteering in pursuit of scientific truth is reminiscent how Dr. Barry Marshall infected himself
with bacteria to prove a cure for stomach ulcers that more mediocre
minds had violently resisted and ridiculed. That spirit of selfless courage in pursuit of truth reminded me too of Andre Geim's quip how
"It's better to be wrong than be boring."[65]

Andre Geim is a man who does not seem to be wrong much, and
like other great spirits, he is seldom boring. *"Don't take yourself too seriously,"* Geim said in a slide show to an audience of scientists[65]; *"In my
experience, if people don't have a sense of humor, they are usually not very good
scientists either."*[66] In video clip after video clip, I found myself laughing out loud at Sir Andre's often self-deprecating jokes, learning all
the while by connecting to the funny spirit of this otherwise serious

scientist. *"I've often heard it said a preacher might learn with a comedian for a teacher,"* Goethe said in *Faust*[67], and it is true how we all learn as we all laugh together.

Journalist Giles Whittell had the privilege of interviewing Sir Andre for a 2014 article for *The Economist* publications, and he described Geim as *"someone so warm in person and so well-loved by his colleagues."*[58] I was not surprised, for I saw that same fuzzy trait of a great spirit even from *YouTube* videos on the Internet. Spiritual presence can be sensed in person, but it is also can be detected from facial expressions, tones of voice, and body language in a video.

For instance, it was obvious from Geim's formal dinner reception speech to the 2010 Nobel Prize crowd in Stockholm, when he won his award, as he gently touched his right hand to his left chest and said *"From the very bottom of my heart, thank you all."*[59] There was love in Sir Andre Geim's gesture, as if rays of light were shining from his heart. It was a spirit that mere words could not convey, and it reminded me of stories of friendships, like Freundlich and Eddington, and a quotation posted on Sir Michael Berry's blog, attributed to literary legend Dr. Samuel Johnson, how *"Kindness is in our power even when fondness is not."*[70] There is incredible healing power of forgiveness when given without judgment or opinion—forgive yourself and forgive others—and this same spirit reminds us how false judgments and misguided opinions often prevent more meaningful connection to *truth*.

Connection is at the heart of wellness, as connection is at the heart of all truth—but we must remember that *connection* is also at the heart of science. Sir Michael Berry stressed that point when accepting the 2014 Richtmyer Award from the American Association of Physics Teachers. *"The underlying theme is connections,"* said Sir Michael, reminding his audience of science educators how *"many people in many walks of life have made the same point, encouraging connections."*[71] To prove his point, Berry offered the wisdom of a retiring colleague, the late Sir Charles Frank, a pioneer in liquid crystal physics research, on how *"Physics is not just concerning the nature of things, it concerns the 'connections' between the natures of different things.'*[72]

For the sake of your wellness, remind yourself how *"connection"* is lost if you cling to your opinions or judgments. Your opinions or judgments may have elements of truth or may depend on narrow defi-nition for their truth, yet somehow you lose the deeper meaning of *truth* by stubbornly insisting you are right. Look how many physicians clung to their false opinions that stomach ulcers were not caused by bacteria and how many insisted that beriberi was caused by a bacte-rial infection. Look how many scientific skeptics still cling to a Royal Commission's false judgment from 1784 that there is no such thing as animal magnetism and how many falsely insist that *spirit* is not relevant for medicine. These opinions and judgments, and countless more like them today, all prevent meaningful connection to *truth*. There can be no *truth* without connection—for it's all connected, *everything to every-thing else.* That's true for health, as it is true for history, science, and your self; all connected in unity.

Albert Einstein intuitively understood how everything was con-nected, and Einstein searched for these unifying connections through-out his life—even coining the term *"unified field theory"* as the Holy Grail of physics.[73] 1905 was a *"miracle year"* for Einstein because he found "connections" between the natures of so very many different things that year. In this *Annus Mirabilis*, he found connections between matter and energy, between time and space, and between atomic par-ticles and light—but as said earlier in this section, Einstein found one more obscure connection in that miracle year that matters most for your health and wellness.

Einstein helped explain a mysterious natural phenomenon that had puzzled scientists since 1827, when a Scottish botanist named Robert Brown observed the strange motion of a speck of pollen on the water of his microscope's slide, describing how the pollen moved to and fro across the water in erratic nonlinear patterns. Botanist Brown tested to see if this odd motion could be scientifically explained by living biological functions of the pollen, so he used pollen from long-dead plants, but the motion of the pollen always stayed the same, like a dot dancing haphazardly on the water. One by one, Brown tested for other physical causes of the pollen's motion—water currents, evaporation, light, vibrations, and so forth—but none offered an explanation for the pollen's oddly familiar zigzagging motion.

Most likely, you have already seen this phenomenon of Brownian motion with your own eyes, as dots of dust dancing in a ray of light. The ancient Roman philosopher poet Lucretius described this commonplace motion in 60 BC in his classic treatise *On the Nature of Things*, which Lucretius understood as a visible manifestation of a universal force normally hidden from sight:

> *Observe what happens when sunbeams are admitted into a building and shed light on its shadowy places. You will see a multitude of tiny particles mingling in a multitude of ways in the empty space within the actual light of the beam...*
>
> *To some extent a small thing [like these tiny particles dancing in the sunlight] may afford an illustration and an imperfect image of great things. Besides, there is a further reason why you should give your mind to these particles that are seen dancing in a sunbeam: their dancing is an actual indication of underlying movements of matter that are hidden from sight.*[74]

In his fourth *Annus Mirabilis* paper, Albert Einstein said that atomic particles jostling and colliding accounted for Brownian motion, normally hidden from sight.[75] Einstein's *Aha!* connection between atomic particles and Brownian motion helped prove to skeptical scientists of the early 1900s how atomic particles were real—not merely imagination—and could make the dust dance in a sunbeam and a speck of pollen zigzag across a slide. In other words, Einstein's paper served as the scientific foundation for the future study of particle physics, including the imaginary *"clariton"* that Sir Michael Berry quipped was the *"elementary particle of sudden understanding."*[76]

Sudden understanding does not come from a particle; as Sir Michael said, it comes from connection. That was true for Einstein in 1905, and it remains true for you and me today too. There are some things we cannot understand until we see the connection, and then understanding seems simple, as if we should have known it all along.

Perhaps now, ready to turn a page in your own life and ready to end this last chapter of the book, you are ready to make a scientific connection that Einstein did not; that Einstein *could not* in 1905. You can make this connection now for yourself—perhaps you already have—but again, remember this connection was always there, patiently waiting for your understanding.

In 1905, although Einstein helped explain Brownian motion with atomic particles, Einstein and the scientists of his time could not understand the erratic zigzagging patterns of the motion itself, describing the movement as a "random walk."[77] The motion was unpredictable, nonlinear, and immeasurable; it was as amorphous as the rough natural shapes of coastlines, clouds, lungs, or lightning. Without the geometry to explain Brownian motion, its oddly self-similar natural patterns remained mathematically inexplicable. Decades after Einstein died in 1955, Benoît Mandelbrot would formulate fractal geometry, specifically revealing in 1982 how Brownian motion had a fractal dimension. Still unexplained, however, was the actual force that physically moved the dots of pollen, sunlight, or other physical objects into these familiar fractal patterns—but that connection of physics needed to wait until 2013.

You don't need a dot to see the connection! Decades before the data was published in 2013 in the prestigious journal *Nature*, Douglas Hofstadter had already predicted how magnetic fields invisibly expanded into stunningly beautiful fractal patterns, resembling a psychedelic butterfly with self-similar features at every scale of the pattern. His prediction became known as *"Hofstadter's butterfly"* among physicists, many of whom raucously ridiculed the notion that magnetic fields could behave this way.

The idea first came to Hofstadter as a doctoral student in physics in the early 1970s, and Hofstadter recalled how his PhD advisor was *"scornful,"* calling his prediction *"mere numerology"* and dismissively chiding Hofstadter that he *"would be unable to get a PhD for this kind of work."*[77] Hofstadter received his physics doctorate for other work, but fortunately for science and for all of humanity, he honored the strivings of his spirit and in 1976 made his prediction public in a scientific journal known as Physical Review B.[78]

Although Douglas Hofstadter was a brilliant visionary physicist, and the son of Nobel Prize-winning physicist Robert Hofstadter, he left the study of physics, unwilling to inanely wait for others to find the dots validating his theory of a magnetic butterfly with a self-similar geometric shape. Back in 1976, when Douglas Hofstadter made his prediction public, this shape could not yet be described mathematically—that dot would of course not appear until 1982. Temporarily discouraged perhaps, but undaunted in his quest for truth, Douglas Hofstadter would continue to find connections, discovering how lines blurred between physics, philosophy, cognitive consciousness, and comparative literature, eventually winning Pulitzers and other prizes for books like 1979's *Gödel, Escher, Bach: An Eternal Golden Braid* and 2007's aptly-named *I Am a Strange Loop.*

The points of proof would come for Hofstadter's butterfly in 2013, like Eddington eventually arrived to prove Einstein's relativity, but it took new tools for scientists to see a magnetic field closely enough to find his fractal butterfly. By far the most important of these new tools was the development of *graphene*[79]—think of a bee's hexagonal honeycomb lattice made of a single layer of carbon atoms—which, as you may recall, won a Nobel Prize in Physics in 2010 for Sir Konstantin Novoselov and his friend and mentor Sir Andre Geim.

"An interesting part of this story," explained Sir Andre Geim to an audience of research scientists gathered to hear him in the Netherlands, *"is that the [graphene] paper was rejected twice by [the prestigious Journal] Nature."*

As Geim told the story, this rejection teaches us how scientific research can sometimes be so meaningful and *"so nice that it does not require actually publication in a high profile journal."*[80] The good-natured and jovial Geim was being sarcastic, and his punch line made the audience of research scientists—themselves striving for high profile publication—burst into laughter, understanding the ironic truth of what Sir Andre was saying. They applauded him loudly as Geim urged them to carry on, to keep going even in the face of ridicule and rejection.

"Don't give up," Andre Geim urged, for *"it can still be a Nobel Prize winning paper."*[81] He smiled broadly, knowingly, with his life's experience of perseverance and eventual vindication through the taunts and jeers of institutional groupthink. *"Don't tell this to science ministers,"*[82] Geim further cautioned his audience, with the hushed tones sometimes used to speak truth to power, and with the wisdom of someone who discovered that the path towards *truth* does not move in a smooth, straight line.

Regardless of its place of publication or its scientific politics, the discovery of the fractal shape of a magnetic field has profound meaning for your health and wellness. It helps explain, scientifically speaking, *how an invisible connection can physically move the dots into place in your own life.* Even for hardened skeptics, it now proves how dots of matter can float and dance in the dynamic universal magnetic field as if on the wings of an infinitely expanding invisible butterfly.

Early on in his distinguished career, Andre Geim observed this phenomenon with his very own eyes. He tells a funny story how one evening, during his outside-the-box free-spirited "Friday Night Experiments," he poured water into a very large and powerful laboratory magnet. *"You'd expect water would wind up somewhere on the floor,"* Geim said—but it did not.[83] What he observed instead was astounding, propelling his scientific voyage to discover flying frogs and graphene alike. "Recently people have asked me, why did I do it?" and an amused Andre answered, *"I have no idea… it's so unscientific,"* chuckling to himself how *"it was just pouring water."*[84]

Geim watched as the water he poured into the strong magnetic field floated and danced in the air, in patterns that made *"beautiful...images you can watch for minutes and hours and hours...very therapeutic in fact,"* Sir Andre added.[85] His "therapeutic" description triggered another connection in a mind forever connecting, and Geim explained how physics influences medical sciences and how water levitating as if alive in a magnetic field was truly *"a therapeutic phenomenon."*[86] *"If you are angry,"* he thoughtfully continued, *"look at the water and it will help."*[87]

These wise words of wellness from a Nobel laureate in physics may seem odd to you if you are accustomed to rigid lines between academic disciplines. Perhaps then you need to blur your own illusory lines about scientists and how scientists should think and feel, how scientists should investigate the truth.

Even if you are not able to see the levity and levitation in Geim's magnetic lab, you may have already experienced this "therapeutic phenomenon" in your own life, perhaps by looking at a rainbow in the sky or the twinkle in an eye. Think how you can measure the wellness of others by the twinkle in their eye—even for a loved one sick in bed—and how the twinkle in another's eye can help you feel well yourself, in the way that spirit is contagious in its connection. Realize too how the beautiful sight of a rainbow is somehow uplifting and healing, though it is merely water droplets floating in the air, diffracting and curving the light in magnetically mesmerizing ways.

A rainbow can teach something else fundamental about your wellness. You may perceive lines and borders in a rainbow, sharply separating the colors in your mind, but that is just an illusion. In fact, there are no lines or borders in a rainbow, and the spectrum of healing light you see is indivisibly connected together in perfect unity. It is an urgent lesson for the world's wellness, for beyond the lines and borders we pretend to see in the light, we are all connected together by universal and ubiquitous magnetic spirit.

"I don't divide the world by religions or countries,"[88] Andre Geim says, well knowing how some people yearn to narrowly separate and categorize him too. They draw lines and label him as Russian or German, English or Dutch, Jew or Gentile, yet Sir Andre is somehow all of these, and yet none, for his boundless spirit knows no lines nor limits. In his storied research labs, Geim puts this healthful attitude into practice. There are *"Ukrainians and Russians, Israelis and Iranians, Pakistanis and Indians"*[89] all working together in his lab, although Geim knows their home nations are all self-righteously angry at one another, even hatefully at war. So Sir Andre makes sarcastic jokes that make some cringe until they laugh out loud.

His warm and honest humor is surely a "therapeutic phenomenon" too, indivisibly connected to higher *truths* like kindness, creativity, empathy, and love. *"It gives great joy to break prejudices and biases against each other,"* he says, his laughter blurring the illusory lines that seem to separate us. *"It's really OK,"* says Sir Andre, describing the process of healing the wounds of these age-old divisions; *"for two or three months there is tension, and out of respect for each other, people try to put a smile on their faces...then finally after six months all my racist jokes and politically incorrect jokes are actually taken as jokes,"* making Nobel-winner Sir Andre Geim, in his own words, *"a great ambassador for peace."*[90]

———

Peace is a Nobel-worthy goal at the heart of wellness too, but peace ultimately requires a change in perception.[91]

It requires that you blur your rigid lines and stop proving points to make your self feel right. Peace comes neither from self-validation nor ego-gratification. What peace requires is genuine connection to *spirit* and its higher *truths*. It requires connection to *"the better angels of our nature,"* to borrow words of President Abraham Lincoln, spoken on the eve of the Civil War, who ensured a bitterly divided nation's peace by seeking the divine spiritual truths that connect and unify us all.[92]

It may seem that peace and the wellness it brings cannot be yours, because you are too busy struggling to overcome obstacles, reach achievements, fight adversaries, or vanquish infirmities, but those are mere dots of measurement. Fixating on these dots can never bring you peace. You may believe that you are undeserving of peace, but whether you have made bad errors or done bad things, whether you feel like a victim or villain, whatever guilt you've gathered or sins you've suffered, in *truth*, those are more dots waiting to be gently moved toward the forgiving light of connection.

Focus on connection, and you might be amazed to see how the dots can miraculously move into place for you. The dots can magically appear as people in your life, as resources or opportunities, lessons or signs, synchronicities or coincidences—all of which may seem strangely part of the connection you feel. You'll soon notice how the more you connect, the more the dots will appear.

Even before these dots fall into place, though, peace can be yours, because peace comes with the connection, not the dots.

If you still do not understand how to find connection for yourself, then it may be helpful to think of your *self* as a magnetic field—which you truly are, scientifically speaking. Some of your own magnetic fields revolve around you in strange loops and recurring patterns that prevent more meaningful connection to *truth*. Without judgment or opinion, carefully observe your own recurring patterns. Some of your own strange loops keep you from *truth* and prevent your wellness, but with forgiveness and love, you can gently and consciously correct these self-limiting patterns and release them to the *infinite*.

Correct them by connecting them to the other fields within you, the ones that do not loop around you, but instead—as is the scientific property of all magnetic fields—extend into *infinity*. It is these *infinite* fields in which your true *spirit* and all its shining *truths* are found.[93] This true *spirit* is boundless, and it soars in freedom and joy. Extending endlessly beyond your body, it makes you feel vibrantly alive, as big as a mountain, as high as a cloud, as bright as a galaxy of stars, and connects you indivisibly together with all of nature and God and the transcendent, transformational miracles of the *infinite*.

You can live your life in magnetic ways that give you purpose and meaning, recognizing your self-limiting recurring closed loops and connecting to unlimited infinite miracles that bring the important dots of your life into view. Or not. The choice is yours. As Albert Einstein is said to have said, *"There are only two ways to live your life. One is as though nothing is a miracle. The other is as though everything is a miracle."*

When I was uncertain how to end this chapter, knowing it would be the last chapter of this book on the heart of wellness, I asked for wisdom and guidance from *spirit*.

I ask for its wisdom and guidance often, for I know it is the best part of my *self*, connecting me to everything and everyone and the *infinite*, giving me meaning and purpose. I always try to ask with gratitude for the answer I will receive, whenever I receive it. When I receive an answer, somehow it always seems obvious to me that *spirit* has brought it, and though it might not be the answer I expected, I graciously and gladly accept it. I know that however the answer moves me forward, I am happy for the journey of self-discovery and learning.

When I asked *spirit* how to end this book, I was walking on the streets of midtown Manhattan, in the neighborhood of Times Square and the Port Authority, which some describe as the beating heart of New York City. As I walked along after a long day of business meetings and legal appearances, I knew I was finally headed home, and in my mind, I was already thinking again about writing the end of this chapter. At the time, I was pondering the many scientific stories of this last chapter, because somehow I sensed that a story on *science* (even of the science-meets-spirituality variety) did not seem a good way to end a story of *spirit*. That is why I asked for help and assistance from *spirit*.

Near Ninth Avenue, I came upon a vendor selling fruits from a street-corner stand. I decided to buy a bunch of bananas for my son Jason, who was living at home that summer and diligently studying for the bar exam, having recently graduated law school from the University of Texas at Austin. Part of Jason's daily study routine was concocting fruit smoothies or juices in our kitchen blender, and I knew that our supply of bananas was low. I was happy to help Jason *"eat healthy"* to use Jason's expression, although I knew vodka or other distilled spirits would sometimes go into the blender (and would eventually birth Jason's entrepreneurial journey to create a flavored vodka ice pop—creating what he calls Vice Pops®). Regardless, it did not matter to me, for I enjoyed seeing my son Jason happy and well, which is why I stopped at the fruit stand to buy bananas.

As I approached the fruit stand, I saw the vendor attending to a little customer, a boy probably two or three years of age, with pale white freckled skin and a big head of curly orange hair. The little boy was gleeful, tightly clutching in each of his two little hands an over-size plastic bag filled with fruits. His attention was fixed intently on the vendor as his proud mother and father watched their toddler son, great joy radiating from their hearts. *"What else? What else?"* the vendor would say to the little boy. *"But you have no strawberries! Do you want strawberries?"* The child was beaming and squealed *"Yes!"* with delight as the vendor placed a container of ripe red strawberries into one of the plastic bags. *"And peaches? Do you want peaches?"* the vendor asked. *"Yes!"* the boy squealed again as the vendor held up two big bright orange peaches, placing one in each of the two bags.

This continued with several more fruits, and I watched the boy's parents, still elated by their little son's happiness, become increasingly concerned about the cost of all this fruit. As the boy's bags began to bulge too big to hold more, his little arms straining from the weight of the fruit, his parents dutifully asked the vendor, *"How much do we owe you?"* their joy turning to apprehension. *"Nothing,"* replied the vendor, a brown-skinned Middle Eastern man in his late twenties, who gave the appearance he was trying to make a living to support his own small children. The boy's parents, uplifted by the kindness of the gesture, promised to bring the vendor gifts from their own lives, enthusiastically saying they would return soon. It was apparent to me that something more than mere money had been exchanged, something special that would not soon be forgotten, but could never be quantified.

As the little child and his parents departed the stand with their fruit, I took my turn as next in line and asked the vendor for a bunch of bananas. *"That was a wonderful thing you just did,"* I said to him, handing him a bill much larger than the cost of the bananas. *"I do that for all the children,"* he said selflessly and nonchalantly as he offered me my change. I waved the change aside, thanking him for what he had just done, feeling enriched and energized by the experience in the way that giving love away makes love grow inside you too. He smiled and thanked me, and as I walked away, I realized in that shining moment how I had just received the ending to this book.

How easily peace and joy can be ours when we honor the beautiful *spirit* that connects us together—all of us joining with something bigger than ourselves! Though the vendor was probably a Muslim from Pakistan or Bangladesh, like many of the street fruit sellers in New York, and though the little boy and his parents appeared to be Jewish, like many families who lived on the West Side of Manhattan, peace between them was not any more difficult. I shook my head in awe and amazement at the small miracle that had just taken place, and it gave me hope how new recurring patterns can transform the world, growing in degrees over time.

Some might see that moment of grace and goodwill as a random coincidence, even though I saw the magical moment as another dot moved by connection and another reason to believe in the power of the *infinite*. Even in this new Age of Awareness, even as we begin to sci-entifically recognize how spirit extends like a magnetic matrix through the universe and deep within ourselves, providing us with source and purpose, some truths will still remain beyond measure, for doubters to doubt. As the iconic Sir Isaac Newton had said, *"these are things that cannot be explained in few words, nor are we furnished with that sufficiency of experiments which is required to an accurate determination and demonstration of the laws by which this electric and elastic Spirit operates."*[94]

These truths though they may be doubted as beyond measure are no less valid. Indeed, they are the best part of a good life, the part that gives life its purpose and meaning. For me, these truths have long seemed a shining beacon, felt deep in my heart, though I realize how skeptics might ridicule and dismiss some of the unseen inner truths most important to me in my own life.

How could I possibly prove the whispered feelings I felt when diagnosed with lung cancer that I needed to survive for the sake of my youngest son Nicholas, not knowing then that I would stage a life-affirming intervention for him almost eight years later? How could I prove my inner sense that I needed to write a book during this inter-vention, how that perceived purpose would give my life much-needed peace and clarity, and how the intervention ultimately saved me as much as it saved my son? How could I ever convince a skeptic that my lung cancer was triggered from the toxic release of an emotionally-scarring memory stored in my upper lung about a long-forgotten dog, after my own dog tragically died after being hit by a delivery van, but that the post-surgical remembrance, reconciliation, and healing release of this painful buried childhood memory led me to better health, hap-piness, and awareness? Indeed, for the most hardened skeptic, how could I ever prove the love I feel and the wellness I share, though I know these truths beyond measure are true too?

Verily, these are all things that cannot be explained in few words, nor are there sufficiency of experiments to determine and demonstrate what I already know in my heart to be true. For me, proof did not matter for these and other personal moments of spiritual synchronicity, revelation, and faith. Regardless of proof, these miraculous moments of insight gave me comfort and guidance, filled me with determination and strength, provided me with wisdom and knowing, or just made me smile with wonder and awe. Through all the doubt, I embraced and celebrated these marvelous moments beyond measure, and that made me feel well.

NOTES ON SOURCES

<u>Back Cover</u>

1. Dates are important in history, because history tries to understand events by examining how one event leads to another. Historians record the date of events chronologically, graphing cause and effect between these events on timelines, but seldom pause to ask bigger questions about whether a line on a graph can truly measure time? That important question about the nature of *time* leads to even more unfathomably deep questions, like what is the source of time?

Of course, *source* is important for history too, for it is a test of the authenticity of a story's facts and of history's truths. Good history books are filled with notes on these sources—and this book conforms to that historical custom—but here too the bigger question is what is the *source* of these truths?

At its heart, this book believes truth can be found through source, and that an awareness of source is what defines this new historical Age. An awareness of source is not merely philosophical or abstract, for source affects our everyday lives, both the sublime aspects of life as well as the mundane. Through this awareness of source, we learn too that time is no obstacle, for source reveals its truths without regard to cause, effect, or timelines.

That was all true in the story of this book's cover. When I first searched for cover art for this book on the heart of wellness, I found a beautiful, insightful painting that my daughter Melissa had already completed years before, when just a student in college studying art. After I discovered her painting, there was no question in my mind what the cover would be (though Melissa further adapted her work for my book, for which I am grateful). Truth inspires awe, and to this day I am amazed how her painting *predated* my own book, as if there was some bigger purpose and meaning behind both events—some might say it was *meant to be*. Perhaps this story about time and source as illustrated by the cover of a book is not all that remarkable; the same thing also happened with the cover of my first book (again to my amazement!), where my daughter's painting (of a man and a dog staring into the horizon) captured the essence of the book long before it was ever written.

Whatever meaning you ascribe this historical timeline of which came first—a book or its cover—the story says something intriguing about the quantum entanglements of time and source. What makes the entangled story of book and cover all the more remarkable to me, and what inspired me to add this back cover note on sources, is a dream Melissa described to me just as I was about to publish this book, my second. Though a dream inspired my first book, I seldom remember my own dreams, but Melissa has always remembered and vividly described her dreams since she was a child. She told me that this particular dream really startled her, and that she was still wondering what the dream meant.

In Melissa's dream, she was hiking in a forest with some friends and came upon a marvelous hidden tree house, which she suddenly realized was her secret, long-forgotten childhood hiding place (our family had no such tree house). She then went into the tree house to explore it, and discovered her secret, long-forgotten diaries and journals (she did have personal journals as a child). In flipping through the pages of one forgotten childhood journal of the dream, she came upon an anatomical picture showing blood and guts and internal organs, and the picture horrified her—she found its literal imagery grotesque—which is when she awoke from the dream, and Melissa said the dream disturbed her still.

As she described the dream to me, an eerie feeling swelled inside, and I showed her the epigraph dedication of this book, which she had never seen before. The epigraph asks whether an anatomically-precise picture of the heart could ever accurately describe the true complexion of our beating hearts? To me, Melissa's dream was more than mere coincidence, and it filled me with wonder and awe for the source of these symbols of truth. Somehow, that same unseen source of truth inhabited my waking consciousness and my daughter's unconscious without regard to time or its illusory lines.

2. A bildungsroman is a spiritual journey that leads from pain and disappointment to moral growth and psychological healing; said another way, it is an unlikely hero's story about finding meaning and purpose in life. Bildungsroman was a new word for me when I first came across it while writing this book. Used to describe a literary genre of novels, I realized the word applied to my own life's story, beginning with an intervention for my teenage son Nick, that launched us both on a sometimes terrifying adventure of self-discovery, eventually leading to a deeper sense of wellness and peace for us both. It may be a new word for you too, but the thesis of this book is that discovering the heart of wellness for yourself can send you on a bildungsroman of your own—a personal journey to a new age of awareness.

Introduction: Why Wellness?

1. *"Now, About My Operation in Peking"* (a/k/a *"Now, Let Me Tell You About My Appendectomy in Peking..."*), New York Times, July 26, 1971, pg. 1 (column 8) to pg. 6 (column 3), quote on page 6 under the sub-heading of "Hardly a Journalist Trick"

2. *Ibid.*, pg. 6

3. *Future Shock*, by Alvin Toffler (1970), New York: Random House, on pg. 414 (in chapter entitled "Strategies for Survival"). Toffler quotes psychologist Herbert Gerjuoy, who states: "The new education must teach the individual how to classify and reclassify information, how to

evaluate its veracity, how to change categories when necessary, how to move from the concrete to the abstract and back, how to look at problems from a new direction — how to teach himself." Toffler is cited instead of Gerjuoy, whom Toffler himself credits in *Future Shock*, because of Toffler's influence to this book beyond the lines of the specific quotation. Nonetheless, I thank Gerjuoy (not to be confused with Gurdjieff, who said much the same thing but in a more mystical way and who I thank too). Gratitude teaches lessons about learning how to learn too.

Chapter One: Start with Simplicity

1. Verse 64, *Tao Te Ching*, by Lao Tzu. The entire verse (in four paragraph stanzas) is well worth a read, so quoted here in its entirety:

> What is at rest is easily managed.
> What is not yet manifest is easy to prevent.
> What is rooted is easy to nourish.
> What is brittle is easy to break.
> What is small is easy to scatter.
>
> Put things into order before they exist.
> Prevent trouble before it arises.
> The giant pine tree grows from a tiny seedling.
> A tower nine stories high starts with a single brick.
> A journey of a thousand miles begins with a single step.
>
> Rushing into action, you fail.
> Trying to grasp things, you lose them.
> By forcing a project to completion,
> you ruin what was almost ripe.
> People usually fail when they are on the verge of success.
> So give as much care at the end as at the beginning,
> and there will be no failure.

The Master takes action
by letting things take their course.
He does not collect precious things;
he learns not to hold onto ideas.
He helps people find their true nature
but does not venture to lead them by the nose.

Chapter Four: The Meaning of a Word

1. *"High-Level Wellness for Man and Society,"* Halbert L. Dunn. M.D., Ph.D., F.A.P.H.A., American Journal Public Health Nations Health, June 1959; 49(6); pgs. 786–792, available online at: http://ajph.apha-publications.org/doi/pdf/10.2105/AJPH.49.6.786.

2. *Ibid.,* pg. 786.

3. *Following the Equator: A Journey Around the World* (1897), by Mark Twain a/k/a Samuel L. Clemens (Hartford, Connecticut, The American Publishing Company), pg. 605 (Chapter LXI)

4. *"High-Level Wellness for Man and Society,"* Halbert L. Dunn, pg. 790.

5. *The Story of My Life* (1903), by Helen Keller, Chapter IV

6. *The Work of Teachers in America: A Social History Through Stories* (1997), by Rosetta Marantz Cohen and Samuel Scheer, pg. 168, with Anne Sullivan journal entry from March 20, 1887.

7. *The Restored Classic: The Story of My Life* (1903), by Helen Keller, edited by Roger Shattuck with Dorothy Herrmann, with supplementary accounts by Anne Sullivan, her teacher, and John Macy (W.W. Norton & Company, Inc., New York), pg. 200 (excerpt from Anne Sullivan's 1891 report).

8. *Ibid.,* pg. 368 (excerpt from Anne Sullivan's 1891 report).

9. *Ibid.,* pg. 28 (excerpt from *The Story of My Life,* Chapter IV).

10. There are countless ways to kindle a miracle; for some readers, it might be *A Course In Miracles,* published by the Foundation for Inner Peace (first published in three volumes in June 1976). My good friend Gary Lahti gave me this book as a gift, as I was recovering from lung cancer surgery and ventured to a social event outside my home for the

very first time. Though I had never heard of the book before, I was somehow drawn to read it over the course of more than a decade, and it slowly helped evolve my perception of the world and myself.

11. *Following the Equator: A Journey Around the World*, by Mark Twain, pg. 605.

Chapter Five: Who's in Charge of Change?

1. *"High-Level Wellness for Man and Society,"* Halbert L. Dunn. M.D., Ph.D., F.A.P.H.A., American Journal Public Health Nations Health, June 1959; 49(6); pg. 786.
2. *Ibid.*, pg. 787.
3. *Ibid.*, pg. 786.
4. *Ibid.*, pg. 786-7.
5. *Ibid.*, pg. 790.
6. *Ibid.*, pg. 790.
7. *"Just What the Doctor Ordered: During Prohibition, an odd alliance of special interests argued beer was vital medicine,"* by Beverly Gage, Smithsonian Magazine (History & Archaeology), April 2005, pgs. 2-3, available online at: http://www.smithsonianmag.com/history-archaeology/Just_What_the_Doctor_Ordered.html
8. *"Proton Pump Inhibitor Use and the Risk of Chronic Kidney Disease,"* by Benjamin Lazarus, Yuan Chen, Francis P. Wilson, Yingying Sang, Alex R. Chang, Josef Coresh, and Morgan E. Grams, published in JAMA Internal Medicine Feb. 2016, 176(2), available online at: http://archinte.jamanetwork.com/article.aspx?articleid=2481157; see also *"Common heartburn drugs linked with kidney disease,"* by Dennis Thompson, published by CBS News (HEALTHDAY), Jan. 11, 2016, available online at: http://www.cbsnews.com/news/common-heartburn-drugs-linked-with-kidney-disease/

Chapter Six: Taking Charge of Your Health

1. Quote from home page of the Office of the Nobel Laureates in Western Australia, published by the Government of Western Australia,

Department of the Premier and Cabinet Office of Science, found at http://www.helicobacter.com

2. *"Systematic review: are probiotics useful in controlling gastric colonization by Helicobacter pylori?"* by M. Gotteland, O. Brunser, and S. Cruchet, published in Alimentary Pharmacology & Therapeutics 23, 1077-1086 (Institute of Nutrition and Food Technology, University of Chile, Santiago, Chile), at pg. 1085.

3. *Ibid.*, pg. 1077.

4. *Ibid.*, pg. 1077.

5. *Ibid.*, pg. 1077.

6. *"Trends in Alternative Medicine Use in the United States, 1990-1997: Results of a Follow-up National Survey,"* by David M. Eisenberg, Roger B. Davis, Susan L. Ettner, Scott Appel, Sonja Wilkey, Maria Van Rompay, and Ronald C. Kessler, in JAMA (Journal of American Medical Association), November 11, 1998, Vol. 280(No. 18), pgs. 1569-1575, online at http://jama.jamanetwork.com/article.aspx?articleid=188148

7. *"Alternative Medicine is Booming, Study Shows: Americans Spend $27 Billion a Year on Herbs, Massages, and other Elective Treatments,"* by William J. Cromie, the Harvard University Gazette, November 12, 1998, pg. 1 (of 4) at http://news.harvard.edu/gazette/1998/11.12/altmed.html

8. *Ibid.*, pg. 1.

9. *"High-Level Wellness for Man and Society,"* Halbert L. Dunn, pg. 797.

10. *"Alternative Medicine Goes Mainstream,"* by Alicia Waltman and Chatterjee Camille, published in Psychology Today, March 1, 2000, pg. 1 at http://www.psychologytoday.com/articles/200003/alternative-medicine-goes-mainstream

11. *"Alternative Medicine is Booming, Study Shows: Americans Spend $27 Billion a Year on Herbs, Massages, and other Elective Treatments,"* by William J. Cromie, the Harvard University Gazette, November 12, 1998

12. *"Alternative Medicine Goes Mainstream,"* pg. 2.

13. *((((Tuning Jack FM))))*, by S.J. Spiegel (published by CreateSpace 2013), pg. 21-22 (Chapter 3, *"Hot Showers…And Other Sources of Inspiration"*).

Chapter Seven: What Makes You Feel Well?

1. Kenneth H. Cooper, MD, from his website at http://cooperaerobics.com/About/Our-Leaders/Kenneth-H-Cooper,-MD,-MPH-Full-Bio.aspx, at pg. 2, cited as the "Cooper philosophy" which it says "has been proven valid in scientific research."
2. http://www.uu.nl/en/research/christiaan-eijkman
3. *"British India and the 'Beriberi Problem', 1798-1942"* by David Arnold, published in Cambridge Journal of Medical History (An International Journal for the History of Medicine and Related Sciences), July 2010; 54(3), 295-314, found online at http://www.ncbi.nlm.nih.gov/pmc/articles/PMC2889456/, at pg. 10 of 20.

Chapter Eight: Learning What Makes You Feel Well

1. *"The Poison Squad: An Incredible History,"* by Bruce Watson, published June 27, 2013, by Esquire online at http://www.esquire.com/blogs/food-for-men/poison-squad
2. *"Mrs. Winslow's Soothing Syrup For Children Teething; Letter From A Mother In Lowell, Mass. A Down-Town Merchant,"* first published by the New York Times on December 1, 1860, available online at http://www.nytimes.com/1860/12/01/news/mrs-winslow-s-soothing-syrup-for-children-teething-letter-mother-lowell-mass.html
3. *"Mrs. Winslow's Soothing Syrup – oooh so soothing"* by Ferdinand Meyer V, published January 5, 2013 on Peachridge Glass (Your comprehensive resource for the latest antique bottle and glass news), with reproduced labels and advertisements, online at http://www.peachridgeglass.com/2013/01/mrs-winslows-soothing-syrup-oooh-so-soothing/
4. *"Patent Medicines & Miracle Cures: Original Documents from the Archives of the New York City Bar,"* featured in the library of the New York City Bar Association in September 2011, published online at http://www.nycbar.org/library/featured-exhibitions/patent-medicines-and-miracle-cures
5. *"Use Only As Directed,"* by Jeff Gerth and T. Christian Miller, with design/development by Krista Kjellman Schmidt, Lena Greoger, and

Al Shaw, published September 20, 2103, by ProPublica, online at http://www.propublica.org/article/tylenol-mcneil-fda-use-only-as-directed

6. *Organon of the Medical Art*, by Samuel Hahnemann, edited and annotated by Wenda Brewster O'Reilly, 6th edition based on a translation by Steven Decker (Birdcage Books 2001), §82, pg. 130.

7. *Ibid.*, §81b, pg. 128.

8. *The Autobiography of Mark Twain*, arranged and edited, with introduction and notes, by Charles Neider (Harper & Row Publishers, Inc. 1959), Chapter 19, pgs. 131-132.

9. *Ibid.*, pg. 132.

10. Kenneth H. Cooper, MD, from his website at http://cooperaerobics.com/About/Our-Leaders/Kenneth-H-Cooper,-MD,-MPH-FullBio.aspx, at pg. 2, cited as the "Cooper philosophy" which it says "has been proven valid in scientific research."

11. *"High-Level Wellness for Man and Society,"* Halbert L. Dunn. American Journal Public Health Nations Health, June 1959; 49(6); pgs. 786–792, at pg. 787.

12. Quote from home page of the Office of the Nobel Laureates in Western Australia, published by the Government of Western Australia, Department of the Premier and Cabinet Office of Science, found at http://www.helicobacter.com

13. *The Autobiography of Mark Twain,* arranged and edited, with introduction and notes, by Charles Neider (Harper & Row Publishers, Inc. 1959), Chapter 26, pgs. 174.

14. *Ibid.*, pg. 174.

Chapter Nine: Taking Good Care

1. *"Happy Birthday, Pete Seeger!"* by Lydia Hutchinson, published on May 3, 2013, in Performing Songwriter, available online at http://performingsongwriter.com/pete-seeger-flowers-gone/

2. *Devotions Upon Emergent Occasions,* by John Donne, Meditation number XVII.

3. *Ibid.*, Meditation number XVII.

4. *Bible*, Luke 23:34.

5. *Essay on Civil Disobedience*, by Henry David Thoreau, originally published as *"Resistance to Civil Government"* in *Aesthetic Papers*, pgs. 356-387, quote from pg. 358, essay available online with historical commentary at https://www.walden.org/Library/About_Thoreau's_Life_and_Writings:_The_Research_Collections/Civil_Disobedience. This Essay is a treasure worth reading, and it profoundly influenced Dr. Martin Luther King, Jr., Mohandas Karamchand ("Mahatma") Gandhi, Count Lev Nikolayevich ("Leo") Tolstoy, among many others.

6. *Ibid.*, pg. 358.

7. Constitution of the World Health Organization (first signed July 22, 1946 and formally adopted April 7, 1948), available online at http://www.who.int/governance/eb/who_constitution_en.pdf

8. *"High-Level Wellness for Man and Society,"* Halbert L. Dunn. American Journal Public Health Nations Health, June 1959; 49(6); pgs. 786–792, at pg. 788.

9. *Ibid.*, pg. 788.

10. *Ibid.*, pg. 787.

11. *"Turning Point 1936: Hans Selye 'invents' stress (or at least gives it its name),"* McGill Reporter, Aug. 2, 2011 (internally quoting from Selye's 1979 memoir *The Stress of My Life*), available online at http://publications.mcgill.ca/reporter/2011/08/hans-selye-invents-stress/.

12. *Ibid.*

13. *"The legacy of Hans Selye and the origins of stress research: A retrospective 75 years after his landmark brief 'Letter' to the Editor of Nature,"* by Sandor Szabo, Yvette Tache, and Arpad Somogyi, *Stress*, Sept. 2012; 15(5): 472-478, published by Informa Healthcare USA, Inc., online at: http://www.selyeinstitute.org/wp-content/uploads/2013/06/The-legacy-of-Hans-Selye44.pdf.

14. *The Voice of Genius: Conversations with Nobel Scientists and Other Luminaries*, by Denis Brian (published by Basic Books 2002), pg. 263 (in Chapter Thirteen, on Hans Selye). Interestingly, the first scientist interviewed and profiled by Mr. Brian in this book was Linus Pauling, who won two unshared Nobel prizes (for chemistry and peace, and many said should have won a third for medicine)—yet who was widely

called a "quack" by his fellow scientists and physicians for some of Pauling's unconventional views (Dr. Dan Bernstein and I had spoken about Linus Pauling, as recounted in chapter six). In *Voice of Genius*, pg. 1, Denis Brian tells the story of a University of Chicago scientist under sworn testimony who was asked to name the greatest chemist and unhesitatingly said "Linus Pauling" and was then rebuked for naming a "fraud"—to which the professor replied, "I was under oath. I had to tell the truth."

15. *"Stress Can Kill—and Dr. Selye Tells How to Survive,"* by Christopher P. Andersen, *People Magazine*, Nov. 4, 1974 (Vol. 2, No. 19), available online at http://www.people.com/people/archive/article/0,,20064643,00.html

16. *"The legacy of Hans Selye and the origins of stress research: A retrospective 75 years after his landmark brief 'Letter' to the Editor of Nature,"* by Sandor Szabo, Yvette Tache, and Arpad Somogyi, *Stress*, Sept. 2012; 15(5): 472-478, published by Informa Healthcare USA, Inc., online at: http://www.selyeinstitute.org/wp-content/uploads/2013/06/The-legacy-of-Hans-Selye44.pdf.

17. *"The pursuit of happiness: The social and scientific origins of Hans Selye's natural philosophy of life,"* by Mark Jackson, published in Hist. Human Sci. 2012 Dec., 25(5): 13-29, available online at http://www.ncbi.nlm.nih.gov/pmc/articles/PMC3724273/

18. *"Scientific Research On Laughter And Humor,"* Dr. Madan Kataria (including research by Hans Selye), found online at: http://www.laughteryoga.org/english/laughteryoga/details/312

19. *Address to the White House Correspondents' Association,* President Franklin D. Roosevelt, Feb. 12, 1943, available online at: http://www.presidency.ucsb.edu/ws/?pid=16360

20. *Ibid.*

21. Dr. Reinhold Niebuhr's serenity prayer has different versions, but this is the best known:

> God grant me the serenity
> to accept the things I cannot change;
> courage to change the things I can;
> and wisdom to know the difference.

Living one day at a time;
Enjoying one moment at a time;
Accepting hardships as the pathway to peace;
Taking, as He did, this sinful world as it is,
not as I would have it;
Trusting that He will make all things right
if I surrender to His Will;
That I may be reasonably happy in this life
and supremely happy with Him
Forever in the next.
Amen.

22. *First Inaugural Address*, President Franklin D. Roosevelt, March 4, 1933, available online at: http://historymatters.gmu.edu/d/5057/

Chapter Ten: Be Connected

1. *"The Many Causes of America's Decline in Crime,"* by Inimai M. Chettiar, Atlantic Magazine, Feb. 15, 2015, quote at pg. 2 of 13, available online at: http://www.theatlantic.com/politics/archive/2015/02/the-many-causes-of-americas-decline-in-crime/385364/
2. *The Wellness Revolution: How to Make a Fortune in the Next Trillion Dollar Industry*, by Paul Zane Pilzer (published by John Wiley & Sons, Inc., New York 2002)
3. *"Galileo Trial: 1616 Documents,"* Inquisition Minutes of Feb. 25, 1616, available from the University of Minnesota online at: http://www.tc.umn.edu/~allch001/galileo/library/1616docs.htm; these documents further reference *The Galileo Affair: A Documentary History*, edited and translated by Maurice A. Finocchiaro (Berkeley: University of California Press, 1989); transcribed by Craig Stillwell.
4. *The Tragedy of Hamlet, Prince of Denmark*, by William Shakespeare; Hamlet was written circa 1600, when Galileo was still a professor at the renowned University of Padua, and when Galileo's unorthodox astronomical views began attracting attention well beyond academia.

5. The phrase *"Eppur si muove—And yet it moves"* is now part of the popular culture, though historians still debate whether or not Galileo ever uttered the phrase. Whether or not Galileo said it (or not) does not diminish the phrase's symbolic importance and its applicability to a scientist like Galileo told to recant his views under penalty of death or imprisonment, who nonetheless had the courage to believe in *truth*, and still see the humor in those who foolishly denied it.

6. *"The Prairie Dog Wars: Is the prairie dog a grass-eating varmint that threatens cattle, or a vital keystone species? The federal government must soon decide,"* by Ted Williams, Mother Jones magazine, Jan./Feb. 2000, available online at: http://www.motherjones.com/politics/2000/01/prairie-dog-wars; see also *"Can Prairie Dogs Save Mexico's Prairie From the Desert?"* Living on Earth radio air date, Jan. 25, 2013, in PRI's Environmental News Magazine, available online at: http://www.loe.org/shows/segments. html?programID=13-P13-00004&segmentID=8 and *"Prairie Dogs and Soil Impacts,"* by Great Plains Restoration Council (with detailed bibliography), available online at: http://gprc.org/research/prairie-dogs-the-truth/prairie-dogs-and-soil-impacts/#.U1qhd825HVQ.

7. *"Prairie dogs' language decoded by scientists: Human-animal translation devices may be available within 10 years, researcher says,"* CBS News June 21, 2013, available online at: http://www.cbc.ca/news/technology/prairie-dogs-language-decoded-by-scientists-1.1322230.

8. Per the book cover for *Systema Naturae*, by Carl Linnaeus, available online at: http://www.biodiversitylibrary.org/item/10277#page/3/mode/1up

9. *The Structure of Scientific Revolutions: 50th Anniversary Edition*, by Thomas S. Kuhn (Univ. of Chicago Press), pg. 10 (Ch. II, "The Route to Normal Science")

10. *Ibid.* pg. 24. (Ch. III, "The Nature of Normal Science")

11. *Ibid.*

12. *"Linnaeus's Asian elephant was wrong species: Molecular sleuths crack 300-year-old mystery over the identity of the Asian elephant type specimen,"* by Ewen Callaway, *Nature*, Nov. 4, 2013, available online at: http://

www.nature.com/news/linnaeus-s-asian-elephant-was-wrong-species-1.14063, Dr. Tom Gilbert quotes on pg. 12 of 17 (podcast available).

13. *Ibid.*

14. *"Human Biodiversity: Genes, Race and History,"* by Jonathan M. Marks (Aldine Transaction, 2nd printing 2009), pg. 50 (Ch. 3, "Physical Anthropology as the Study of Human Variation"). Marks also recognized the "Long shadow of Linnaeus's human taxonomy" in Nature 447, 28 (3 May 2007)(published online 2 May 2007)

15. *Ibid.*

16. *The Autobiography of Mark Twain,* arranged and edited, with introduction and notes, by Charles Neider (Harper & Row Publishers, Inc. 1959), Chapter 26, pgs. 174.

17. As Paul W. Barada, of the *Rushville Republican*, wrote in his weekly newspaper column on Oct. 8, 2013, which he entitled *"Top ten of the second millennium,"* "Most of us, I think, have probably heard of most of the individuals on this Top Ten list. The guy in 10th place, however, was completely new to me. It turns out that William Harvey was an English physician who lived from 1578 to 1657… His most famous writing was a book published in 1628 titled 'On the Motion of the Heart and Blood'." Barada's column available online at: http://www.rushvillerepublican.com/columns/x1442580860/Top-ten-of-second-millennium.

18. The fame and influence of historian Arthur Schlesinger, Jr., including numerous obituaries and remembrances following his death in 2007, was the subject of History News Network's *"Arthur Schlesinger, Jr.'s Legacy"* on Nov. 27, 2007, available online at: http://historynewsnetwork.org/article/35985.

19. *"An Interview With Arthur M. Schlesinger Jr.,"* by Robert van Gelder, published March 10, 1946, in New York Times (Book Section), available online at: http://www.nytimes.com/books/00/11/26/specials/schlesinger-talk46.html

20. *"On the Motion of the Heart and Blood in Animals,"* by William Harvey, Ch. XVI ("The Circulation of the Blood is Further Proved from Certain Consequences"), available online at: http://www.bartleby.com/38/3/16.html

21. *"An Anatomical Disquisition on the Motion of the Heart and Blood in Animals,"* by William Harvey, Introduction, from *"The Works of William Harvey, M.D., translated from the Latin with A Life of the Author,"* by Robert Willis, M.D. (published by the Sydenham Society, London 1847), available online at: https://archive.org/stream/worksofwilliamha00harvia la#page/8/mode/2up
22. *Ibid.*
23. *"On the Motion of the Heart and Blood in Animals,"* by William Harvey, Introduction, available online at: http://www.bartleby.com/38/3/1000.html
24. The full translated quote from Linnaeus: "I well know what a spendidly great difference there is [between] a man and a bestia [beast] when I look at them from a point of view of morality. Man is the animal which the Creator has seen fit to honor with such a magnificent mind and has condescended to adopt as his favorite and for which he has prepared a nobler life" (citing T. Fredbärj (ed.), Menniskans Cousiner (Valda Avhandlingar av Carl von Linné nr, 21) (1955), 4. Trans. Gunnar Broberg, 'Linnaeus's Classification of Man', in Tore Frängsmyr (ed.), Linnaeus: The Man and his Work (1983), 167), featured in *"Carolus Linnaeus Quotes on Animal,"* in Today in Science History, available online at: http://todayinsci.com/L/Linnaeus_Carolus/LinnaeusCarolus-Animal-Quotations.htm
25. *"Empathy and Pro-Social Behavior in Rats,"* by Peggy Mason, Jean Decety, and Inbal Ben-Ami Bartal (each associated with the University of Chicago), Science, Dec. 9, 2011, Vol. 334, pg. 1427-1430, available online at: http://science.sciencemag.org/content/334/6061/1427; see also *"Cagebreak! Rats will work to free a trapped pal,"* by Nell Greenfieldboyce, NPR.org (with podcast), Dec. 8, 2011, available online at: http://www.npr.org/2011/12/09/143304206/cagebreak-rats-will-work-to-free-a-trapped-pal, and *"Jailbreak Rats: Selfless Rodents Spring theirs Pals and Share their Sweets,"* by Ferris Jabr, Scientific American, Dec. 8, 2011, available online at: http://www.scientificamerican.com/article/jailbreak-rat/
26. *"Rats demonstrate helping behavior toward a soaked conspecific,"* by Noboya Sato, Ling Tan, Kazushi Tate, and Maya Okada, published in Animal Cognition, Sept. 2015, Vol. 18, Issue 5, pfa. 1039-1047, available online

at: http://link.springer.com/article/10.1007/s10071-015-0872-2; see also *"The Intriguing New Science that could change your mind about Rats,"* by Brandon Keim, Wired magazine, Jan. 28, 2015, available online at: http://www.wired.com/2015/01/reconsider-the-rat/.

27. *The Merchant of Venice*, by William Shakespeare, Act IV, Scene 1 (a court of justice in Venice), delivered by Salerio, full play available online at: http://www.pubwire.com/DownloadDocs/PDFiles/ SHAKESPR/COMEDY/MERCHANT.PDF

28. *Ibid.*, Act III, Scene 1 (a street in Venice), delivered by Shylock.

29. *Ibid.*

30. *Coriolanus*, by William Shakespeare, Act I, Scene I (a street in Rome), delivered by Menenius, available online at: http://www.shakespeare-online.com/plays/corio_1_1.html

31. *Elizabeth I's Golden Speech*, Nov. 30, 1601, available online at: http:// www.emersonkent.com/speeches/golden_speech.htm; official State biography of Queen Elizabeth I available online at: https://www. royal.gov.uk/HistoryoftheMonarchy/KingsandQueensofEngland/ TheTudors/ElizabethI.aspx

32. Text of the Act for the Relief of the Poor available online at: http:// www.workhouses.org.uk/poorlaws/1601act.shtml; see also *"The 1601 Elizabethan Poor Law,"* by Marjie Bloy, Ph.D., posted on VictorianWeb. org, on Nov. 12, 2002, available online at: http://www.victorianweb. org/history/poorlaw/elizpl.html

33. *Henry IV*, by William Shakespeare, Act IV, Scene 4, delivered by Hotspur.

34. *"High-Level Wellness for Man and Society,"* Halbert L. Dunn. American Journal Public Health Nations Health, June 1959; 49(6); pgs. 786–792, at pg. 789.

35. *"The Project Gutenberg eBook of William Harvey,"* by D'Arcy Power. pg 20 of 132, available online at: http://www.gutenberg.org/ files/46664/46664-h/46664-h.htm

36. *Ibid.*

37. *"Apothecaries—Our History,"* published by the Society of Apothecaries (incorporated as a City Livery Company by royal charter from James I on 6 Dec. 1617 in recognition of apothecaries' specialist skills in

compounding and dispensing medicines), on its official website, available online at: http://www.apothecaries.org/society/our-history/

38. Charter Granted by Queen Elizabeth to the East India Company, 31 Dec. 1600, available online at: http://www.sdstate.edu/projectsouthasia/loader.cfm?csModule=security/getfile&PageID=857407

39. *"Adam Smith,"* available online at: http://www.libertarianism.org/people/adam-smith; see also http://www.adamsmith.org/adam-smith.

40. *"East India Company: The Original Too-Big-to-Fail Firm,"* by Nick Robins, published in BloombergView, Mar 12, 2013, and available online at: http://www.bloombergview.com/articles/2013-03-12/east-india-company-the-original-too-big-to-fail-firm.

41. *"The East India Company: The Company that ruled the waves (As state-backed firms once again become forces in global business, we ask what they can learn from the greatest of them all),"* published in the print edition of The Economist, Dec. 17, 2011, and available online at: http://www.economist.com/node/21541753/print.

42. *"Adam Smith: An Enlightened Life,"* by Nicholas Phillipson (published by the Penguin Group 2010), footnote 27.

43. *"East India Company: The Original Too-Big-to-Fail Firm,"* by Nick Robins, published in BloombergView, Mar 12, 2013, and available online at: http://www.bloombergview.com/articles/2013-03-12/east-india-company-the-original-too-big-to-fail-firm.

44. *"Growth Strategies/ Ben Cohen & Jerry Greenfield: Caring Capitalists,"* published by *Entrepreneur*, Oct. 10, 2008, available online at: http://www.entrepreneur.com/article/197626; *"Ben & Jerry's Caring Capitalism,"* by Jennifer J. Laabs, Personnel Journal Vol. 71, Issue 11, Nov. 1992, published by Questia, available online at: http://www.questia.com/magazine/1P3-717430/ben-jerry-s-caring-capitalism

45. *Ebay Domestic Holdings, Inc. v. Craig Newmark and James Buckmaster and craigslist, INC.,* 16 A.3d 1, 34 (Court of Chancery of Delaware, Civil Action 3705-CC, May 14, 2010).

46. *Ibid.*, 16 A.3d at 34.

47. *Ibid.*, 16 A.3d at 35.

48. Focusing on the qualitative metrics of "value" has its place in business, as it has its place in every aspect of life, and I would be remiss not to cite the master of such philosophy of value and quality: *Zen and the Art of Motorcycle Maintenance: An Inquiry Into Values,* by Robert M. Pirsig, first published 1974 (HarperCollins)

49. *"Nelson Mandela's legacy is economic, too,"* by Mitchell Hartman, published in Marketplace, Dec. 5, 2013 (citing/linking *No Easy Victories: African Liberation and American Activists Over a Half Century,* edited by Wlliam Minter, Gail Hovey, and Charles Cobb Jr., with a Foreword by Nelson Mandela; quote from Mandela's Foreword), available online at: http://www.marketplace.org/topics/world/nelson-mandelas-legacy-economic-too.

50. List of those who made the *"Giving Pledge"* available online at: http://givingpledge.org/index.html.

51. *Plumstead Theatre Society v. Commissioner,* 675 F.2d 244 (1982)(per curiam), affirming 74 T.C. 1324 (1980).

52. *The Merchant of Venice,* by William Shakespeare, Act III, Scene 1 (a street in Venice), delivered by Shylock, full play available online at: http://www.pubwire.com/DownloadDocs/PDFiles/SHAKESPR/COMEDY/MERCHANT.PDF

53. *Renaissance Art: A Topical Dictionary,* by Irene Earls (Greenwood Press 1987), pg. 263 (with definitions of "sfumato" and "perspective" on pg. 224).

54. *Leonardo da Vinci Notebooks (Oxford World's Classics),* selected by Irma A. Richter, edited with an introduction and notes by Thereza Wells, preface by Martin Kemp, Oxford University Press first published 1952, new ed. 2008) at pg. 168. See also *"The Art and Science of Leonardo da Vinci: Excerpts from his Notebooks,"* available online at http://employees.oneonta.edu/farberas/arth/arth200/artist/leonardo.htm and *"Leonardo and Pliny,"* by Jonathan Kline (Temple University), published by Univ. of Virginia, McIntire Dept. of Art in *Leonardo da Vinci: Between Art and Science,* edited by Francesca Florani and Ann Marazeula Kim, and available online at http://faculty.virginia.edu/Fiorani/NEH-Institute/essays/kline. This ongoing publication of Univ. of Virginia is also a wonderful source of scholarship on Leonardo da Vince; *see*

http://faculty.virginia.edu/Fiorani/NEH-Institute/essays/resources/ leonardos-writings/manuscripts-a-m. In da Vinci scholarship, translations are numerous and his notebooks have been disassembled and reassembled in many ways.

55. *"Leonardo da Vinci on atherosclerosis and the function of the sinuses of Valsalva,"* by B. Boon, published in Neth Heart J. Dec 2009; 17(12): pg. 496–499, crediting medical physician and scholar Kenneth D. Keale in footnote 7, available online at: http://www.ncbi.nlm.nih.gov/pmc/articles/PMC2804084/

56. *"Leonardo's Vision of Flow Visualization,"* by M. Gharib, D. Kremers, M.M. Koochesfahani, and M. Kemp, with thanks to Dr. Mehrdad Zarandi, Springer-Verlag's Experiments in Fluids journal, Experiments in Fluids 33 (2002) 219–223 (published Springer-Verlag 2002 available online at: http://www.gharib.caltech.edu/art_and_sciences/leonardo/leonardo-vision-of-flow.pdf

57. *"Da Vinci clue for heart surgeon: A UK heart surgeon has pioneered a new way to repair damaged hearts after being inspired by artist Leonardo da Vinci's medical drawings,"* published by BBC News, Sept. 28, 2005, available online at http://news.bbc.co.uk/2/hi/health/4289204.stm.

58. *"7 Steps to Think like Leonardo da Vinci: The Guide to Everyday Genius,"* by Andrea Balt (published 2014 and available online at: http://www.andreabalt.com/7-ways-to-think-like-leonardo-da-vinci/), enthusiastically reviewing *How to Think Like Leonardo da Vinci: Seven Steps to Genius Every Day*, by Michael J. Gelb (Dell republish 2000)—a book I also enjoyed and tried to apply to my own life. Andrea Balt referenced this common Leonardo da Vinci quote about the earth moved by a tiny bird, on pg. 33 of 49, and also offered her own insights on pg. 31 of her review: "500 years before the Wellness Revolution of our day, Da Vinci offered...timeless pieces of advice on holistic health and healthy living." The quote from Leonardo is also referenced in a review of another excellent da Vinci book, *Da Vinci's Ghost: Genius, Obsession, and How Leonardo Created the World in His Own Image* by Toby Lester (Free Press 2012), entitled *"Words on Books... And a Few Other Things from Time to Time,"* by Tony Miksak (published March 1, 2012, available online at: http://wordsonbooks.blogspot.com/2012/03/da-vincis-ghost.html

59. *"The Russian Enigma,"* BBC broadcast by Winston Churchill on Oct. 1, 1939, reprinted by Churchill Society of London, available online at: http://www.churchill-society-london.org.uk/RusnEnig.html

Chapter Eleven: Belief

1. *Leonardo da Vinci Notebooks (Oxford World's Classics)*, selected by Irma A. Richter, edited with an introduction and notes by Thereza Wells, preface by Martin Kemp, Oxford University Press first published 1952, new ed. 2008) at pg. 168. See footnote 54 to Ch. 10 above.

2. For those who doubt that the ear is drawn to the quiet rest between musical notes, I offer decades of experience as a musician and these two excellent books: *This Is Your Brain on Music: The Science of a Human Obsession* by Daniel J. Levitin (Penguin Group 2006), and *The Music Lesson: A Spiritual Search for Growth through Music* by Victor L. Wooten (Penguin Group 2006). Daniel Levitin is a Professor of Psychology and Behavioral Neuroscience at McGill University, as well as a musician, recording engineering, and producer. Victor Wooten is a multi-dimensional bass player and multi-Grammy® winner, including for his work with Béla Fleck and the Flecktones. In different ways, both men say the same thing about how we are drawn to the silent spaces; "allow the silence to speak louder than your thoughts" writes Wooten at pg. 215, who then explains how this approach holds for musicians learning to improve their craft: "Learn how to make a rest speaker louder than a note. Play a musical line and then start leaving notes out, putting the emphasis on the rest."

3. *"Fact or Fiction?: An Opera Singer's Piercing Voice Can Shatter Glass (Can the high C of a trained soprano quiver glass into dissolution?),"* by Karen Schrock, published in Scientific American, Aug. 23, 2007, available online: http://www.scientificamerican.com/article/fact-or-fiction-opera-singer-can-shatter-glass/

4. *"The Powerful Placebo,"* by Henry K. Beecher, M.D., published in J.A.M.A. Dec. 24, 1955, Vol. 159, No. 17, pg. 1602-1606, available online at: http://jama.jamanetwork.com/article.aspx?articleid=303530 or http://jgh.ca/uploads/Psychiatry/Links/beecher.pdf

5. *Ibid.*, pg. 1603.

6. *Ibid.*, pg. 1605.

7. *Ibid.*, pg. 1606.

8. As Descartes himself wrote, "as I made it my business in each matter to reflect particularly upon what might fairly be doubted and prove a source of error, I gradually rooted out from my mind all the errors which had hitherto crept into it. Not that in this I imitated the sceptics who doubt only that they may doubt, and seek nothing beyond uncertainty itself; for, on the contrary, my design was singly to find ground of assurance..." *Discourse on the Method of Rightly Conducting the Reason, and Seeking Truth in Sciences* by René Descartes, Part III, produced by Ilana and Greg Newby, and available online at: http://www.gutenberg.org/files/59/59-h/59-h.htm (with quote at pg. 7 of 22).

9. *Ibid.*, Part II; this translation of Descartes' *Discourse on the Method* is by Jonathan Bennett in 2007, and available online at: http://www.earlymoderntexts.com/assets/pdfs/descartes1637.pdf at pg. 9 (emphasis in original).

10. *"René Descartes: The Mind-Body Distinction,"* by Justin Skirry, published by The Internet Encyclopedia of Philosophy: A Peer-Reviewed Academic Resource (edited by founder James Fieser, Ph.D. and Bradley Dowden, Ph.D., available online at: http://www.iep.utm.edu/descmind/ (Descartes quote found at "3. The Real Distinction Argument...The Second Version").

11. Descartes' *Discourse on the Method*, transl. by Jonathan Bennett (2007), available online at: http://www.earlymoderntexts.com/assets/pdfs/descartes1637.pdf, at pg. 17.

12. *Ibid.*, at pg. 15 (emphasis in original).

13. *Ibid.*, at pg. 15.

14. *Ibid.*, at pg. 17.

15. *Ibid.*, at pg. 18-19 (Part V).

16. *See, e.g., Descartes' Dream: The World According to Mathematics* by Philip J. Davis and Reuben Hersh, published by Dover Books on Mathematics (2005); *"Descartes' Dream: From Method to Madness,"* by Peter Chojnowski, published by *Life Issues.Net (Clear Thinking about Critical Issues)*, and available online at: http://www.lifeissues.net/writers/cho/cho_14descartesdream.html

17. *"Beyond the pineal gland assumption: A neuroanatomical appraisal of dualism in Descartes' philosophy,"* by Moncef Berhouma, Clinical Neurology and Neurosurgy (2013), available online at: http://dx.doi.org/10.1016/j. clineuro.2013.02.023, at pg. 6, §3.2 (quote from a letter from Descartes to Princess Elizabeth, May 21, 1643).

18. *Ibid.,* at pg. 7. §3.2 (quote from Desartes' *The Passions of the Soul*).

19. *Discourse on the Method of Rightly Conducting the Reason, and Seeking Truth in Sciences* by René Descartes, Part V, produced by Ilana and Greg Newby, and available online at: http://www.gutenberg.org/ files/59/59-h/59-h.htm (with quote at pg. 13 of 22).

20. *See, e.g., "Nonvisual photoreceptors of the deep brain, pineal organs and retina,"* by Vigh B, Manzano MJ, Zádori A, Frank CL, Lukáts A, Röhlich P, Szél A, Dávid C., published in Histology and Histopathology, 2002 Apr;17(2):555-90, and available online at: http://www.ncbi. nlm.nih.gov/pubmed/11962759 and at http://www.hh.um.es/ pdf/Vol_17/17_2/Vigh-17-555-590-2002.pdf; *see also "Descartes and the Pineal Gland,"* first published 2005 and revised 2013 in Stanford Encyclopedia of Philosophy, available online at: http://plato.stanford. edu/entries/pineal-gland/

21. *Discourse on the Method of Rightly Conducting the Reason, and Seeking Truth in Sciences* by René Descartes, Part V, produced by Ilana and Greg Newby, and available online at: http://www.gutenberg.org/ files/59/59-h/59-h.htm (with quote at pg. 13 of 22).

22. *"Descartes Dissected His Wife's Dog To Prove A Point,"* by Morris M., published KnowledgeNuts, and available online at: http://knowledge- nuts.com/2013/09/29/descartes-dissected-his-wifes-dog-to-prove-a- point/ (citing among other sources, "Richard Dawkins on vivisection: *But can they suffer?"* published on BoingBoingNet at http://boingboing. net/2011/06/30/richard-dawkins-on-v.html)

23. *"Profiles in Cardiology: René Descartes,"* by J. Willis Hurst, M.D. and W. Bruce Fye, M.D., M.A., published in Clin. Cardiol. 26, 49–51 (2003), and available online at: https://www.researchgate.net/pub- lication/264596483_Rene_Descartes; *see also "Mind-Body Dualism and the Harvey-Descartes Controversy,"* by Geoffrey Gorham, published in Journal of the History of Ideas, Vol. 55, No. 2 (Univ. of Penn. Press,

Apr., 1994), pp. 211-234, available online at: http://www.jstor.org/stable/2709897.

24. *"The Powerful Placebo,"* by Henry K. Beecher, M.D., published in J.A.M.A. Dec. 24, 1955, Vol. 159, No. 17, pg. 1602-1606, available online at: http://jama.jamanetwork.com/article.aspx?articleid=303530 or http://jgh.ca/uploads/Psychiatry/Links/beecher.pdf, at pg. 1605.

25. *Ibid.*

26. *"Is Broken Heart Syndrome Real?"* published by the American Heart Association (April 15, 2013), available online at: http://www.heart.org/HEARTORG/Conditions/More/Cardiomyopathy/Is-Broken-Heart-Syndrome-Real_UCM_448547_Article.jsp; see also *"'Broken heart syndrome' no longer a myth,"* published by Northeastern University News (July 2009), available online at: http://www.northeastern.edu/news/stories/2009/07/broken_heart.html

27. *"Apical ballooning syndrome or takotsubo cardiomyopathy: a systematic review,"* by Monica Gianni, Francesco Dentali, Anna Maria Grandi, Glen Sumner, Rajesh Hiralal and Eva Lonn, published in European Heart Journal (2006) 27 (13): 1523-1529. doi: 10.1093/eurheartj/ehl032, available online at: http://eurheartj.oxfordjournals.org/content/27/13/1523.full

28. *"High-Level Wellness for Man and Society,"* Halbert L. Dunn. M.D., Ph.D., F.A.P.H.A., American Journal Public Health Nations Health, June 1959; 49(6); pgs. 788–789.

29. *"The Powerful Placebo,"* by Henry K. Beecher, M.D., at pg. 1605.

30. *"Neurobiology of Placebos with Fabrizio Benedetti (BSP 77),"* published by Brain Science Podcast on Sept. 19, 2011, available online at: http://brainsciencepodcast.com/bsp/neurobiology-of-placebos-with-fabrizio-benedetti-bsp-77.html; see also Ginger Campbell, M.D. follow-up interview, *"Placebo Research Update with Fabrizio Benedetti (BSP 127),"* published on March 01, 2016, available online at: http://brainsciencepodcast.com/bsp/2016/127-benedetti

31. *"Open versus hidden medical treatments: The patient's knowledge about a therapy affects the therapy outcome,"* by Fabrizio Benedetti, Giuliano Maggi, Leonardo Lopiano, Michele Lanotte, Innocenzo Rainero, Sergio

Vighetti, and Antonella Pollo, published in the journal Prevention and Treatment of the American Psychological Institute, Vol 6(1), Jun 2003, No Pagination Specified Article 1a, available online at: http://psycnet. apa.org/index.cfm?fa=buy.optionToBuy&id=2003-07872-001

32. *"Placebos Are Getting More Effective—Drugmakers Are Desperate to Know Why,"* by Steve Silberman, published in Wired Magazine, 17:09, Aug. 24, 2009, available online at: http://archive.wired.com/medtech/drugs/magazine/17-09/ff_placebo_effect.

33. *"The Importance Of Increasing Our Knowledge Of Placebo Neurophysiology,"* by Harriet Hall, M.D., published in Better Health, Oct. 3, 2011, available online at: http://getbetterhealth.com/the-importance-of-increasing-our-knowledge-of-placebo-neurophysiology/2011.10.03.

34. *"The Placebo Phenomenon: An ingenious researcher finds the real ingredients of 'fake' medicine,"* by Cara Feinberg, published in Harvard Magazine, Jan/Feb 2013, pgs. 36-39, at pg. 36, available online at: http://harvardmagazine.com/2013/01/the-placebo-phenomenon

35. *Ibid.* at pg. 39.

36. *"Early Palliative Care for Patients with Metastatic Non–Small-Cell Lung Cancer,"* by Jennifer S. Temel, M.D., Joseph A. Greer, Ph.D., Alona Muzikansky, M.A., Emily R. Gallagher, R.N., Sonal Admane, M.B., B.S., M.P.H., Vicki A. Jackson, M.D., M.P.H., Constance M. Dahlin, A.P.N., Craig D. Blinderman, M.D., Juliet Jacobsen, M.D., William F. Pirl, M.D., M.P.H., J. Andrew Billings, M.D., and Thomas J. Lynch, M.D., published in New England Journal of Medicine 2010; 363:733-42, at pg. 733, available online at: http://www.nejm.org/doi/pdf/10.1056/NEJMoa1000678.

37. *The Autobiography of Mark Twain,* arranged and edited, with introduction and notes, by Charles Neider (Harper & Row Publishers, Inc. 1959), Chapter 19, pgs. 131-132.

38. *"High-Level Wellness for Man and Society,"* by Halbert L. Dunn, at pg. 789.

39. *Ibid.*

40. *"Frederic the Great's Eulogy on Julien Offray de la Mettrie,"* available online at: http://bactra.org/LaMettrie/Eulogy/

41. *Man a Machine,* by Julien Offray de La Mettrie (source: Cosma Rohilla Shaliz, *L'Homme Machine*, March 31, 1995, translated by Bussey,

rev. by Mitch Abidor), available online at: https://www.marxists.org/reference/archive/la-mettrie/1748/man-machine.htm, quote at pg. 6 of 40.

42. *"Beyond the pineal gland assumption: A neuroanatomical appraisal of dualism in Descartes' philosophy,"* by Moncef Berhouma, Clinical Neurology and Neurosurgy (2013), available online at: http://dx.doi.org/10.1016/j.clineuro.2013.02.023, at pg. 6, §3.2 (quote from a letter from Descartes to Princess Elizabeth, May 21, 1643).

43. *Man a Machine*, by Julien Offray de La Mettrie, pg. 1 of 40.

44. *Ibid.*, at pg. 35 of 40.

45. *Ibid.*, at pg. 38 of 40.

46. *Ibid.*, at pg. 38 of 40.

47. *"The development of quantum mechanics,"* by Werner Heisenberg, Nobel Lecture delivered Dec. 11, 1933, published by Nobel Prize organization, and available online at: http://www.nobelprize.org/nobel_prizes/physics/laureates/1932/heisenberg-lecture.pdf; *see also "How Quantum Suicide Works,"* by Josh Clark, published in How Stuff Works: Science, Oct. 12, 2007, available online at http://science.howstuffworks.com/innovation/science-questions/quantum-suicide.htm, at pg. 3 ("Heisenberg's Uncertainty Principle"); *"How Does Observing Particles Influence Their Behavior?"* published in Futurism, July 28, 2014, available online at: http://futurism.com/where-did-the-big-bang-happen-wheres-the-center-of-the-universe/

48. *"High-Level Wellness for Man and Society,"* by Halbert L. Dunn, at pg. 787.

Chapter Twelve: Be Spirited

1. *"Testing the Claims of Mesmerism: The First Scientific Investigation of the Paranormal Ever Conducted"* with an introduction by Michael Shermer, published by eSkeptic: Examining Extraordinary Claims and Promoting Science, Sept. 22, 2010, from archives of Skeptic Magazine, Vol. 4, No. 3, and available online at: http://www.skeptic.com/eskeptic/10-09-22/, at pg. 2 of 42.

2. *Ibid.*, at pg. 12 of 42.

3. *Mesmerism: The Discovery of Animal Magnetism*, by Franz Anton Mesmer (1779), translated by Joseph Bouleur (published Holmes

Publishing Group LLC, Joseph Bouleur and Universite de Lyon, 1998, with new material 2006, available online at: http://www.amer-ican-buddha.com/cult.mesmerismmesmer.htm, at pg. 6 of 24. [See also *Mesmerism*, by Doctor Mesmer (1779), being the first translation of Mesmer's historic *M6moire sur la decouyerte du Magnetisme Animal* to appear in English, with an Introductory Monograph by Gilbert Frankau (published by Macdonald & Co. London 1948), avail-able online at: https://www.woodlibrarymuseum.org/rarebooks/item/567/mesmer-fa.-mesmerism-by-doctor-mesmer,-1779:-being-the-first-translation-of-mesmer's-historic-memoire-sur-la-decouverte-du-magnetisme-animal-to-appear-in-english-(with-an-introductory-monograph-by-gilbert-frankau),-1948.]

4. *Ibid.*, at pg. 6 of 24.

5. *Ibid.* at pg. 6 of 24.

6. *Ibid.*, at pg. 9 of 24 (emphasis in original).

7. *Ibid.*, at pg. 21 of 24.

8. *Ibid.*, at pg. 21 of 24.

9. *Ibid.*, at pg. 13 of 24.

10. *Ibid.*, at pg. 20 of 24.

11. *Ibid.*, at pg. 9 of 24.

12. *"Mesmeromania, or, the Tale of the Tub,"* by Christopher Turner, pub-lished by Cabinet Magazine, Issue 21 Electricity Spring 2006, and avail-able online at: http://www.cabinetmagazine.org/issues/21/turner.php (describing and picturing the baquet tub, as well as other thera-peutic practices of Mesmer).

13. *Mesmerism: The Discovery of Animal Magnetism*, by Franz Anton Mesmer (1779), translated by Joseph Bouleur (published Holmes Publishing Group LLC, Joseph Bouleur and Universite de Lyon, 1998, with new material 2006, available online at: http://www.american-buddha.com/cult.mesmerismmesmer.htm, at pg. 21 of 24.

14. *Ibid.*, at pgs. 9-10 of 24.

15. *Ibid.*, at pg. 21 of 24.

16. *Ibid.*, at pg. 5 of 24.

17. *Ibid.*, at pg. 5 of 24.

18. *Ibid.*, at pg. 5 of 24.

19. Description of exhibition of *MIT Libraries Special Collections: Animal Magnetism (Vail Collection)*, available online at: http://libraries.mit.edu/collections/vail-collection/topics/animal-magnetism/. In 1784, the year that the Royal Scientific Commission investigated Dr. Mesmer, the exhibition noted how "Mesmer was the talk of Paris in 1784, as evidenced by the large quantity of material published that year: the Vail Collection has roughly seventy-five items printed in 1784."

20. *"Mesmer's Secret: The Scientific Rhetoric of Mesmerism in the Enlightenment,"* by Usui (published by Tempus: the Harvard College History Review Feb. 18, 2013), available online at: http://www.hcs.harvard.edu/tempus/archives_files/Usui.pdf. This Harvard historian argued that by 1784, "the advancement of science became the noblest of aims, and scientific rationalism, the most obvious means to reach it. In this intellectual climate, where reason was so valued, Mesmer faced obstacles establishing a foothold" (pg. 2 of 17)—yet Mesmer and his followers tried. Indeed, as the author wrote, "Mesmerism did not exist outside the discourse of reason, but rather within it. Those who believed in mesmerism were neither irrational nor romantics. Mesmer's followers valued reason, and it was because mesmerism appealed to their reason that it gained their faith." (pg. 5 of 17).

21. *Dissertatio physico-medica de planetarum influx* (1766), available online at: https://www.woodlibrarymuseum.org/rarebooks/item/566/mesmer-fa.-dissertatio-physico-medica-de-planetarum-influxu,-1766.Mesmer; see also *"The Super-Enlightenment Authors: Franz Anton Mesmer (1734-1815),"* by Jessica Riskin, published Stanford Univ. (The Super-Enlightenment), available online at: http://collections.stanford.edu/supere/page.action?forward=author_franz_anton_mesmer&section=authors

22. *Mesmerism: The Discovery of Animal Magnetism*, by Franz Anton Mesmer (1779), translated by Joseph Bouleur (published Holmes Publishing Group LLC, Joseph Bouleur and Universite de Lyon, 1998, with new material 2006, available online at: http://www.american-buddha.com/cult.mesmerismmesmer.htm, at pg. 20 of 24.

23. *Ibid.*, at pg. 4 of 24.

24. *Ibid.*, at pg. 20 of 24.

25. *Ibid.*, at pg. 21 of 24.

26. *Ibid.*, at pg. 3 of 24.

27. In fact, as Usui argues in *"Mesmer's Secret: The Scientific Rhetoric of Mesmerism in the Enlightenment"* (footnote 20 above), Mesmer very much wanted to use the tools of the Enlightenment—rational observation and measurement—to prove his theory. His method of rational scientific and medical proof was the subject of *"Mesmer's 1780 proposal for a controlled trial to test his method of treatment using 'animal magnetism',"* by I.M.L. Donaldson (Div. of Neuroscience, Univ. of Edinburgh), published in the Journal of the Royal Society of Medicine, Dec 2005; 98(12): 572–575, and available online at: http://www.ncbi.nlm.nih.gov/pmc/articles/PMC1299353/.

28. *"Testing the Claims of Mesmerism: The First Scientific Investigation of the Paranormal Ever Conducted"* with an introduction by Michael Shermer, published by eSkeptic: Examining Extraordinary Claims and Promoting Science, Sept. 22, 2010, from archives of Skeptic Magazine, Vol. 4, No. 3, and available online at: http://www.skeptic.com/eskeptic/10-09-22/, at pg. 10 of 42.

29. *Ibid.*, at pg. 12 of 42.

30. *Ibid.*, at pg. 12 of 42.

31. *Ibid.*, at pg. 13 of 42.

32. *Ibid.*, at pg. 23 of 42.

33. *Ibid.*, at pg. 23 of 42.

34. *Ibid.*, at pg. 34 of 42.

35. *Ibid.*, at pg. 30 of 42.

36. *"The Super-Enlightenment Authors: Franz Anton Mesmer (1734-1815),"* by Jessica Riskin, published Stanford Univ., see footnote 21 above, noted that one of the commissioners dissented from the final report condemning Mesmer because "imagination" itself seemed an inexplicable basis: "Judging an immaterial power of imagination to be unintelligible and insufficient, the botanist and doctor Antoine-Laurent de Jussieu, having served on the commission from the Royal Society of Medicine, dissented from its final report." (at pg. 3 of 4)

37. *"Testing the Claims of Mesmerism: The First Scientific Investigation of the Paranormal Ever Conducted,"* published by eSkeptic, at pg. 19 of 42.

38. *Ibid.*, at pg. 35 of 42.

39. *Ibid.*, at pg. 35 of 42.

40. *Ibid.*, at pg. 36 of 42.

41. *Ibid.*, at pg. 35 of 42.

42. *Ibid.*, at pg. 41 of 42.

43. *"Investigating Mesmer (Part 2 o 2),"* by Romeo Vitelli (published on weblog Providentia: A biased look at psychology in the world, Oct. 7, 2012), available online at:

http://drvitelli.typepad.com/providentia/2012/10/investigating-mesmer-part-2-of-2.html; as Dr. Vitelli describes, the royal commission "report led to the Parliament banning the use of animal magnetism for physicians" as well as "moral outrage" at unproven accusations of Mesmer "taking sexual advantage of the younger women while they were in a suggestible state."

44. *"Testing the Claims of Mesmerism: The First Scientific Investigation of the Paranormal Ever Conducted,"* published by eSkeptic, at pg. 3 of 42.

45. *Ibid.*, at pg. 38 of 42.

46. *History of the Guillotine* by Hon. John Wilson Croker (published in London by John Murray, Albemarle Street 1853), and available online at: http://en.wikisource.org/wiki/History_of_the_Guillotine, at pg. 7 of 35.

47. *Lavoisier: Chemist, Biologist, Economist* by Jean-Pierre Poirier, translated by Rebecca Balinski (published by Univ. of Pennsylvania Press, reprinted 1998), at pg. 159.

48. *Franz Anton Mesmer: His Life and Teaching*, by Richard Basil Ince (published London, William Rider & Son, Ltd. 1920), available online at: http://www.woodlibrarymuseum.org/museum/item/564/ince-rb.-franz-anton-mesmer:-his-life-and-teaching,-1920, at pg. 44.

49. *Mesmerism*, by Doctor Mesmer (1779), being the first translation of Mesmer's historic *M6moire sur la decouyerte du Magnetisme Animal* to appear in English, with an Introductory Monograph by Gilbert Frankau (published by Macdonald & Co. London 1948), available online at: https://www.woodlibrarymuseum.org/rarebooks/item/567/mesmer-fa.-mesmerism-by-doctor-mesmer,-1779:-being-the-first-translation-of-mesmer's-historic-memoire-sur-la-decouverte-du-magnetisme-animal-to-appear-in-english-(with-an-introductory-

monograph-by-gilbert-frankau),-1948, in the introductory monograph by G. Frankau, at pg. 21.

50. *General Scholium to Isaac Newton's Principia mathematica*, published first as an appendix to the 2nd (1713) ed. of the Principia, republished in the 3rd (1726) ed. with some amendments/additions, translated Andrew Motte (London 1729), pgs. 387-93, and available online at: http:// isaac-newton.org/general-scholium/ at pg. 4 of 4.

51. *Ibid.*, at pg. 4 of 4.

52. *"Hans Berger: from psychic energy to the EEG,"* by David Millett, published in Perspectives in Biology and Medicine (The Johns Hopkins Univ. Press), Vol. 44, No. 4, Autumn 2001, pgs. 522-542, available online at: https://methodsinbraincomputerinterfaces.wikispaces. com/file/view/BergerBiography.pdf at pg. 535.

53. *Entangled Minds: Extrasensory Experiences in a Quantum Reality*, by Dean Radin, Ph.D. (published by Paraview Pocket Books 2006), pg. 21, citation in ftnt. 2 to Hans Berger (1940), Psyche, 6.

54. *"Hans Berger: from psychic energy to the EEG,"* by David Millett, at pg. 541.

55. *New revelations about Hans Berger, father of the EEG, and his ties to the Third Reich,"* by Lawrence A. Zeidman, MD, James Stone, MD, and Daniel Kondziella, MD, PhD, published in Neurology, Feb. 12, 2013, Vol. 80 No. 7 Supp. S57.006, available online at: http://www.neurology.org/content/80/7_Supplement/S57.006.short

56. *"From Mesmer to Freud: Magnetic Sleep and the Roots of Psychological Healing,"* by Adam Crabtree (published by Yale University Press 1993).

57. In the entangled timelines of history, Georg Groddeck wrote *Book of the It* in 1923, the same year Sigmund Freud wrote *The Ego and the Id*.

58. *The Doctor and the Soul: From Psychotherapy to Logotherapy*, by Viktor E. Frankl, translated by Richard Winton and Clara Winton (published by Vintage / Random House, 3rd edition 2010), in Introduction, pg. xxv.

59. *"Man's Search For Meaning,"* by Viktor E. Frankl, with a new foreword by Harold S. Kushner (published by Beacon Press / Penguin Random House 1st digital ed. 2006); Kushner writes in the Foreword: "Several times in the course of the book, Frankl approvingly quotes the words of Nietzsche: 'He who has a Why to live for can bear almost any How.'"

60. *"Man's Search For Meaning,"* by Viktor E. Frankl, though translations vary as do editions and publishers; Frankl's adoption of Nietzche as a motto for his psychotherapy appeared in a 1962 rewrite of the book's introduction, explaining logotherapy, which Dr. Frankl entitled *"The Will To Meaning."*

61. *Ibid.*

62. *Ibid.*

63. *The Doctor and the Soul: From Psychotherapy to Logotherapy,* by Viktor E. Frankl, preface to the third edition, page xii.

64. *Ibid.,* page xvi.

65. *"Man's Search For Meaning,"* by Viktor E. Frankl, the 60th Anniv. edition (published by Pocket Books / Simon & Schuster), pg. 166

66. *The Doctor and the Soul: From Psychotherapy to Logotherapy,* by Viktor E. Frankl, Introduction pg. xvii.

67. *The Fractal Geometry of Nature,* by Benoit B. Mandelbrot (published by W.H. Freeman and Company, First Ed. Edition 1982), in Introduction: Theme, pg. 1.

68. *Ibid.,* in Introduction: A Scientific Casebook, pg. 3.

69. *Ibid.,* Introduction: Theme, pg. 1

70. *"New York Times Obituary: Benoît Mandelbrot, Novel Mathematician, Dies at 85,"* by Jascha Hoffman (published New York Times Oct. 16, 2010)

71. *"How Long Is the Coast of Britain? Statistical Self-Similarity and the Fractal Dimension,"* by B. B. Mandelbrot, published in *Science,* 156, 1967, pg. 636-638, available online at: http://users.math.yale.edu/~bbm3/web_pdfs/howLongIsTheCoastOfBritain.pdf; this explanation of a "Trojan Horse" appeared in "Annotations" on the online publication.

72. *Ibid.,* pg. 636.

73. *Ibid.,* pg. 637.

74. *Ibid.,* pg. 637.

75. *Ibid.,* pg. 636.

76. *Ibid.,* pg. 636.

77. *Ibid.,* pg. 636.

78. *Ibid.,* pg. 636.

79. *Ibid.,* pg. 638.

80. TED® talk filmed February 2010, and available online at: http://www.ted.com/talks/benoit_mandelbrot_fractals_the_art_of_roughness; Transcript at: https://www.ted.com/talks/benoit_mandelbrot_fractals_the_art_of_roughness/transcript?language=en The cauliflower image is first seen at 1:34 on a rebroadcast of this TED® video on YouTube.

81. *Ibid.*, the quote appears at the beginning of the video, after 00:11 in the online transcript.

82. *The fractalist: Memoir of a Scientific Maverick*, by Benoît B. Mandelbrot, published by Vintage Books, a div. of Random House, LLC 2012).

83. TED® talk filmed February 2010, after 4:31 in the online transcript.

84. TED® talk filmed February 2010, after 5:58 in the online transcript.

85. TED® talk filmed February 2010, after 5:58 in the online transcript.

86. TED® talk filmed February 2010, after 16:33 in the online transcript.

87. *See, e.g., "Who Discovered the Mandelbrot Set? Did the father of fractals 'discover' his namesake set?"* by John Horgan, published by Scientific American, March 13, 2009 (originally appearing in April 1990 in Scientific American under the title "Mandelbrot Set-To"), and available online at http://www.scientificamerican.com/article/mandelbrot-set-1990-horgan/.

88. *Mesmerism: The Discovery of Animal Magnetism*, by Franz Anton Mesmer (1779), translated by Joseph Bouleur (published Holmes Publishing Group LLC, Joseph Bouleur and Universite de Lyon, 1998, with new material 2006, available online at: http://www.american-buddha.com/cult.mesmerismmesmer.htm, at pg. 6 of 24.

89. *"How Long Is the Coast of Britain? Statistical Self-Similarity and the Fractal Dimension"* by B. B. Mandelbrot, at pg. 636.

90. *"Boston and the History of Biomagnetism,"* by David Cohen, Massachusetts Institute of Technology and Massachusetts General Hospital, published in Neurology and Clinical Neurophysiology 2004:114 (Nov. 30, 2004), available online at: http://davidcohen.mit.edu/sites/default/files/documents/NCNP_Hist9May28.pdf; quote at pg. 2 of 4.

91. *Ibid.*

92. *See, e.g., "Jim Zimmerman and the SQUID,"* by R.L. Kautz, published in Applied Superconductivity, IEEE Transactions on (Vol:11, Issue: 1), available online at: http://ieeexplore.ieee.org/xpl/login.jsp?tp=&arnumber=919524&url=http%3A%2F%2Fieeexplore.ieee.org%2Fxpls%2Fabs_all.jsp%3Farnumber%3D919524.

93. *"SQUID Magnetometry: Harnessing the Power of Tiny Magnetic Fields,"* by Brian Fishbine, published by Los Alamos National Laboratory, Research Quarterly Spring 2003, available online at: http://www.lanl.gov/quarterly/q_spring03/squid_text.shtml.

94. A good example is *"A review of Energy Medicine: The Scientific Basis,"* by Harriet Hall, MD (published in Skeptic Magazine, Vol. 11, Nr. 3, 2005 and republished in Confessions of a Quackbuster, Jan 14, 2006), pgs. 1-9, available online at: http://quackfiles.blogspot.com/2006/01/review-of-energy-medicine-scientific.html. Dr. Hall reviews the book *"Energy Medicine: The Scientific Basis,"* by James L. Oschman, Ph.D. , with a forward by Candace Pert, Ph.D., Prof. Dept of Physiology and Biophysics Georgetown Univ. School of Medicine, who discovered the opiate receptors in the brain among Dr. Pert's many other accomplishments. *Energy Medicine: The Scientific Basis* published by Churchill Livingstone / Elsevier Ltd (2000). Dr. Hall concludes her review of Dr. Oschman's book by saying, *"Science is not a matter of cherry picking whatever supports your hypothesis. Rather it is a self-correcting methodology where all the evidence is considered and critiqued, and competing hypothesis are tested. The book masquerades as science, but it amounts to little more than speculation and polemic in support of a preconceived belief."* (pg. 7 of 9)

Dr. Hall's own words should be subjected to the same tests, so that her own polemic does not masquerade as science. In other words, does she consider all the evidence or does she cherry-pick only what supports her preconceived beliefs? Hall says this of Mesmer: *"In the case of Mesmer, no documented phenomenon was there to exclude"* yet she ignores that an animal's magnetic biofield (indeed, a plant's or a human's too) can now be measured and observed, even though such phenomenon could not be documented back in 1784. (pg. 2 of 9) For other historical figures she derives her "proof" from conformist peers (*"On the Quackwatch website Dr. Stephen Barrett says, in red warning letters"* she says about technologies of Reinhold Voll, pg. 2 of 9), or derives her "proof" from regulatory officials who crown genius (*"The FDA officials who banned those devices would disagree"* she says about another electrotherapy device, pg. 2 of 9), or finds her "proof" in the vicissitudes and shifting fortunes of business (*"Of course, a device doesn't have to be effective to be patented, and no one uses this device today"* she says about Harold Saxton Burr's invention detecting the oscillating electrical field of the ovaries, pg. 2 of 9).

Even Dr. John Zimmerman, inventor of the SQUID and one of the fathers of biomagnetism (along with his friend Dr. David Cohen at MIT), is maligned by Dr. Hall in this same speculative and polemical fashion. She criticizes Zimmerman's detection of magnetic fields from a healing hand thusly: *"Dr. John Zimmerman used a superconducting quantum interference device (SQUID) to detect a large biomagnetic field emanating from the hands of a practioner during therapeutic touch...The study was published in 1990 in the journal of the Bio-Electo-Magnetics Institute, whose founder and president just happens to be...John Zimmerman!"* (pg. 3 of 9). In maligning Dr. Zimmeman's reputation, Dr. Hall neglects to mention that the International Federal of Medical and Biological Engineering (IFMBE) sponsors the James Zimmerman Prize in the late SQUID pioneer's memory, which has been awarded to prominent scientists such as Dr. Andrei Matlashov of the Department of Energy's Los Alamos National Laboratory (Dr. Matlashov himself pioneered the use of SQUIDs for the "first ever ultra-low field MRI of the brain" in 2008). *"Andrei and his Superconducting Quantum Interference Devices,"* published in DOE Pulse: Science and Technology Highlights from the DOE National Laboratories, Oct.8, 2012, available on line at http://web.ornl.gov/info/news/pulse/no373/profile.shtml.

Finally, it is worth noting that Dr. Harriet Hall is dismayed by the growing use of quantum physics to explain what was previously scientifically inexplicable: *"Pseudoscience and new age philosophies frequently invoke quantum theory out of context. Oschman's book is no exception. If there is a God of Quantum Physics, he ought to smite those who take his name in vain."* (pg. 7 of 9) Again, Dr. Hall asks us to cherry-pick what supports her hypothesis by saying *"Physicists such as Victor Stenger assure us that quantum theory does not apply to large objects or to human consciousness.*" (pg. 7 of 9) You can choose to believe Victor Stenger (at least as interpreted by Dr. Harriet Hall) on whether quantum science is relevant to a new Age of Awareness, or you can choose to believe James Oschman and Candace Pert and James Zimmerman and a growing body of other scientists, all of whom Hall criticizes or ignores. Hall also ignores new tools of quantum science, such as the superconducting quantum interference device (SQUID) invented by Dr. Zimmerman.

Of course, it is up to you to believe which scientists you want to believe—but remember that your belief does matter, as Royal Scientific Commissioners would agree.

Chapter Thirteen: Beyond Measure

1. "*Universal, primordial magnetic fields discovered in deep space by UCLA, Caltech physicists,*" published by UCLA Newsroom Sept. 21, 2010, available online at: http://newsroom.ucla.edu/releases/universal-primordial-magnetic-171824; "*Evidence for Gamma-Ray Halos Around Active Galactic Nuclei and the First Measurement of Intergalactic Magnetic Fields,*" by Shin'ichiro Ando (Caltech) and Alexander Kusenko (UCLA/Tokyo), published in The Astrophysical Journal 722, L39 (2010), available online at: http://arxiv.org/abs/1005.1924.
2. "*The Prince of Mathematics: Carl Friedrich Gauss*" by M.B.W. Tent (AK Peters Ltd. 2006)
3. "*Clerk Maxwell's Influence on the Evolution of the Idea of Physical Reality*" by Albert Einstein in *Einstein's Essays in Science* (1934), republished by Dover Publications 2009, at pg. 40, available online at: https://openlibrary.org/books/OL23153101M/Einstein's_essays_in_science
4. *See, e.g.,* "*Hofstadter's Butterfly*" in Wikipedia; first described in "*Energy levels and wave functions of Bloch electrons in rational and irrational magnetic fields,*" by Douglas R. Hofstadter, Phys. Rev. B 14, 2239 (published 15 September 1976).
5. TED® talk filmed February 2010, and available online at: http://www.ted.com/talks/benoit_mandelbrot_fractals_the_art_of_roughness;

Transcript at: https://www.ted.com/talks/benoit_mandelbrot_ fractals_the_art_of_roughness/transcript?language=en
The cauliflower image is first seen at 1:34 on a rebroadcast of this TED® video on YouTube; and quote from Benoît Mandelbrot at 1:30 in transcript.

6. *Cuno Engineering Corp. v. Automatic Devices Corp.*, 314 US 84, 91 (1941) ("That is to say, the new device, however useful it may be, must reveal the flash of creative genius, not merely the skill of the calling")

7. *"Lightning-Induced Magnetic Anomalies on Archaeological Sites,"* by Geoffrey Jones and David L. Maki, Archaeological Prospection, Vol. 12, Issue 3, 2005, pgs. 191-197.

8. *"The Bee Essay,"* by Mark Twain, first published in *What is Man? and Other Essays* (1917 ed. Harper & Brothers), pg. 283, republished by Cornell Univ. Library 2010.

9. *Faust*, by J. W. von Goethe, Part One, Scene IV (The Study, Mephistopheles to Student), lines 1937 to 1939, though English translations from the German vary.

10. *Faust*, by J. W. von Goethe, Part One, Prelude on Stage (Comedian), line 179, though English translations of the German vary.

11. *"Bibliography of Harold Saxton Burr,"* published in Yale Journal of Biology and Medicine, Dec. 1957; 30(3), pgs. 163-167, available online at: http://www.ncbi.nlm.nih.gov/pmc/articles/PMC2603696/

12. *"Electrical Characteristics of Living Systems,"* by H.S. Burr and C.T. Lane, Yale Journal of Biology and Medicine Oct. 1935, 8(1): 31-35, available online at: http://www.ncbi.nlm.nih.gov/pmc/articles/ PMC2601305/

13. *Blueprint For Immortality: The Electric Patterns Of Life* by Harold Saxton Burr, published by C.W. Daniel (1972), Chapter One ("An Adventure in Science"), pg. 12.

14. *Ibid.*, at pg. 12-13.

15. *"Harold Saxton Burr,"* in Wikipedia, available online at: https:// en.wikipedia.org/wiki/Harold_Saxton_Burr; quote attributed to Ruby Khoo in New Straits Times, Dec. 7, 1991, in *"Wondrous Whole of Science and Spirituality"*.

16. *"Boy Soldier"* by Martin Lifschultz (published Amazon Digital Services LLC Jan. 2009).

17. *"Pharmaceutical Company Grunenthal Apologizes 50 Years After Drug Pulled Off Market,"* by Syndney Lupkin via World News, published ABC News, Sept. 1, 2012, available online at: http://abcnews.go.com/Health/drug-manufacturer-apologizes-thalidomide-victims/story?id=17135262.

18. *"The Project Gutenberg eBook of William Harvey,"* by D'Arcy Power. pg 20 of 132, available online at: http://www.gutenberg.org/files/46664/46664-h/46664-h.htm.

19. *Being Mortal: Medicine and What Matters in the End*, by Atul Gawande, M.D. (Metropolitan Books / Henry Holt and Company 2014), Epilogue, pg. 259.

20. *Ibid.*, at pg. 39-40

21. *Ibid.*, at pg. 41.

22. *Ibid.*, at pg. 41.

23. Historians can utilize a record of Wikipedia revisions to study how thought evolves. See: https://en.wikipedia.org/wiki/Help:Page_history.

24. *The Body Electric: Electromagnetism and the Foundation of Life*, by Robert O. Becker, M.D., and Gary Selden, published by William Morrow 1985, in the "Introduction: the Promise of the Art" at pg. 21.

25. *"Bioelectromagnetic Energy Fields Accelerate Wound Healing and Activate Immune Cell Function,"* by Lisanne D'Andrea-Winslow, Don Johnson, and Amy Novitski, published in Journal of Medical and Biological Sciences, Vol. 2, Issue 1, 2008, at pg. 13 of 15, available online at: https://www.researchgate.net/publication/237822820_Bioelectromagnetic_Energy_Fields_Accelerate_Wound_Healing_and_Activate_Immune_Cell_Function

26. *"Vitalism"* in Wikipedia, as of April 1, 2016, 1st paragraph, available online at: https://en.wikipedia.org/wiki/Vitalism

27. *Living Energies: Viktor Schauberger's Brilliant Work with Natural Energy Explained*, by Callum Coats, AA Dipl, ARAIA, ARIBA, published by Gateway Books, Bath UK 1996, at pg. 64.

28. *See, e.g., "Implosion: Viktor Schauberger and the Path of Natural Energy,"* compiled by Riley Hansard Crabb and Thomas Maxwell Thompson, from *Implosion Instead of Explosion*, published 1985 and available online at: http://bluestarenterprise.com/articles/viktor-schauberger/vitor-schauberger-implosion-the-path-of-natural-energy.

29. *"Viktor Schauberger: Austrian Patents (Water Control by Vortex Action),"* by Robert A. Nelson, published by RexResearch, available online at: http://www.rexresearch.com/schaub/schaub.htm#112144

30. *See, e.g., Nature as Teacher: How I Discovered New Principles in the Working of Nature*, by Viktor Schauberger and Callum Coats, ed. and translated by Callum Coats, published by Gateway 1999.

31. *"IgNoble Prize 2000: Levitation without Meditation,"* by Professor Sir Michael Berry, Oct. 5, 2000, available in https://michaelberryphysics.wordpress.com/ignobel/; a video of the award presentation and Sir Andre Geim's prize acceptance speech is available online, beginning at 52:52 of 1:44:41, at http://www.improbable.com/ig/2000/.

32. *"About the IgNoble® Prizes,"* posted on http://www.improbable.com/ig/

33. Dr. Han Selye, the physician who discovered the connection between stress and disease (see, *supra*, Chapter Nine: Taking Good Care), even wrote a poem on the topic, published in his 1979 memoir *The Stress of My Life (2nd Edition)*, pg. 230-231, reprinted in The American Institute of Stress, available online at http://www.stress.org/the-poem/, entitled *"From Dream to Discovery"*:

> *I think I have the instinctive feeling*
> *And patiently, through the years, I have acquired the kind of knowledge*
> *Needed to explore Your law.*
> *But my faith was weakened by this apprenticeship.*
> *No longer can it steer me steadily towards my goal.*
> *For I have come to distrust faith and overvalue proof.*
> *So, let reverence for the unfailing power of all Your known laws*
> *Be the source of my faith in the world of discovering the next commandment...*

I cannot know whether You listen
But I do know that I must pray:
Almighty Drive who, through the ages,
Have kept men trying to master Nature by understanding.
Give me faith now—for that is what I need most.

34. *"My contribution to particle physics,"* by Professor Sir Michael Berry, FRS, Melville Wills Professor of Physics (Emeritus), University of Bristol, Research, available online at: https://michaelberryphysics. wordpress.com/about-2/

35. *Ibid.*

36. *Ibid.*

37. *Tesla: Inventor of the Electrical Age,* by W. Bernard Carlson, published by Princeton University Press 2013, Chapter Two: Dreaming of Motors, at pg. 51, reprinted from *My Inventions: The Autobiography of Nikola Tesla.*

38. *Ibid.*

39. *Ibid.*

40. *"Telsa biography: Nikola Tesla, The Genius Who Lit the World"* on the Tesla Memorial Society of New York website, available online at: http://www.teslasociety.com/biography.htm

41. *"The Theory Behind the Equation"* by Michio Kaku, posted 10.11.05, on NOVA (PBS), and available online at: http://www.pbs.org/wgbh/nova/ physics/theory-behind-equation.html; see also *Einstein's Mistakes: The Human Failings of Genius* by Hans C. Ohanian, published by W.W. Norton & Co. 2009, Ch. 4: A Storm Broke Loose in My Mind, at pg. 86-7.

42. *Darkness at Night: A Riddle of the Universe* by Edward Harrison, published by Harvard University Press 1989, footnote 2 to pgs. 177-178 (Chapter 16 "The Expanding Universe"), at pg. 253.

43. *The Work of Teachers in America: A Social History Through Stories* (1997), by Rosetta Marantz Cohen and Samuel Scheer, pg. 168, with Anne Sullivan journal entry from March 20, 1887.

44. *"The Nobel Prize in Physics 1921: Albert Einstein,"* published on the official website of the Nobel Prize, available online at: http://www. nobelprize.org/nobel_prizes/physics/laureates/1921/

45. *Blueprint For Immortality: The Electric Patterns Of Life* by Harold Saxton Burr, published by C.W. Daniel (1972), Chapter One ("An Adventure in Science"), pg. 12-13.

46. *Ibid.*, in book's Foreword; see also *"The Electrical Patterns of Life; The Work of Dr. Harold S. Burr,"* by World Research Foundation (WRF) staff, available online at:
http://www.wrf.org/men-women-medicine/dr-harold-s-burr.php

47. *Ibid.*, in Chapter Seven: The Continuing Adventure, section 9, at pg. 132.

48. *Ibid.*, in book's Foreword.

49. *Ibid.*, in Chapter Seven: The Continuing Adventure, section 9, at pg. 132.

50. *Ibid.*, in Chapter Seven: The Continuing Adventure, section 10, at pg. 133.

51. *Ibid.*, in Chapter Seven: The Continuing Adventure, section 9, at pg. 130.

52. *"Friendship between Nikola Tesla & Mark Twain"* by Dragoljub A. Cucić, Bratislav Stojiljković, and Aleksandar S. Nikolić, conference paper 2012, curating the letters between Twain and Tesla, which can be found at ResearchGate.net, available online at: http://www.research-gate.net/publication/232807620; excerpt appears in a letter from Twain to Telsa dated November 17, 1898 (which the authors cite as appearing also *Empires of Light: Edison, Tesla, Westinghouse, and the Race to Electrify the World* by J. Jonnes, published by Random House Publishing Group 2004.

53. *"The Transmission Of Electrical Energy Without Wires As A Means For Furthering Peace"* by Nikola Tesla, Electrical World and Engineer, Jan. 1905, pp. 21-24, available online at: http://www.tfcbooks.com/tesla/1905-01-07.htm

54. *"The Dark Side of the Nobel Prizes,"* by Marc Lallanilla, published in LiveScience Oct. 4, 2013, available online at: http://www.livescience.com/40188-dark-history-alfred-nobel-prizes.html; see also *"How 'merchant of death' Alfred Nobel became a champion of peace,"* by Marc Preel, published in TheLocal SE Oct. 4 2010, available online at: http://www.thelocal.se/20101004/29406

55. *"Alfred Nobel's Will: The Establishment of the Nobel Prize"* on the official website of the Nobel Prize, available online at http://www.nobel-prize.org/alfred_nobel/will/.

56. *See, e.g., "Did Researchers Cook Data from the First Test of General Relativity? (Rumors of data mishandling in an historic eclipse study don't gibe),"* by JR Minkel, published in Scientific American, March 6, 2008, and available online at: http://www.scientificamerican.com/article/did-researchers-cook-data-from-first-general-relativity-test/

57. *See, e.g.,* the official St. Andrews biography of Freundlich, available online at http://www-history.mcs.st-andrews.ac.uk/Biographies/Freundlich.html, in which it notes how the last years of Freundlich's life were "unhappy" in his forced retirement, denied access to the very telescope he established at St. Andrews. To me, it is another example of mistaken attachment to hard lines of administrative policy, without considering the spirit of the matter.

58. *The Nature of the Physical World (Gifford Lectures of 1927),* by Arthur Eddington, annotated and introduced by H.G. Callaway, based on Gifford Lectures delivered in the Univ. of Edinburgh in 1927, reprinted in Everyman's Library by arrangement with the author and Cambridge Univ. Press, at pg. 324 (Chapter 15, "Science and Mysticism").

59. *See, e.g., "Astrophysics and Mysticism: the life of Arthur Stanley Eddington,"* by Ian H Hutchinson, Prof. of Nuclear Science and Engineering, at Massachusetts Institute of Technology, Dec. 2002, available online at: http://silas.psfc.mit.edu/eddington/. "He is a mystic" bluntly concluded MIT Professor Hutchinson, after reviewing Eddington's own writings—including his 1929 Swarthmore essay on spiritual matters entitled *"Science and the Unseen World."* Hutchison's conclusion of mysticism was not meant to tarnish Eddington's legacy, because "whatever these blemishes may be, Eddington's greatness of intellect and spirit outshines them."

60. *"Science and the Unseen World (Swarthmore Lecture 1929)"* by Arthur Eddington, published by MacMillan, NY (1929), excerpted in *"Astrophysics and Mysticism: the life of Arthur Stanley Eddington,"* by Prof. Ian H. Hutchinson (MIT 2002), *supra.*

61. *The Nature of the Physical World (Gifford Lectures of 1927)*, by Arthur Eddington, annotated and introduced by H.G. Callaway, especially pgs. 274-280 (Chapter 13, "Reality"); Eddington explains, on pg. 278-280, how the duality between science and spirit is uncomfortable, a "mere shelving of the inquiry into the nature of the world of experience. This view of the relation of the material to the spiritual world per-haps relieves to some extent a tension between science and religion. Physical science has seemed to occupy a domain of reality which is self-sufficient, pursuing its course independently of and indifferent to that which a voice within us asserts to be a higher reality. We are jealous of such independence. We are uneasy that there should be an apparently self-contained world in which God becomes an unneces-sary hypothesis."

62. *Ibid.*, at pg. 324 (Chapter 15, "Science and Mysticism")

63. *Leonardo da Vinci Notebooks (Oxford World's Classics*, selected by Irma A. Richter, edited with an introduction and notes by Thereza Wells, preface by Martin Kemp, Oxford University Press first published 1952, new ed. 2008) at pg. 168. See note 54 to Ch. 10 above.

64. *"IgNoble Prize 2000: Levitation without Meditation,"* by Professor Sir Michael Berry, Oct. 5, 2000, available in https://michaelberryphysics. wordpress.com/ignobel/.

65. *"The Deliberate Amateur: How outlandish experimentation and 'grazing shallow' led to a Nobel Prize win"* by Sarah Lewis, published *Slate* May 21, 2014, in Slate issue themed *"How Failure Breeds Success"* (adapted from *The Rise: Creativity, the Gift of Failure, and the Search for Mastery*, by Sarah Lewis, published Simon & Schuster 2014), available online at: http://www.slate.com/articles/business/how_failure_breeds_suc-cess/2014/05/nobel_prize_in_physics_andre_geim_went_from_lev-itating_frogs_to_science.single.html, pg. 5 of 5.

65. *Physics@FOM Veldhoven 2011, Andre Geim, Tuesday evening lecture*, posted on YouTube, available online at https://www.youtube.com/watch?v=GidsDtpKsMM, at 21:48 et. seq. of 1:08:11.

66. *"The Deliberate Amateur: How outlandish experimentation and 'grazing shallow' led to a Nobel Prize win"* by Sarah Lewis, at pg. 3 of 5.

67. *Faust: A Tragedy by Johann Wolfgang Von Goethe*, English translation by Bayard Taylor, published by Houghton Mifflin Co. 1870, available online at: https://www.stmarys-ca.edu/sites/default/files/attachments/files/Faust.pdf, in Part I, Scene I, spoken by character Wagner, at pg. 23.

68. *"COVER STORY: The godfather of graphene. When Andre Geim discovered graphene, he went from winning the Ig Nobel prize to the Nobel. Giles Whittell meets the quirky Russian physicist who may be the new James Watt"* by Giles Whitell, published in Intelligent Life Magazine (a/k/a 1843 Magazine / The Economist Unwinds, a publication of The Economist), Sept./Oct. 2014, available online at:

http://www.intelligentlifemagazine.com/content/features/giles-whittell/andre-geim, at pg. 6 of 10.

69. *Andre Geim Nobel Prize dinner speech Dec. 10, 2010*, posted on YouTube, available online at https://www.youtube.com/watch?v=7FlqJdxM2Wg, at 5:05 of 5:17.

70. *"Quotations"* on weblog of Sir Michael Berry, available online at: https://michaelberryphysics.wordpress.com/quotations/

71. *Richtmyer Memorial Lecture - Sir Michael Berry - WM2014*, posted on YouTube, available online at: https://www.youtube.com/watch?v=tUyoCrBx37s, at 5:30 of 49:54.

72. *Ibid.*, at 5:51 of 49:54.

73. *"Einstein's Quest for a Unified Theory,"* published in APS News, American Physical Society, Dec. 2005, Vol. 14, No. 11, available online at: https://www.aps.org/publications/apsnews/200512/history.cfm

74. *On the Nature of the Universe*, by Lucretious, translated by R. E. Latham, revised with an introduction and notes by John Godwin, published by Penguin Books (translation first published 1951, revised translation with new introduction and notes published 1994), at pg. 40 (lines 115-118) and pg. 41 (lines 123-128).

75. It was the fourth in terms of popular recognition (compared to his celebrated papers on time/space, energy/matter, and photoelectricity), but it was not the fourth paper chronologically. Einstein submitted his paper on Brownian motion on May 11, 1905, making it his second paper of the miracle year (after his first paper on photoelectricity, and

followed sequentially by his third paper on time/space and his fourth on matter/energy). Indeed, his Brownian motion paper was technically not even about Brownian motion, although scientists and scholars later reclassified it as such. It was entitled *"On the Motion of Small Particles Suspended in a Stationary Liquid, as Required by the Molecular Kinetic Theory of Heat,"* and Einstein himself speculated how "It is possible that the movements to be discussed here are identical with the so-called 'Brownian molecular motion'; however," as Einstein readily and humbly admitted on the first page of his paper, "the information available to me regarding the latter [the phenomenon of Brownian motion] is so lacking in precision, that I can form no judgment in the matter." With the growing popular recognition of Einstein's genius, the paper was later translated and republished in English as *Investigations on the Theory of the Brownian Movement* (by Albert Einsein, edited with notes by R. Fürth, translated by A.D. Cowper, and published by Dover Publications 1926, republished 1956), and is available online at: http://users.physik.fu-berlin.de/~kleinert/files/eins_brownian.pdf. Einstein quote at pg. 1.

76. *"My contribution to particle physics,"* by Professor Sir Michael Berry, see ftnt. #36, *supra*. It is worth noting that the properties of a field differ from those of a particle, even to particle physicists.

77. See, e.g., *"Random Walk and the Theory of Brownian Motion,"* by Mark Kac, published in The American Mathematical Monthly, Vol. 54, No. 7, Part 1 (Aug.-Sept. 1947), pg. 369-391, available online at: http://math.hawaii.edu/~xander/Fa06/Kac--Brownian_Motion.pdf

78. *"Physicists net fractal butterfly: Decades-old search closes in on recursive pattern that describes electron behaviour"* by Devin Powell, published in Nature (News), 501, 144-145, Sept. 12, 2013 (online story Sept. 10, 2013), available online at: http://www.nature.com/news/physicists-net-fractal-butterfly-1.13717, at pg. 2 of 5.

78. *"Energy levels and wave functions of Bloch electrons in rational and irrational magnetic fields,"* by Douglas Hofstadter, published in Physical Review B, 14, 2239, Sept. 15, 1976, available online at: http://journals.aps.org/prb/abstract/10.1103/PhysRevB.14.2239

79. *"Hofstadter's butterfly spotted in graphene,"* by Hamish Johnston (editor, physicsworld.com), published May 15, 2013 in PhysicsWorld.com, and available online at http://physicsworld.com/cws/article/news/2013/may/15/hofstadters-butterfly-spotted-in-graphene; see also *"Hofstadter's butterfly and the fractal quantum Hall effect in moiré superlattices"* by C. R. Dean, L. Wang, P. Maher, C. Forsythe, F. Ghahari, Y. Gao, J. Katoch, M. Ishigami, P. Moon, M. Koshino, T. Taniguchi, K. Watanabe, K. L. Shepard, J. Hone & P. Kim, published in Nature 497, 598–602 (May 30, 2013), and available online at http://www.nature.com/nature/journal/v497/n7451/full/nature12186.html.

80. *Physics@FOM Veldhoven 2011, Andre Geim, Tuesday evening lecture,* posted on YouTube, available online at https://www.youtube.com/watch?v=GidsDtpKsMM, at 44:00-44:30 of 1:08:11.

81. *Ibid.,* at 44:45 of 1:08:11.

82. *Ibid.,* at 51:56 of 1:08:11.

83. *Ibid.,* at 15:10-15:53 of 1:08:11.

84. *Ibid.,* at 15:10-15:53 of 1:08:11.

85. *Ibid.,* at 16:13-16:50 of 1:08:11.

86. *Ibid.,* at 16:48 et. seq. of 1:08:11.

87. *Ibid.,* at 16:50 et. seq. of 1:08:11.

88. *"COVER STORY: The Godfather of Graphene. (When Andre Geim discovered graphene, he went from winning the Ig Nobel prize to the Nobel. Giles Whittell meets the quirky Russian physicist who may be the new James Watt)"* by Giles Whitell, published in Intelligent Life Magazine (now 1843 Magazine), a publication of The Economist, Sept./Oct. 2014, available online at: http://www.intelligentlifemagazine.com/content/features/giles-whittell/andre-geim, at pg. 9 of 12.

89. *Ibid.,* at pg. 8 of 12.

90. *Ibid.,* at pg. 7-8 of 12.

91. Readers may be interested in *The Anatomy of Peace: Resolving the Heart of Conflict,* by The Arbinger Institute, published by Berrett-Koehler Publishers, Inc., First Edition ed. (2006). The book was life-changing required reading for my son Nicholas and me, in the wilderness program that followed his intervention.

92. *First Inaugural Address*, by Abraham Lincoln, delivered Monday, March 4, 1861. Lincoln's closing remark to a nation bitterly divided over the issues of slavery was this: "We are not enemies, but friends. We must not be enemies. Though passion may have strained it must not break our bonds of affection. The mystic chords of memory, stretching from every battlefield and patriot grave to every living heart and hearthstone all over this broad land, will yet swell the chorus of the Union, when again touched, as surely they will be, by the better angels of our nature."

93. In the conclusion of *Blueprint For Immortality: The Electric Patterns Of Life*, published by C.W. Daniel (1972), Chapter 7 ("The Continuing Adventure"), Section 10, pg. 133, Harold Saxton Burr writes: "The experimental findings recorded in these pages are the first stepping-stones on a long journey into the unknown—guide-posts for further adventures in science. They indicate that the Universe is an ordered system, the human organism an ordered component. Law and order prevail from the biggest to the smallest; and to suggest that there is any chaos is merely to display our lack of information. In short, the Universe has meaning and so have we. Though we do not understand it, the meaning is there. The continuing adventure of science and of ourselves is to seek, through the Field Concept, an ever-greater understanding of the changing, growing meaning of life."

94. *General Scholium to Isaac Newton's Principia mathematica*, published first as an appendix to the 2nd (1713) ed. of the Principia, republished in the 3rd (1726) ed. with some amendments/additions, translated Andrew Motte (London 1729), pgs. 387-93, and available online at: http://isaac-newton.org/general-scholium/ at pg. 4 of 4; see ftnt. #51, Ch. 12, *supra*.